A SHORT HISTORY OF
MEDICINE

STEVE PARKER

Penguin
Random
House

DK LONDON

Senior Editor Angela Wilkes
Editors Hugo Wilkinson,
Andy Szudek, Victoria Pyke,
Anna Fischel, Georgina Palffy
Senior Art Editors Michael Duffy,
Helen Spencer
Art Editors Mark Lloyd,
Jane Ewart
Editorial Consultant Martyn Page
Managing Editors Stephanie Farrow,
Gareth Jones
Senior Managing Art Editor Lee Griffiths
Picture research Luped Media Research

Jacket Designer Laura Brim,
Surabhi Wadhwa-Gandhi
Jacket Editor Emma Dawson, Manisha Majithia
Jacket Design Development Manager
Sophia M.T.T.
Senior Producer, Pre-production Andy Hilliard
Producer, Pre-production Lucy Sims
Senior Producer Rachel Ng
Production Controller Mandy Inness
Publisher Andrew Macintyre
Art Directors Phil Ormerod, Karen Self
Associate Publishing Director Liz Wheeler
Publishing Director Jonathan Metcalf

DK INDIA

Senior Art Editor Chhaya Sajwan
Managing Art Editor Sudakshina Basu
Jacket Designer Suhita Dharamjit
Jackets Editorial Coordinator Priyanka Sharma
DTP Designer Rajdeep Singh, Rakesh Kumar, Md. Rizwan
Managing Jackets Editor Saloni Singh
Pre-production Manager Sunil Sharma
Production Manager Pankaj Sharma

Previously published in 2013 as *Kill or Cure*
This edition first published in Great Britain in 2019
by Dorling Kindersley Limited,
80 Strand, London WC2R 0RL

Copyright © 2013, 2019 Dorling Kindersley Limited
A Penguin Random House Company

2 4 6 8 10 9 7 5 3 1
001–314177–May/19

ISBN 978-0-2413-7965-3

Printed in the United Kingdom

A WORLD OF IDEAS:
SEE ALL THERE IS TO KNOW

www.dk.com

Contents

240   MODERN MEDICINE 1920–2000

336   GENES AND FUTURE DREAMS 2000–PRESENT

Introduction

What is a doctor? In ancient Egypt, healing was the perogative of sorcerers, while in early Greece doctors were considered itinerant curiosities more likely to harm than help. By the 16th century, innovative doctors were practising an eclectic mix of medicine, alchemy, astrology, herbalism, mineralogy, psychotherapy, and faith-healing, while in the modern world medicine has evolved to make it possible for doctors to operate on patients remotely from another continent.

Today, there is a complex array of scanning and imaging options with which to view the inside of the body, but in ancient Egypt such information would have been deemed utterly irrelevant: examining the patient was unheard of at a time when illness was considered to be the work of the gods. Hippocrates, who practised in ancient Greece and was considered by many to be the father of modern medicine, found himself imprisoned for many years when he rejected the idea that illness was the whim of deities. Yet by the time he died, he had revolutionized the practice of medicine and established the basic foundations of the role of the physician.

Many others contributed, of course – Imhotep of Egypt, Chakara in India, Galen in Rome, and Zhang Zhongjing of China in ancient times. Islam's medieval Golden Age boasted al-Rhazi and Ibn Sina (Avicenna), and the Renaissance had anatomist Andreas Vesalius and the groundbreaking Paracelsus, who founded many of the principles of modern medicine. All these figures contributed to medicine, often in ways that challenged the conventional views of the time.

Of course, there were many wildly inaccurate theories, and some – to our eyes – outlandish remedies, from boiled newborn puppies to the ashes of a burnt swallow (used to "cure" hirsuitism). So popular was bloodletting by leech that at one point doctors were actually known as "leeches". And so established were Galen's theories on human anatomy that for centuries, no one questioned the fact that his findings had been gathered by dissecting the bodies of dogs and monkeys, rather than humans. Alongside the more spectacular "medicines", however, were herbs and minerals that to this day form the basis of tried-and-tested drug cures, and in amongst the quacks and charlatans were many diligent and painstaking innovators.

Rigorous observation and detailed detective work have played a huge part in the development of medicine. Before English physician William Harvey published his momentous book on the heart and circulation in 1628, for example, he spent over 20 years dissecting and experimenting on the pulsing hearts of thousands of animals from more than 60 species. Building on concepts and evidence dating back to ancient times, Harvey also wove theory and practice into a scientifically sound, evidence-based

ENGRAVING OF MALE MUSCULATURE
Andreas Vesalius's great work *De Humani Corporis Fabrica*, 1543, established a new standard of clarity and accuracy in the study of human anatomy.

description of the circulatory system. Armed with this knowledge, physicians were able to make major improvements in the way they diagnosed and treated disease. There are, of course, famous instances where chance has also played an important role. Had the weather not been unseasonably cold when Scottish medical researcher Alexander Fleming left his messy laboratory to go on holiday, for example, he might not have discovered penicillin, which has since prevented immeasurable suffering and saved countless lives. It took the stimulus of World War II, however, to fully realise the potential of this, the first antibiotic.

War and conflict have given impetus to many branches of medicine, acting as a catalyst for innovation and learning. One of the earliest medical documents, the 3,600-year-old Smith Papyrus of ancient Egypt, describes treatment of wounds probably sustained on the battlefield; in ancient Rome, gladiators' injuries provided valuable medical insight at a time when human dissection was forbidden. In the 16th century, French army surgeon Ambroise Paré used innovative procedures, such as poultices and ligatures, that then filtered from the battlefield through to general surgery. Another French surgeon, Baron Dominique Jean Larrey, pioneered the use of ambulances and triage in the 19th century. During World War I, doctors noted that mustard gas affected fast-multiplying cells in the body, which ultimately led to the development of anti-cancer chemotherapy drugs. Medicine even benefited from the most deadly weapon of all, the atomic bomb: its effects indirectly led to bone marrow transplants and one of medicine's newest areas of research – stem cell therapy.

The journey made by the science of medicine is an astonishing one. Nowadays we take for granted our modern operating theatres with their rigorously germ-free environments and sterilized equipment, but it is worth remembering that the notion of germs as transmittors of infection has only existed since the 19th century. It is also hard to imagine that there was a surprising amount of surgery already taking place millennia ago: holes were being drilled in patients' heads from prehistoric times through to the 18th century, for example. And while in ancient Greece it was rare for the skin to be deliberately broken, surgeons in ancient Rome developed tools, equipment, and procedures not dissimilar to those in use today. However, modern surgery is also making use of robots, lasers, and mind-boggling technology. Just as we struggle to imagine prehistoric brain surgery, it is equally hard to imagine just how much has been achieved by modern medicine. It has waged war on age-old killers such as cholera, smallpox, and tuberculosis, decoded our DNA, mapped the human genome, and created the potential for nanotechnology and tissue-engineering. The future ambition for medicine is phenomenal, but the challenges are not to be underestimated.

Better nutrition, improved public health and hygiene, safety awareness, and health education have accompanied medicine in bringing immense strides in life quality and longevity over the past century. Prominent medical advances have included vaccinations, antibiotics, new drugs and medicines, safer surgery, improved care during pregnancy and childbirth, and recognition of health hazards such as carcinogens, pollutants, occupational issues, and risk factors for heart disease, stroke, and other major killers. However, medicine is now big business, with economics preventing equality from keeping pace with technology, so that millions of people still have little, if any, access to healthcare.

The episodes in this book have been selected to illustrate how medicine has changed from the inspired, dedicated, but often isolated individuals of the past to today's specialist teams equipped with the latest technology. Anecdotal rather than encyclopedic, the book aims to give non-technical insights into the intrinsically fascinating, occasionally horrifying, and always captivating subject of medicine.

Beliefs and Traditions

TO 900

Medicine is as old as humankind. More than 50,000 years ago, stone-age, cave-dwelling humans first crushed and infused herbs for their curative properties. Traditional forms of medicine — sadly, few of which are known to written history — evolved on all continents, from the deserts and jungles of Africa to North American plains, South American rainforests, and balmy Pacific islands.

Earliest records in West Asia, the Middle East, North Africa, China, and India document myriad diseases, healing plants, and surgical procedures. Ancient Egyptians had complex, hierarchical methods of medicine integrated into their religious beliefs. Gods and spirits were in charge of mortal disease, and priest-physicians — Imhotep is one of the first great names in medical history — mediated with the supernatural realm to ease human suffering.

The civilizations of Greece and Rome had their respective medical giants in Hippocrates and Galen. Hippocrates set standards for patient care and the physician's attitudes and philosophy that persist today. Galen wrote so extensively and authoritatively that his theories and practices attained quasi-religious status and effectively stalled medical progress in Europe for 1,400 years. After the Roman Empire ended, the murky arts of alchemy, sorcery, exorcism, and miracle cures flourished in Western Europe.

Ancient India and China also developed sophisticated medical systems with outstanding contributors. In India, in the centuries before and after Hippocrates, Susruta and Chakara produced encyclopaedic founding works of Ayurvedic medicine. Chinese physician Zhang Zhongjing, a contemporary of Galen, also compiled works that described hundreds of diseases and prescribed thousands of remedies.

Prehistoric Medicine

TIME: **30,000 YEARS AGO**, approaching the depths of the last great ice age. Place: a clearing next to a rock cavern, in the Iberian Peninsula, Western Europe. As dusk falls, a band of stocky, thick-set humans, draped in rough, furry cloaks, gathers around a bed of ferns, heathers, and moss. On the bed lies the oldest of the group – a male aged about 40 years. His eyes are closed as if he is asleep, his skin is pale, and his breathing is weak. The onlookers murmur and chant with guttural sounds, occasionally raising their heads to gesture at the setting sun. In the flickering firelight, one of the younger females raises her voice to a passionate howl, leaps up, and comes forward to press a bitter-smelling paste into the old man's mouth. He stirs slowly, opens his eyes – and smiles.

The scene, of course, is fictional. But something like this may have happened at El Sidron, a well-studied archaeological site in northwest Spain. Here, hundreds of fossilized bones and teeth were found that once belonged to some 13 Neanderthals (*Homo neanderthalensis*) – our "sister" species of human, which died out 30,000–25,000 years ago. In 2012, scientists analysed teeth from five of the Neanderthals, using an advanced technique known as pyrolysis gas-chromatography mass spectrometry. Trapped in the hardened plaque layer (called "calculus") on each tooth were microfossils and other remains of plants that their owners had eaten. Evidence of wood smoke and starchy cooked plants was found, and one individual had eaten bitter-tasting plants, including yarrow and chamomile. These herbs have no real nutritional value, and their bitter taste must have been off-putting. So why were they eaten? One possibility is that the plants were used as natural medications. Yarrow has long been known as a traditional tonic and astringent, and chamomile as a relaxant and anti-inflammatory.

The evidence at El Sidron points to some of the earliest known human medicine – the prevention, identification, treatment, and curing of illness and disease. Our understanding of prehistoric times depends on the study of preserved human remains, artefacts such as tools and adornments, and natural objects like plant seeds and animal fossils. Cave paintings and rock art also help. Several prehistoric images show human forms with the heart included, but there seems to be little other graphic evidence of anatomical

THE FIRST TASTE OF MEDICINE
The fossilized teeth of Neanderthals who lived up to 30,000 years ago have been found to contain traces of various herbs, including chamomile and yarrow. Such herbs are thought to have been the very first medicines.

SOOTHING HERB
The plant species *Nepeta cataria* — commonly known as catnip — was used in prehistoric treatments for settling the stomach.

awareness. Vital insights into prehistoric medicine also come from modern anthropology — gathering information from native cultures, especially in the Americas, Africa, Asia, and Australasia. Studies of these cultures suggest that prehistoric peoples had a mix of religious and spiritual beliefs about the causes of disease — typically attributing them to possession by evil spirits, or revenge for sinful behaviour. To effect healing, they combined mystical and supernatural actions, such as making offerings to the spirits, sacrifices to the gods, and pleas to lift a curse, with practical treatments such as poultices, ointments, and concoctions made from herbs, minerals, and animal body parts such as blood and powdered bones. In hunter-gatherer times, before the advent of agriculture and settlement, long-distance organized trade was very limited, so all forms of medication came from the local environment.

Anthropologists have also suggested that one member of a group would have held a special position in medical matters — a man variously referred to as a healer, shaman, or medicine-man (see pp.88–89), whose duties included being a priest, a soothsayer, an oracle, an advisor, or even a ruler. This shaman was believed to hold special powers, such as the ability to communicate with the gods and spirits, and was also proficient at preparing herbal potions and administering hands-on treatments such as massage.

Working back from modern anthropological knowledge, and using preserved evidence such as bones and artefacts, the following treatments are thought to date back to prehistoric times: fractured or broken bones were put back in their natural positions to heal; clay or mud was plastered onto broken limbs and left to dry hard, as a prehistoric version of a plaster-cast; splints, made of wood, bone, or horn secured with plant vines and fibrous bark, were bound to broken limbs; wounds were dressed with poultices of healing herbs and covered with rudimentary bandage strips cut from animal hides; stomach and digestive problems were eased by chewing orchid bulbs or drinking their extracts; certain types of willow bark — the original source of acetylsalicylic acid, better known as aspirin — were chewed to relieve pain and reduce swelling; witch hazel and saps from various trees and plants were used to soothe burns and scalds; and some types of clay or soil were eaten (in a practice known as "geophagy") to neutralize harmful substances in contaminated foods and provide minerals lacking in the diet.

Dentistry was also practised. Among the tens of thousands of objects found at the prehistoric site of Mehrgarh, near Sibi in west-central Pakistan, were 11 human teeth — all molars, and probably from nine individuals — that had apparently been drilled using a device tipped with a sharp-pointed flint. Researchers have reconstructed the device — essentially an arrow with a bow-saw used to rotate it (see p.20) — and estimated that the holes were made in less than a minute. The condition of the teeth and the subsequent wear marks in the holes show that they were drilled while the owners were still alive — although, oddly, only four of them show signs of decay.

Drills were also used for trepanning (see pp.20–21) — a radical form of surgery that involved breaching the skull to expose the layers of tissue covering the brain (meninges), and sometimes even the brain tissue itself. The earliest known trepanning procedures were performed using the cracked edges of flints, which were used as chippers or scrapers to remove the bone, either fragment by fragment, or to gouge a channel around a central area of bone that could then be lifted clear. More sophisticated techniques involved using bow-saw rotary drills — larger ones than those employed at Mehrgarh. As for the purpose of

PREHISTORIC DEER DOCTOR
This 20,000-year-old cave painting in Ariège, France, shows a figure believed to be a healing priest. Dressed in a deer skin and antlers, he may be dancing to drive away evil spirits.

trepanning, the oldest explanations centre on the notion of releasing evil spirits from the patient, who would then keep the removed piece of bone as a talisman to prevent the spirits returning. Modern interpretations suggest that these prehistoric patients may have been incapacitated by the unbearable pain of migraine, or the involuntary seizures of epilepsy. Other possibilities include intense depression and severe bipolar disorder, or internal bleeding causing intracranial pressure, compressing the brain tissue and causing life-threatening damage. As indicated by Hippocrates (see pp.30–39), trepanning was also useful as a drastic first-aid measure in the case of head wounds – again, to help relieve intracranial pressure by releasing the blood from a haemorrhage beneath the skull.

In 1991, a naturally preserved, mummified, and frozen male human body was found in the European Alps, near the border between Austria and Italy. He became known as Ötzi the Iceman, and is now one of the most studied of all human bodies. Ötzi was about 45 years old when he died 5,300 years ago. He had sophisticated leather garments and shoes under a woven-grass cloak, and carried a knife, axe, bow, arrows, bark containers, and what might have been a simple prehistoric medical kit. Two of Ötzi's possessions were thumb-sized lumps of a fungus or mould known as *Piptoporus betulinus* (birch polypore, razor strop, or birch bracket fungus). Each lump was holed to thread onto a leather strip so that it could be secured, probably to clothing. The medicinal properties of this fungus feature in many folklore traditions and have been supported by scientific analysis. It is a laxative, and eating it can bring on diarrhoea. It also shows antibiotic action, and contains substances that are poisonous to intestinal parasites such as whipworm, *Trichuris trichura*. It so happens that Ötzi had whipworm, as revealed by detailed medical examination of his remains that showed worm eggs in his large intestine.

LIFE EXPECTANCY IN PREHISTORIC TIMES

25–40 YEARS

Perhaps even more intriguing were Ötzi's tattoos. There were more than 50 of these scattered over his body – on the left wrist, left calf, right knee, both ankles, right foot, and on both sides of his

ICE AGE TATTOOS
A pathologist examines the remains of Ötzi the Iceman, whose tattoos may have been part of a prehistoric treatment similar to acupuncture or acupressure.

lower backbone – all arranged in groups of parallel lines. They were probably made by rubbing charcoal into incisions made in his skin, and being so widespread, and mostly hidden by clothes and shoes, it is unlikely that they were for decoration.

X-rays and CT scans show Ötzi's skeleton suffered from degenerative bone and joint conditions of the back, knees, and ankles. Some tattoos were positioned over these possibly painful areas. Perhaps they were some kind of symbolic therapy for relief. Another idea is that they were related to a form of acupuncture or acupressure therapy; many of the lines correspond to the acupuncture lines known as channels or meridians in Chinese medicine (see pp.64–73). Ötzi's full medical mystery is yet to be solved, but he does support the growing evidence that prehistoric medicine was more sophisticated than many modern experts have assumed.

Trepanning

As long ago as 10,000 BCE, in places ranging from France and western Asia to South America, surgeons practised trepanning – cutting or drilling holes in patients' skulls using flint tools. This treatment is the oldest known surgical procedure, and it may have been intended to relieve the pressure caused by depressed skull fractures, to treat seizures or mental health disorders, or to release evil spirits from the patient's head.

Prehistoric trepanning

Many of the earliest trepanning operations were carried out using a wooden bow drill. To spin the drill, the surgeon wound the leather thong around the drill shaft and moved the bow with a sawing motion.

TREPANNED PREHISTORIC SKULLS HAVE BEEN FOUND WITH HOLES DRILLED IN VARIOUS LOCATIONS ON THE HEAD

Parietal bone of the skull

BRONZE AGE SKULL
ISRAEL, 2200–2000 BCE
Excavated at Jericho (now in the West Bank, western Asia), this skull has a cluster of holes made by trepanning. The holes are circular, showing that the surgeon used a drill – incisions made by a knife are usually square or irregular in shape.

Flint drill tip

Shark's tooth drill tip

Bow

REPLICA NEOLITHIC TREPANNING BOW DRILL
BRITISH, 1930–70
British researcher Dr T.W. Parry used this bow drill and other tools in experiments to investigate ancient trepanning techniques.

At the edges of the holes, the bone is beginning to grow back, showing that this patient survived the risky operation – many did not

Frontal bone of the skull

Later tools

Trepanning was still common in the 18th century, and surgeons used sharp metal trepanning tools to treat head wounds and conditions such as epilepsy. However, high mortality rates, especially when the surgeon pierced the tissue beneath the bone, meant that the practice declined during the 19th century.

TREPANNING DRILL
BRITISH, 18TH CENTURY
The typical trepanning drill was shaped like a carpenter's brace and bit. The surgeon held the wooden top piece firmly and rotated the drill by turning the bulbous handle in the middle of the metal crank.

DRILL BITS
BRITISH, 18TH CENTURY
The drill came with metal bits of different sizes. Each has a central spike to help the surgeon position it precisely, and serrations designed to cut into bone.

The Priest-Physicians of Egypt

A S PREHISTORY SHADED INTO HISTORY, medicine developed into a more sophisticated art. Glimpses of this development can be seen in the early civilizations of West Asia's "Fertile Crescent", or Mesopotamia – the land of the Tigris–Euphrates river system, now mainly Iraq plus adjoining parts of Turkey, Syria, and Iran. From some 5,300 years ago, the wedge-like cuneiform writing of Sumeria and the following Akkadian, Assyrian, and Babylonian cultures provide tantalizing snapshots of physicians and their craft. Some medical practitioners of the time, known as ashipus, decreed that ailments were caused by spirits and could be cured by sorcery. They would divine which particular evil sprite was responsible for the problem, and then try to drive it away by means of chants, spells, and curses. Another class of practitioners, the asus, were more involved in practical treatments, such as preparing herbal potions, washing, massage, and bandaging balms onto affected parts of the body. Ashipus and asus often worked together, one helping the other, although they kept their trades distinct and carefully guarded their most precious secrets.

Hammurabi (meaning Kinsman Healer) was ruler of Babylon from around 3,800 to 3,760 years ago. His famous Law Code, written in cuneiform script on a pillar of diorite stone, included several pronouncements on medical care. These held physicians responsible both for success and failure. Rewards and punishments depended partly on the standing of the patient. Saving the life of a noble "with a bronze lancet" was worth ten shekels (more than a year's pay for the average tradesperson),

KINSMAN HEALER
Babylonian king Hammurabi (left) receives his royal insignia from the sun god Shamash.

while saving a slave was worth two shekels. However, if a wealthy patient died under the surgeon's knife, that surgeon could lose a hand – and a lost slave would have to be replaced. Frustratingly, the Code gives few descriptions of the type of surgery practised at the time, and no mention is made of the use of herbs or mineral potions for medical treatment – perhaps because the illnesses treated in this way were believed to be caused by evil spirits or sins, and so were not the physician's responsibility.

Gula, or Ninkarrak, was the Babylonian goddess of healing and the patron goddess of physicians. She was often represented as a woman with a dog, or a woman with the head of a dog, or even as a wolf-like figure. Patients dedicated dog statues and even live dog sacrifices to her, hoping to recover from disease. She came to prominence around 3,600 years ago, during the time of the Kassites – an ancient Babylonian civilization – and her main temples were at Isin (modern-day Ishan al-Bahriyat, Iraq) and Nippur (Nuffar in-Afak, also in Iraq). Herbal and other plant remedies were numerous in those times. Recipes for healing poultices included dregs of wine, prunes, and pine sap, all of which have antibacterial properties – although the addition of lizard excrement is less easy to justify.

Ancient Egypt's gods and spirits were deeply woven into the daily routine and working lives of tradespeople and professionals, so it is difficult, from our modern perspective, to disentangle the truly medical parts of the Egyptian physician's job from his religious and spiritual activities. This task becomes even more difficult when the physician in question is Imhotep (also known as Imuthes), who lived in Heliopolis 4,650–4,600 years ago.

Imhotep ("He who comes in peace") lived during the early phase of Egypt's Old Kingdom, and his fame rapidly spread far and wide. Even during his earthly life, he attained demi-god status, which was unique for an ordinary citizen or commoner in Egyptian society, where such honours were reserved for persons of royal descent. By the late New Kingdom, 3,000 years ago, he was regarded as a full

"Eat, drink, and be merry, for tomorrow we shall die"

IMHOTEP

deity and the son of Ptah, the creator-god or fashioner of the universe and the benefactor of craftspeople. Ptah's partner was Sekhmet (Sachmes), the lion-headed goddess of warfare and healing — and held to be the mother of Imhotep. Some historical sources describe Imhotep as a hands-on healer who was skilled at preparing soothing potions to treat conditions such as arthritis and gout. Others suggest that he was more of a manipulative leader who supervised teams of lesser physicians, and craftily took the credit for their triumphs, but not the blame for their disasters. Imhotep's standing as a cult medical practitioner persisted in Ancient Greece, where he was twinned or even merged with Asclepios (see p.32), the Greek god of healing.

Another great physician of Imhotep's day was Hesy-Ra, who served Pharaoh Djoser as Chief Dentist and Physician. He was venerated for his tooth-pulling and other oral skills, and he seems to have recognized what we now call diabetes mellitus by noticing that some patients urinated frequently and copiously.

Much is known about Ancient Egypt from preserved papyri — documents made from a grass-like sedge plant of the Nile known as the papyrus. Only a few papyri deal with medical matters. One is the Smith Papyrus, named after American Egyptologist and collector Edwin Smith, who purchased it in Luxor in 1862. The Smith Papyrus is incomplete, ends in mid-sentence, and dates to some 3,600 years ago, but the hieroglyphic style and phraseology suggest that it was copied from a much older document — possibly written or dictated by Imhotep himself. Dealing mainly with wounds, injuries, general trauma management, and surgery, the Smith Papyrus has little in the way of supernatural or magical content compared to other papyri of the time. There is only one chant or incantation pleading to the gods for assistance and blessing. Instead, the content is organized

DIVINE IMHOTEP
The Egyptian physician Imhotep was deified after his death, becoming the god of medicine and the son of the creator-god Ptah.

GODDESS OF HEALING
The lion-headed and cobra-crowned
Sekhmet was a warrior goddess as
well as a goddess of healing. She was
said to be the mother of Imhotep.

in a rational progression from the head to the lower back, and the text demonstrates sound scientific knowledge in its treatment of muscles, bones, joints, and the blood supply. The papyrus discusses 48 case histories, each of which is laid out in a familiar, modern style, including a description of the problem all the way from examination and diagnosis to outlook and treatment. The practice of examining the patient to make a diagnosis is taken for granted today, but in Ancient Egypt, where gods ruled while moving in mysterious ways, interfering in this way was unheard of.

Among the Smith Papyrus cases are the earliest known descriptions of the cranial sutures (the joints between skull bones), the meninges (the layers surrounding the brain), and the cerebrospinal fluid (the liquid that surrounds and cushions the brain). Injuries at particular sites, including the brain and the cervical spine (neck vertebrae), are linked to loss of sensation and paralysis in various parts of the body, and to incontinence and quadriplegia. The Smith Papyrus treatments also include some of the first mentions of closing wounds with sutures (stitches), using raw meat to stem bleeding, and applying honey to prevent or treat infection. For example, Case Three states: "A man having a gaping head wound… penetrating to the bone… perforating his skull… After thou has stitched it, thou should lay fresh meat upon his wound the first day. Thou should not bind it… Thou should treat it afterward with grease, honey, and lint every day, until he recovers…" With its emphasis on trauma, the Smith Papyrus could be considered a manual for treating soldiers wounded in battle, or workers maimed on major construction projects, such as the pyramids – and the authors knew the limits of their craft. Of the 48 Smith Papyrus cases, 14 are classed as "Outcome Unfavourable: An ailment not to be treated... A case which the surgeon cannot cure and which he is led to discuss by his scientific interest alone".

Another valuable document of the time is the Ebers Papyrus, which, like the Smith Papyrus, physically dates from around 3,500 years ago, but was probably copied from much older documents, possibly originating in Imhotep's time. In 1872, it was bought by the German writer and Egyptologist Georg Ebers, who specialized in penning historical novels set in Ancient Egypt, Greece, and Rome. It has about 110 pages, is more than 20m (66 ½ft) long, is 30cm (12in) tall, and currently resides at the University of Leipzig, Germany, where Ebers was professor of Egyptian studies. In contrast to the Smith Papyrus, the Ebers Papyrus details hundreds of spells, chants, and incantations designed to expel evil and disease from the sufferer, as well as many herbal and mineral remedies. Also, the contents are less systematically organized. They begin with magic spells to ward off bad spirits, then describe an extensive array of parasitic gut infestations, bowel diseases, skin problems, ulcers, anal problems, heart conditions, head-based disorders, urinary difficulties, wounds, and gynaecological issues.

Even older is the Kahun Gynaecological Papyrus. Dating from about 3,800 years ago, it is one of the first medical documents known, and is now in the care of University College, London. It is concerned mostly with the female reproductive system, and discusses aids to fertility, conception, pregnancy testing, and contraception. For period pains, it prescribes: "Treatment for a woman who loves bed, she does not rise, and does not shake off...

her gripings or spasms of the womb... Let her drink two henu [about one litre] of khaui, and let

DIVINE PROTECTION
Amulets such as this faience (glazed ceramic) brooch were worn by Ancient Egyptians to ward off evil and to protect against disease.

her spue it out immediately". There is also a recipe for a contraceptive preparation made from honey, sour milk, and crocodile dung, to be inserted into the vagina.

Slightly later than Smith and Ebers came the Hearst, Brugsch, and London Medical Papyri. Together with evidence from tomb carvings and other artefacts, including the equipment used for mummification, these provide a good account of history's first comprehensive system of medicine. Mummy preparation (see p.29) gave Egyptian physicians a patchy knowledge of the body's insides, and practice in the use of instruments such as saws, hooks, drills, and forceps. However, treatment by surgery – apart from traumatic injuries – was rare.

The Ancient Egyptians attached great importance to diet and hygiene. False eyes, false teeth, and similar prostheses were also being developed. Yet the spiritual and magical side of healing remained central. Neck, upper-arm, wrist, calf, and ankle amulets were worn to repel visits from demons or vengeful spectres that might bring disease and suffering. And if the demons did make it into the body, then the first recourses were spells and invocations, rather than rational examination and treatment.

Surgery in Ancient Egypt

The priest-physicians of Ancient Egypt were held in great esteem. They conducted surgery mainly for the treatment of traumatic injuries: doctors stitched wounds, performed simple operations to mend broken bones, and amputated limbs, using willow-leaf bandages for their antiseptic properties. They also cut out and cauterized tumours, and may even have performed delicate procedures such as tracheotomy (opening the airway), using a wide range of tools, including scalpels and knives made of flint or the glass-like rock obsidian, which they could hone to a razor-sharp edge.

Ancient prostheses

Archaeologists have found artificial toes from Ancient Egypt – one made of wood and leather, another from plaster, glue, and linen. These are the oldest known prosthetic devices. They would have been invaluable to people who had lost a toe through injury, or as a result of gangrene caused by a condition such as diabetes, helping them to balance and walk more easily when wearing traditional Egyptian sandals.

PROSTHETIC BIG TOE OF WOOD AND
LEATHER, 15TH CENTURY BCE

Saw blade

Scoop probe

Flask

Tooth forceps

Cupping vessels

Shears

RELIEF SHOWING SURGICAL TOOLS
EGYPT, 2ND CENTURY CE

This Roman-period carved relief from the temple of the crocodile-god Sobek, at Kom Ombo, illustrates a range of surgical tools, together with items used in diagnosis and in the preparation of medicines.

Catheter

Knife

Bowl

Weighing scales

Scalpel

Sponge

Mummification

When important Egyptians died, their bodies were preserved by mummification. The process involved removing the internal organs and treating the body with preservatives – the Egyptians did not place a taboo on the handling of corpses, as some later cultures did. However, embalmers made only small incisions in the corpse, so their work did not give them a detailed knowledge of anatomy.

Bronze hook inserted through nostril

EXTRACTING THE BRAIN AND ORGANS
A long hook was used to pull the brain out through the nose, while the intestines, liver, stomach and lungs were removed through a cut in the left side of the body, before they could decompose. The heart – centre of emotion and intelligence – was left in for the afterlife, but all the other organs were dessicated.

ORGAN CONTAINERS
The embalmer either returned the dehydrated organs of the deceased to the body or placed them in containers called canopic jars. These jars, shaped to resemble miniature coffins and bearing the heads of guardian deities, were put in the tomb alongside the mummified body.

Hippocrates and
Greek Medicine

SOME 2,700 YEARS AGO, the original Olympic Games were being established, and Greek civilization and influence were spreading throughout much of Europe. Within 200 years or so, Greece had entered its Classical phase, which saw glorious achievements in politics, art, philosophy, and literature. In this centre of the ancient world, Hippocrates of Cos (c.460–c.370 BCE) – perhaps the most important figure in the history of medicine – was born.

Greek medicine borrowed much from preceding Egyptian beliefs and practices (see pp.22–29), but it shifted away from the previous view of disease as some kind of punishment from the gods. Greek physicians moved towards the idea that illness was a natural phenomenon of the body, caused by imbalances in what were known as the four "humours" (see pp.106–107) – an idea that remained central to medicine for 2,000 years. Humorism, as it is called, may have reached Greece from Egypt or Mesopotamia, or it may have come from the Greek idea of the four elements – earth, air, fire, and water – as crystallized by the philosopher Empedocles a few decades before Hippocrates. Whatever its origin, humorism held that the body contained, or was even made of, four fluids: blood, yellow bile, black bile, and phlegm. In a healthy body, these humours were calm and well balanced, but if something happened to disturb their equilibrium, illness ensued. The type of humoral imbalance, and the particular humours involved, defined the disease. This was because each humour had its own special qualities, linked not only to one of the classical elements, but also to a particular part of the body, and even to a season of the year. Blood was associated with air, the liver, spring, warmth, and moisture; yellow bile was related to fire, the spleen, summer, warmth, and dryness; black bile was linked to earth, the gall bladder, autumn, cold, and dryness; while phlegm was related to water, the lungs, the brain, winter, cold, and dampness. So, for example, if blood as a humour became "excessive", the illness was likely to be warm and moist in character, with symptoms such as redness, swelling, rapid pulse and breathing, perspiration, uneasy sleep, and even delirium – the typical profile of a fever due to infection.

THE FATHER OF WESTERN MEDICINE
Hippocrates, here depicted treating a sick woman,
established medicine as a discipline distinct from
magic and religion.

The treatment would therefore be bleeding to reduce the quantity of
blood and its corresponding sanguine humour. Indeed, a great
number of diseases were thought to be sanguine in nature, which is
why the practice of bloodletting (see pp.132–33) became so common
in Europe. Other ways in which to restore balance to the humours
included taking herbs and foods associated with the particular
humour in question, either to increase or reduce its quantity and
influence, and the use of emetics and purges.

Hippocrates wrote a great deal about the humours in the collection
of works known as the Hippocratic Corpus, which consists of some 60
written documents, ranging from scattered notes and jottings to long,
well-argued theses and sets of case histories. The modern view is that
Hippocrates himself did not write all of these works — which vary not
only in style but in opinion — but that they were added to by students,
disciples, and later followers up to four or five centuries later. Certainly
this explains the vast scope of the Corpus, which ranges from
philosophical excursions into the nature of knowledge and the
standing of medicine within the sciences, to diagnoses of fevers and
epidemic infections, problems associated with fractured bones and
displaced joints, female infertility, veins, teeth, hygiene, dreams,
haemorrhoids, and epilepsy. This last condition was known as the
sacred disease by many Greeks, who saw it as a result of demonic

possession. The Hippocratic view rejected this idea, considering epilepsy to be a problem based entirely on the body: "Men believe only that it is a divine disease because of their ignorance and amazement".

Details of Hippocrates' life are somewhat limited, but he was a contemporary of Socrates and was referred to by various prominent Greeks, including Plato, who was about 35 years younger, and Aristotle, who was a teenager when Hippocrates died. His father may well have been a physician, and the young Hippocrates probably trained at the asclepeion on the isle of Cos, where he was born. The asclepeion was a temple dedicated to Asclepios, the Greek god of healing and medicine, and a place where the sick were treated. Asclepios himself was perhaps a derivation of one of the healing gods of Egypt, maybe the physician-turned-deity Imhotep. His trademark, known as the Rod of Asclepios, was a stick with a snake coiled around it – perhaps because potentially fatal snake venom was used in tiny doses as a therapy, or because the reptile's regular skin-shedding represented the casting off of old problems and illnesses and entering a new phase of life. Whatever its origins, the staff-and-serpent duo has been used as a symbol of medicine and the healing arts throughout the ages. Two of Asclepios's daughters also live on in medical terminology; Hygieia, linked to our word "hygiene", and Panacea, noted as the goddess of the universal cure-all.

Throughout his life, Hippocrates seems to have wandered the shores of the Aegean and inland, both in Greece and what are today Bulgaria and Turkey. He practised as a physician, wrote, lectured, tutored students, and argued about his medical ideas and practices. He was also said to be more than proficient at music, poetry, mathematics, and even athletics. At one stage he was apparently imprisoned for up to 20 years because he rejected the

GOD OF HEALING
Shown here with his snake-entwined staff, Asclepios was the Greek god of physicians, healing, and rejuvenation.

idea that deities and spirits were the causes of illness. He was sentenced by dignitaries who believed that their role was to mediate between humanity and the gods, and who saw that their power was being eroded by Hippocrates' new teachings. Sadly, Hippocrates' whereabouts in later life, and his place of death, are unclear – the latter perhaps being Larissa, northwest Greece.

Many aspects of the Hippocratic approach to medicine are still with us today. We distinguish between illnesses that are described as acute (sudden and short-lived) or chronic (long-term and persistent), and diseases that are endemic (occur frequently in a particular region or population) and epidemic (break out suddenly, then spread rapidly and affect a large proportion of the population). The Hippocratic School of Medicine also pioneered methods of clinical observation, examination, recording, and analysis of patient consultations – procedures we now take for granted in medical practice. Observation was already important at the time, but Hippocrates formalized it into a systematic process. It should be carried out at least once a day, in order to follow the diagnosis and natural history of the disease, which would then enable a doctor to give a prognosis or a prediction: "I believe that it is an excellent thing for a physician to practise forecasting. He will carry out the treatment best if he knows beforehand from the present symptoms what will take place later". Documentation included regular notes of signs and symptoms, such as pulse, breathing, temperature, skin complexion, appearance of the eyes and mouth, palpation of the inner organs, and excretions.

Hippocrates was keen on urine and faeces, since he believed that they offered much guidance on how the body was functioning: "In proportion to what a person eats, he should evacuate bowels two or three times daily... more copiously in the morning." Also: "It is better that flatulence should be passed than that it should be retained". Investigating the lower bowel involved an anal or

"Wherever the art of medicine
is loved, there is also a love
of humanity"

HIPPOCRATES OF COS

REFUSING GIFTS FROM THE ENEMY
According to legend, Hippocrates refused lavish gifts from Artaxerxes, king of the Persians, whose troops were being ravaged by plague. Hippocrates' refusal to help the enemy raised patriotism above the physician's duty to serve all men.

rectal speculum – a tongs-like device that opened the orifice to allow inspection of the interior. This was one of the earliest forms of endoscopy – peering into the body's innards through a natural opening or purpose-made incision. For troublesome haemorrhoids, the treatments ranged from ointments or salves to ligation (tying off).

Hippocrates advised that all records should be written in a clear, objective, and uncluttered fashion, so that the physicians involved could look back and draw from their experiences when dealing with new patients. Crucially, other doctors could also access the records and thereby learn from the information. This was the beginning of the vast health and medical databases that have become so important in the 21st century.

With so much attention paid to ascertaining the patient's condition, it may seem surprising that the Hippocratic attitude towards treatment was restrained, cautious, and even humble. The best remedies were peace, clean conditions, comfortable rest, good nutrition, and continued observation – allowing the body's natural powers of self-healing to do the work. Bandaging, massage, and soothing balms might be required now and then, but powerful medicines and invasive techniques were a last resort. A major edict for the physician was: "First, do no harm". Invasive techniques were rare, since at this time in Greece, as later in Ancient Rome (see pp.40–47), there were bans on most forms of human dissection for anatomical learning or treatment. Surgery was limited to patching up wounds and similar trauma. The skin was rarely broken deliberately, so the human body's insides were mostly a mystery.

Hippocrates had a trusted list of gentle, tried-and-tested remedies, which included olive oil, honey, and a range of more than 200 vegetables and herbs – either to be eaten whole or taken as extracts – from figs, garlic, and onion to parsley, poppy, hibiscus, chamomile, cumin, and saffron. Believing that some long-term conditions resulted from excessive or unwise dietary consumption, he espoused: "Let food be your medicine and medicine be your food".

Another aspect of Hippocratic thought is the notion of the crisis – the observation that a sickness develops, worsens, and reaches a kind of tipping point, at which either the body starts to fight back and the patient's recovery begins, or a downward spiral ensues,

GREEK SURGICAL TOOLS
This marble relief shows a case of knives, lancets, and bone levers flanked by a pair of vessels used for bloodletting.

from which the body can still rally into remission — or fade again, or relapse. These ideas of remission and relapse originate from Hippocrates' time, and probably come from Hippocrates himself.

Many diseases and conditions were first described by Hippocrates and his followers. One is the clubbing of the nails and fingers — a condition sometimes known as "Hippocratic fingers". This can be an important indication of pulmonary problems such as abscesses on the lungs or lung cancer, of heart diseases such as endocarditis, and of various congenital conditions.

The sheer scale of Hippocrates' influence tends to overshadow the achievements of other Greek physicians. One such doctor was Herophilus (c.335–280 BCE), who worked in Alexandria, where he was allowed to found a tradition of dissecting human corpses. He studied the heart, blood vessels, brain, eye, and the nervous system, and is regarded as one of the first true anatomists. Slightly later, Erasistratus (304–250 BCE) was also at Alexandria for a time, where he helped to establish the medical school and had influential ideas on the function of the heart and the blood system (see p.135).

Gradually, the Hippocratic movement changed the public's view of the physician as an itinerant curiosity who had little social standing (and who was likely to cause more problems than he solved) to that of an upstanding member of society. Vital to this transformation was another great Hippocratic health-care instigation — a code of conduct. We know its details under the general umbrella term of the Hippocratic Oath, and its requirements have resonated with patients and the general public through the ages. After all, who wants a doctor who is slovenly, unhygienic, shabby, immoral, unethical, a careless blabbermouth, and not up to speed with the latest advances?

The Hippocratic Corpus' *On the Physician*, and the texts derived from it through history, prescribe what the ideal doctor should be like. He should be upright, honest, stable, and beyond reproach or corruption, and must attend the patient with courtesy and consideration, take

WITNESS ALL THE GODS
The Hippocratic Oath – shown here in a later version, in English – requires a physician to swear that he or she will abide by various ethical principles, including that of confidentiality.

care of the patient's position, and note his symptoms diligently. The doctor's surgery should also inspire confidence by being clean, tidy, well lit, and organized, with each piece of equipment laid out methodically. Another Hippocratic idea was that information about the patient's ailment should remain confidential – and that if other people are involved in the consultation, then they too must respect this privacy. The instructions even go so far as to recommend what the physician should wear and how he should stand and move. This Hippocratic vision of the ideal doctor, so comforting to potential patients, has endured through evolving adaptations of the Hippocratic Oath. Extracts from various translations run approximately:

"I swear by Apollo the healer, Asclepios, Hygieia, and Panacea… Witness all the gods, all the goddesses, to keep according to my ability and my judgment, the following oath… I will prescribe regimens for the good of my patients, in accordance with my ability and my judgement… I will never do harm to anyone… I will give no deadly medicine if asked… I will preserve the purity of my life and my arts… In every house I will enter only for the good of my patients, keeping myself away from all intentional ill-doing and all seduction and especially from the pleasures of love with women or men, be they free or slaves… All that may come to my knowledge in the exercise of my profession or in daily commerce… I will keep to myself, holding such things shameful to be spoken about, and will never reveal…"

Medical students around the world can choose to swear upon their medical authority's version of the Hippocratic Oath. Although rarely used in its original form, the modern adaptations embody the spirit of the upstanding, ethical, moral, careful, clean, and compassionate physician.

Galen and the Rule of Rome

IF THERE WERE AN AWARD FOR the deepest and most enduring influence over Western medicine, then Galen of Pergamon, perhaps with Hippocrates of Cos (see pp.30–39), would head the shortlist. After travelling the eastern Mediterranean during his thirties, Galen settled in Rome – the imperial centre of civilization, with its empire stretching from the Atlantic Ocean east to the Red, Black, and Caspian seas. In Rome, Galen built up a massive body of work and a towering reputation that presided over human anatomy, physiology, and medicine for more than 1,400 years, and in some respects for a few centuries longer.

Claudius Galen (129–c.216 CE) was raised and educated in a well-to-do family in Pergamon – the modern-day city of Bergama, in western Turkey. One of the chief hubs of trade and learning in both Greek and Roman times, Pergamon had a library of approximately 200,000 works, which drew philosophers and other intellectuals from around the Mediterranean and West Asia. Young Galen's father apparently had a dream in which his son was commanded to study medicine by Asclepios (see p.32), the Greek god of healing. This Galen did, from the age of 16, before setting off at the age of 20 on travels that took him around mainland Greece and Turkey, to islands such as Crete and Cyprus, and to the hallowed city of Alexandria, Egypt – home of the ancient world's largest library and foremost medical school. Galen soaked up knowledge and experiences in all areas of medicine as well as philosophy, and returned to Pergamon in about 157 CE. Here he took the prestigious position of physician-surgeon to the gladiators who fought

GALEN OF PERGAMON
Perhaps the greatest physician of antiquity, Claudius Galen made numerous contributions to medicine, particularly in the fields of anatomy and pharmacology.

in front of thousands of baying spectators. His skills with knife, saw, and other surgical tools were soon famous throughout the region — and Galen himself recorded how he was able to treat gladiators' terrible wounds with far greater success than any of his rivals or predecessors. He also noted how gladiatorial injuries, particularly deep gashes and sliced innards, were like windows into the body. This fascination with dissection and anatomy would stay with him for life.

Pergamon soon became too small for a man of Galen's ability and ambition, and in 162 CE he decamped to Rome. He stayed in the Eternal City for the rest of his years, apart from a return to Pergamon between about 166 CE and 168 CE. In Rome, Galen worked his way into the upper echelons of medicine and into the favour of imperial appointees. However, the city's regular medical hierarchy felt threatened by this regional upstart, and their muttered intimidation forced Galen to make his brief return to Pergamon. He was commanded back by Emperor Marcus Aurelius, who wished him to serve as imperial physician, as did the emperor's successors, Commodus and Septimius Severus.

Rome was regularly hit by plagues during this period, most of which were epidemics of smallpox. The epidemic from about 165 CE to 180 CE, known as the Antonine Plague (from the emperor's full name, Marcus Aurelius Antoninus), has also been called the "Plague of Galen". This is because, while other commentators noted how the disease was jeopardizing Rome's military power, the imperial physician wrote extensively about its terrible human cost. Historians point to some five million dead across the Roman world during the Antonine Plague, thought to include co-emperors Lucius Verus in the first surge of 169 CE, and Marcus Aurelius during a later outbreak in 180 CE. Even the start of Rome's decline has been blamed on the plague, since it weakened armies and forced commanders to withdraw from politically unstable territories.

Galen completed most of his immense written work in Rome, during the rule of Commodus. Estimates of his total output range from five to ten million words, with some three million surviving. His language of choice was his native Greek. He dictated at speed to a small army of scribes, and his manuscripts were stored in various stately rooms and temples around the city, particularly the Temple of Peace. Much of the immense Galenic Corpus — the body of work attributed to him and his close helpers — has been copied and handed down relatively unscathed. Other works, however, were lost to much of

BLOOD SPORTS
This Roman mosaic shows gladiators fighting to the
death – a sport that gave Galen, as a physician, plenty
of first-hand experience of human anatomy.

Europe as the western half of the Roman Empire collapsed, although
they survived in the east as the Roman territories there were absorbed
by the Byzantine Empire. Several centuries later, Galen's works were
taken up by Islamic scholars, who translated them into languages
such as Arabic and Syriac (see pp.100–105). From here, many works
made their way back to Europe, especially during the early Renaissance,
where they were translated into Latin, and eventually into regional
European languages such as English, German, French, and Spanish.

Galen's works were so vast (both in scope and volume) that many
have been misinterpreted, poorly translated, and "corrected" along the
way according to the beliefs of later times. Writings that were actually
his have been appropriated by later authors, while scripts from other
writers have been wrongfully attributed to Galen. Today, experts still

disagree over whether Galen even wrote certain pieces, and, if so, how close our versions of them are to his originals. The basis of Galen's medical philosophy was Greek (see pp.30–39). He followed Hippocratic doctrines, such as the idea that the body is made of four humours – namely blood, yellow bile, black bile, and phlegm (see pp.106–107). He explicitly linked these to the four elements – air (gas), water (liquid), earth (solid), and fire (combustion and change) – blood corresponding to air, yellow bile to fire, black bile to earth, and phlegm to water. He also held that there were primary and secondary features of these elements that related to temperature and humidity – air being wet first and hot second; fire being hot and dry; earth being dry and cold; and water being cold and wet. According to Galen, imbalances or improper mixing between these features led to ill health.

Galen also grafted onto the humours and elements a series of behavioural types or personality traits that had been earlier postulated by Aristotle. Galen suggested that an excess of a certain humour in the body produced a particular temperament or disposition in that person. Thus a sanguine (blood) character is typically active, creative, and sociable, if perhaps impatient; a choleric (yellow bile) character is usually driven, passionate, and domineering, if aggressive; a melancholic (black bile) character is generally quiet, pensive, and self-contained, if prone to sadness; while a phlegmatic (phlegm) character is commonly calm, composed, kind, and lethargic.

Some of Galen's writings cover philosophy and philology. He devoured Greek texts and made extensive comments on works by Hippocrates, Herophilus, Erasistratus, and others (see p.37). He was keen on the details of language in medicine, and, concerned that many Greek works had become corrupted, he tried to recover their true medical meanings. To these, he added his own ideas on a huge range of health and medical topics, from diet, hygiene, and staying

"Every animal is sad after coitus, except the human female and the rooster"

CLAUDIUS GALEN

fit, to the causes of disease, examination of the patient, respiration, humours, elements, temperaments, herbal remedies, purging, bloodletting, and, of course, surgery and anatomy.

The practice of human dissection for teaching and demonstration purposes was forbidden by law in Ancient Rome (although surgical treatments were advanced for the time), so Galen resorted instead to opening up animals – from fish and reptiles to dogs, goats, pigs, and allegedly one of the emperor's deceased tame elephants. In particular, he valued "apes" as subjects – although his Barbary ape victims were actually a type of macaque monkey. From these species he confidently and authoritatively (and often erroneously) compiled a map of human anatomy.

Aside from the achievements of Galen, the rule of Rome brought progress in many areas of health and medicine. These included the encouragement of bathing and general hygiene, the provision of clean drinking water, improved sanitation, and advances both in surgery and in herbal and mineral-based remedies. The Roman surgeon's "tool kit" (see pp.46–47) boasted a varied array of scalpels and other blades, drills, and saws for bone removal and amputation, hooks and simple retractors to hold nerves and vessels aside or to close gaping wounds, and urinary catheters to relieve bladder and urethra blockages. Opium, alcohol, and herbs such as henbane provided relief from pain, while alcohol, hot oils, and vinegar were used to clean wounds and incisions. Around this time, general surgery expanded into specialisms such as chest, abdomen, limbs, neck, eyes, ears, and teeth. Dental crowns and false teeth were fashioned from gold, silver, ivory, bone, or wood, depending on the status of the patient.

ROMAN PHARMACIST
This tombstone of Armenian king Mithridates VI depicts a Roman pharmacist and his assistant preparing medicines.

Many plants were used for medicines, as much for religious reasons – being favourites of particular gods or priests – as for any therapeutic effect. These were listed by Greek physician, plant

PHYSICIAN'S JARS
Dating from the 1st century CE, these glass
containers held various ointments and
unguents designed for medicinal use.

expert, and herbalist Pedanius
Dioscorides (c.40–90 CE) in his
De Materia Medica (*On Medical
Substances*). This massive work in
five-volumes was the first to
establish the idea of the pharmacopoeia
– an encyclopaedia of pharmaceutical preparations, healing herbs,
minerals, and other drugs and medications, explaining how they are
produced, what they are prescribed for, and their intended effects.

Another physician from Greece, who preceded Galen, was Soranus
of Ephesus (c.98–140 CE). Among his major works was *Gynaikeia*
(*Gynaecology*), which covered not only gynaecology, but also obstetrics,
midwifery, perinatal care, and paediatrics (care of the infant), with
sections on abortion and birth control. Much of the description is given
in graphic, practical detail. For instance, Soranus spends time detailing
the characteristics he expects of the ideal midwife – including
discretion, literacy, mental ability, good memory, respectability,
soundness of limb, robustness... and long, slim fingers with short nails.

For all its other achievements, however, the medicine of Ancient
Rome will always be dominated by Galen. It was some eleven centuries
later that new trends for dissection were led by Mondino de Liuzzi at
Bologna (see p.117). With the ban on human cadaver dissection then
circumventable, Liuzzi reintroduced the process into his medical
courses. In 1316, he wrote *Anathomia Corporis Humani* (*Anatomy of the Human
Body*) as a manual for his students. A groundbreaking work, it
nevertheless upheld some of of Galen's anatomical errors. This was
followed by the pioneering work of Renaissance anatomists such as
Andreas Vesalius (see pp.116–25), which contradicted many of Galen's
declarations on anatomy. In the following century, Galen's complex
ideas on the physiology of heart and blood were superseded when
William Harvey clarified the process of blood circulation (see pp.134–43).
Such refutations of Galen may hardly seem surprising, given the
immense scope of his work and the strictures under which he worked.
Yet such was his gigantic sway, that even in the 19th century some
medical schools were still reliant on parts of his teaching.

Roman Surgical Tools

One of the most remarkable discoveries made by archaeologists in the Roman city of Pompeii, destroyed by a volcanic eruption in 79 CE, was a collection of surgical instruments in the building called the House of the Surgeon. Made of bronze or iron, these beautifully preserved 1st-century CE tools were typical of those used since the 5th century BCE. The design of such tools changed little until the 19th century.

CUPPING VESSEL
Heated and placed on the skin to draw out the blood, vessels like this were used for bloodletting (see pp.132–33).

SCALPELS
Like modern surgeons, Roman physicians used scalpels in a wide range of shapes and sizes. As well as large-bladed scalpels, they had instruments with smaller blades for making fine incisions or reaching parts of the body to which access was restricted.

SURGICAL SCISSORS
Shears were sometimes used in surgery, but achieving a sharp edge to them was hard. They were most often used to cut hair, which was believed to benefit health.

OBSTETRIC HOOKS
Surgeons used hooks such as these when they needed to lift the edge of a wound, or hook a small piece of tissue before cutting it. They also used hooks to grip or manipulate blood vessels or pieces of tissue during surgery.

VAGINAL SPECULUM
Used during the examination and treatment of vaginal and uterine disorders, this device opens using a lever mechanism with a screw thread. Similar instruments were still in use during the 18th century.

CLYSTER
This syringe-like instrument came in two parts: a vessel with tube, and a piston. It was used to administer enemas, or drain excessive fluids from the patient's body.

BONE LEVERS
Levers such as these were designed to ease a bone into its correct position when setting a fracture. The ends of the levers are curved and ridged so that they grip the surface of the bone well.

The Dark Ages
in Europe

IN THE YEAR 476 CE, A COALITION of Germanic and other tribes, led by warlord Flavius Odoacer, marched through Italy seizing lands and power. In Ravenna, the Roman emperor Romulus Augustus was deposed and exiled. This event commonly marks the end of the western Roman Empire, which had been fading for three centuries. It also signifies the drift of Europe into nearly a thousand years of confused, obscure history called the Middle Ages, which ended with the flowering of the Renaissance in the 14th century. During the earlier phase of the Middle Ages, up until about the year 1000, European societies and cultures fragmented. The rule of law weakened in the face of warring tribes, and much of the progress made by Ancient Greece (see pp.30–39) and Rome (see pp.40–45) was lost or even reversed. Historical records were scant, living conditions declined for many under feudal systems, and fear, poverty, and persecution were widespread. The popular term for this era is the Dark Ages.

It was a dark time for medicine too. Practitioners were often untrained and unlicensed, partly because there were few professional bodies or systems in place to oversee their activities and to rein in their excesses. Diagnoses were spurious, and driven by reward and the promise of influence. Some treatments helped, but others were damaging and even cruel. During these centuries, European medicine still relied on concepts from Ancient Greece and Rome – especially the theory of the four humours (see pp.106–107). Medical care now became the realm of the Church, which was primarily Catholic, and summarily organized courts and self-serving guilds. The lessons of Hippocrates, which had shown that sickness was a natural process within the body, and not the result of divine punishment or demonic possession, were largely discarded. As a result, quackery and charlatanism flourished. If a physician or healer treated a patient who then recovered, then all credit to the practitioner, who could claim a special link to the Almighty. If the outcome was a worsening of the condition, or even death – well, that too was God's will. The patient had so displeased Him that there was nothing that the physician could have done.

TRADITIONAL REMEDIES
A medieval apothecary and his assistant
prepare herbal remedies – treatments
that were often dismissed as witchcraft.

The most recent advances in medieval
medicine were the preserve of the
nobility, the rich, and the Church.
Some religious authorities even
shunned age-old cures, such as the
use of healing herbs, as "witchcraft".
The only way to a true cure, they
said, was total dedication and
obedience to God, who would
dispense reward by banishing the illness. The phenomenon of the
"miracle cure" also came to the fore, with some alleged physicians
claiming saintly powers. However, most peasants in the countryside
were far removed from such matters, and continued to use herbal
recipes and other treatments from ancient times.

From about the 12th century, early versions of hospitals began to
appear. Most of them were attached to monasteries, convents, and
similar religious institutions. Generally clean, with reasonable food
and compassionate staff, they provided much-needed care and
comfort to all manner of sufferers from most levels of society. They
were also stopping places for travellers, retreats for students, and
havens for the destitute, disabled, elderly, "feeble-minded", and
others who were disadvantaged. Worship was incorporated into a
highly organized daily routine, partly to encourage recovery and
partly as an institutionalizing force, and physicians visited regularly.
Nevertheless, a typical consultation with a physician – especially
during the Early Middle Ages – could be a dicey affair. In fact, it might
not even be with a physician, but with a herbalist, a midwife, an
occultist, or even a part-time witch. The practitioner might begin by
studying the skin, taking the pulse (which indicated heart "spasms",
since blood circulation had not been discovered), and noting the
breathing patterns. Perhaps he or she would make a few incisions in a
vein to assess the quality of the blood – runny or sticky, bright or
dark? – and then sniff, prod, decant, and generally scrutinize the
liquid and solid excrement. Tasting blood, urine, and even faeces
might be necessary, as well as swirling them around with various

chemical reagents. All of these observations helped to establish the balance of the humours and whether phlegm, yellow bile, or another humour was at fault. The patient's own account of the problem might also provide clues. For instance, he or she — being mindful of God's ability to punish — might admit to some recent transgression or immorality. If the local physician was not with the patient, all the results were communicated to him, and he would then diagnose remotely and convey the prescription back to the patient and carers.

The great cure-all treatment of the age was undoubtedly bleeding or bloodletting (see pp.132–33). This dated back to Hippocrates and Galen, the latter believing that among the four humors, blood was dominant. Many illnesses involved an excess of blood, a condition known as a plethora, and so removing some reduced the surplus and purged the body. Having no knowledge of the circulatory system, people thought that blood was made in the liver and consumed in the tissues (see pp.134–43). If this turnover became unbalanced, blood might accumulate and stagnate in the extremities. Again, bloodletting was the obvious answer.

Galen and his followers had devised sophisticated sets of instructions for bleeding. The manner of the procedure depended on the symptoms and their severity, details about the patient (such as age and pre-existing conditions), the time of day, week, and year, and even the prevailing weather. There were guidelines on whether to open either an artery or a vein, and where on the body to do so. Venesection (phlebotomy) involved releasing blood from a sizeable superficial vein, especially in the forearm; the blood oozed slowly, was easy to control, and clotted readily. Opening an artery (arteriotomy) was much riskier as the blood spurted out under pressure, was difficult to quantify, and took longer to congeal. The question of which vessel to approach was also highly complex. Theory linked certain internal organs, such as the liver and the lungs, with particular veins, although these were not always easy to access. This led to the practices of "derivation" and "revulsion". In derivation, blood was drawn from near the affected area; revulsion involved bleeding from a site far away. So neck pain might be treated in the revulsion manner by letting blood from the ankle, while a disorder of the spleen might require opening a vein in the left wrist. Medieval physicians added more detail to the bloodletting procedure, including what kind of knife or leech to use, and what the patient should do while

BLEEDING THE EMPEROR WITH LEECHES
This illustration from Boccaccio's *Decameron* shows the Roman
emperor Galerius being bled by leeches. According to the text,
his symptoms included putrefaction and an abominable stench.

the blood flowed – pray, recite poetry, even play a musical instrument.
Some conditions required only an eggcup of the red liquid. Others
stipulated that the patient be bled until they swooned or collapsed – a
positive sign that bad spirits had been expunged and that the humours
were back in equilibrium.

A handy medical reference text for physicians was the "leechbook",
perhaps so-called because physicians were nicknamed "leeches",
from the habit of using these worm-like creatures to drain blood for
almost any ailment. Most leechbooks contained remedies of the time
gathered indiscriminately from a vast array of sources. A well-known
surviving example dating back to the 10th century, perhaps derived

AMOUNT OF BLOOD DRAWN BY A SINGLE LEECH

5—10 ML
(0.17– 0.33FL OZ)

from a 9th-century version, is *Medicinale Anglicum*, commonly known as *Bald's Leechbook*. Its first part covers almost 90 external and infectious problems affecting the ear, face, teeth, and so on, down to the feet; the second part deals with internal disorders such as vomiting, stomach pains, and diarrhoea. Woven into the lists are dog bites, rash from bug stings, hair loss, headache, backache, liver pains, worries about evil spirits, men who lack virility, and women who talk too much.

Bald's Leechbook even has a surgical remedy (very rare for the time) for harelip: "Mash mastic very small, add egg white, mingle as thou dost vermilion, cut with a knife the false lip edges, sew tight with silk, smear all over with the salve, ere the silk rot". A more gentle treatment (if not for the bird involved) is given for excessive hair: "If hair be too thick, take a swallow, burn it to ashes under a tile and have the ashes shed on [the site]". A leechbook was an eclectic compendium covering practical advice, herbs and minerals, rituals, poems, incantations, religious pleas, and philosophical musings, some of which can be traced back to ancient Roman and Arabic teachings.

Without a leechbook, a physician might be inclined to experiment. One such experimenter was Johannes de Mirfield, a respected physician of St Bartholomew's Hospital, London, who recommended the following medicinal bath: "Take blind [newborn] puppies, gut them, and cut off the feet; then boil in water, and in this water let the patient bathe. Let him stay in the bath for four hours after he has eaten, and while in the bath, he should keep his head covered, and his chest completely swathed with the skin of a goat, so he does not catch a sudden chill".

One area of particular ignorance in Medieval Europe was anatomy. The Catholic Church, in particular, was against incisions and invasions of the body, unless it was for life-threatening wounds, and then only for the nobility and members of the ruling class. Those brave doctors who did try to open up patients were hampered on many fronts. Basic anatomical knowledge was scanty, so few doctors had any idea which organs were where and what they did. If the patient was conscious, anaesthesia and pain relief could only be provided by administering alcohol, opium, or something similar in terrifyingly hit-and-miss doses – and with no knowledge of germs or antisepsis, dirt and pus in the innards would almost certainly lead to infection and death.

One of the chief afflictions of the time was leprosy, more recently referred to as Hansen's Disease. Recorded since antiquity, especially on the Indian subcontinent, leprosy generated great fear, not only because it gradually attacked parts of the body until they rotted and fell away, but also because it was reputedly so easy to catch. Consequently, leprosy victims suffered intense social stigmatization, and many were quarantined or confined to leper colonies (otherwise known as leprosaria or lazar houses). Some of the colonies allowed the lepers no rights whatsoever, since Catholic doctrine decreed that people with leprosy had already died and were effectively the "living dead". At the other extreme, some saw leprosy as a pre-death visitation from God – a kind of purgatory and cleansing of sins in preparation for the ascent to Heaven – which gave lepers special sanctified status.

Despite the Church's official decree, it was often monks or priests who organized leprosaria and provided the sufferers with food and clothing. If lepers were allowed out, they had to carry and ring a bell, both to warn others of their coming and as a plea for charity. Few physicians or other healthy people ventured near. For reasons that are not entirely clear, leprosy became much less common during the 14th and 15th centuries in Europe – probably helped by the Black Death (see pp.54–55), which claimed the lives of so many who were already weakened by other forms of disease.

AIDING THE LIVING DEAD
An Augustinian monk brings food to a leper at a leprosarium. At the time, the Church's official doctrine was that lepers were people who had already died.

The Bubonic Plague

A scourge that swept Europe and Asia for centuries, the bubonic plague struck populations swiftly and brutally, killing millions and changing the world map irrevocably. Caused by the bacterium *Yersinia pestis*, carried by rat fleas, its main symptoms are swollen lymph nodes, seizures, and gangrene. It is often fatal, killing two-thirds of its victims within days, and spreads rapidly: pandemics occurred in the 6th–8th, 14th–18th, and 19th–20th centuries. There was no reliable treatment before antibiotics in the 20th century.

18TH-CENTURY PLAGUE DOCTOR WEARING HERB-INFUSED MASK

C.1400 Europe's population is reduced by tens of millions, as the plague **spreads uncontrollably**, exacerbated by poor living conditions and ineffective treatments.

C.1650s–70s So many people die in such a short space of time across Europe that they have to be buried pell-mell in brick-built **plague pits.**

541–42 The plague arrives in **Constantinople**, triggering an outbreak that spreads from Persia across the Roman Empire to Ireland.

1348 The authorities in Venice and Florence enforce strict **sanitary laws**, removing plague victims from the streets.

1377 Ragusa (Dubrovnik) imposes a **30-day quarantine** on travellers to the city.

1647 The **Great Plague of Seville** kills around 150,000 people in Seville and some 350,000 in other parts of Spain.

1346 The outbreak known as the **Black Death** begins, probably in the Russian Steppes; it reaches the Crimea later in the year.

1351 The plague reaches most of Europe and the Middle East, killing **millions of people**.

1439 English Parliament states that **"noble physicians"** advise avoiding contact with plague victims.

1665–66 The Great Plague of London leads to the death of about **100,000** people; many more flee the city.

ESTIMATED
PERCENTAGE OF
THE WORLD'S
POPULATION
KILLED BY THE
BLACK DEATH
DURING THE
14TH CENTURY

20%

1898 French physician Paul-Louis Simond shows that *Xenopsylla cheopis* fleas (oriental rat fleas) **transmit** the plague.

1894 Hong Kong-based scientists Kitasato Shibasaburo and Alexandre Yersin isolate the **plague bacillus** and name it *Yersinia pestis.*

1896 The plague **pandemic** reaches India and Pakistan.

1710-11 Half the population of Riga, Latvia, is **wiped out** by the plague.

1720 The Great Plague of Marseilles is the **last major outbreak** of plague in Europe.

1899 Ships carry the plague to **new territories** such as Egypt and Hawaii.

1707 A *cordon sanitaire* is set up around Prussia, with all visitors **quarantined**.

1855 The **third plague pandemic** begins in Yunnan Province, China.

1945 Scientists carry out the first clinical trials of the antibiotic **streptomycin** against the plague.

1679 The Plague of Vienna is part of a larger outbreak in **Austria, Germany, and Bohemia** (now part of the Czech Republic).

The Alchemists

ALCHEMY CAN BE DIFFICULT TO PIN DOWN. It has long and varied traditions across Asia and Europe and was prominent in medieval times, but its roots go back thousands of years. It combines philosophies and beliefs dealing with magic, spirits, and the supernatural, with intensely practical analytical and laboratory techniques involving elements, minerals, and other substances that would be familiar in chemistry research centres today. Alchemists' aims have varied through time and from place to place. Some of their best-known quests have included: changing "base" metals (common, ordinary, or inexpensive ones) such as lead, into precious metals, especially gold, using an object or formulation known as the Philosopher's Stone; creating a substance that can dissolve any other substance – the Universal Solvent or Alkahest; inventing a potion that confers eternal youth on those who drink it – the Elixir of Life; producing a substance that can cure every disease and ailment – the Panacea or Universal Remedy. These laudable aims have had useful, practical results – but there are many more layers to the curious realm of alchemy. It is essentially concerned with transmuting matter from one form to another, or remodelling one being into another. Physically, this means creating the most valuable substance in existence or achieving immortality. On a spiritual level, it involves the pursuit of fulfilment, completion, or perfection.

Practical or functional alchemy developed from chemical processes such as fermenting beer, tanning leather, smelting ores to extract valuable metals and minerals, preparing medicinal potions and balms, and distilling extracts from plants and the earth. These procedures involved processing and refining commonplace base substances to gain a pure, desired final product. For example, in metallurgy, ordinary rocks were smelted and treated, eventually to yield valuable metals such as glistening gold or the amazing silvery liquid metal mercury (or quicksilver). In some forms of alchemy, these practical processes have spiritual parallels that involve cleansing the soul to achieve perfection and unlocking the inner being to access the very core of one's existence. Indeed, for alchemical medicines to work against disease, it was thought, physical effects such as relief from symptoms can only occur if accompanied by such psychic transformations.

HOPING FOR A CURE
An alchemist fires up a stove to heat one of his
concoctions. Hopeful customers sample his potions
in the background.

The spiritual, mystical, and symbolic aspects of alchemy can be
regarded as "esoteric" – that is, restricted to one or a few individuals
who possess special awareness and privilege. This links alchemy to
the tradition of Hermeticism, which is based on the pronouncements
of Hermes Trismegistus, a semi-mythical figure of Ancient Egypt.
According to legend, he received divine knowledge and insight that
was then passed down through the ages – knowledge that could
enable spiritual or magical forces to affect the physical, material
world. The *Tabula Smaragdina* (*Emerald Tablet*) attributed to Hermes
Trismegistus would have lasting influence on alchemists for centuries.
During the Late Middle Ages and the Renaissance, the Hermetic

"That which is above is from that which is below"

THE EMERALD TABLET

tradition included alchemy as one of its three major components, along with numerology and the "magic of letters" – cryptography. The useful, practical aspects of alchemy, on the other hand, can be seen not as esoteric but as "exoteric", or widely accessible to anyone. From a modern standpoint, the idea of chasing such miraculously unrealistic objectives as the Elixir of Life or the Universal Remedy seems doomed from the start, yet by doing so, alchemists have made immense contributions to the development of mainstream sciences, especially chemistry, materials science, and medicine.

Alchemy and its applications to medicine have long and illustrious histories in Asia, especially China and India. In Europe, it can be traced back to the times of Ancient Egypt, Greece, and Rome. One of its earliest texts was written or compiled by Zosimos of Panopolis, who was probably an Egyptian living in Alexandria at the time of Roman control, some 1,700 years ago. Zosimos expounded at length on the philosophical and mystical aspects of alchemy, saying, for instance, that the transmutation of metals can occur only with a similar spiritual transformation of the soul and its ascent into the divine realm.

With the demise of the Roman Empire, alchemy – like mainstream medicine of the time – faded from historical view in Western Europe. But in common with other scholarly and academic pursuits, the spread of Islam in Eastern Europe, North Africa, and West Asia brought exciting developments. One of these was greater reliance on tests and experiments using an early form of scientific methodology. Jabir ibn Hayyan (c.721–c.815), known in Europe as Geber, was based in Kufa, near Baghdad (in what is now Iraq). The writings attributed to him were extensive and eclectic, ranging from philosophy and astrology to "the behaviour of matter when subjected to forced change". These accounts recorded experiments and analyses using substances varying from mild acetic acid (vinegar) to extremely corrosive sulphuric acid, as well as sulphur and mercury. Jabir's practical work involved distillation, crystallization, precipitation, and other procedures widely used today, employing flasks, burners, filters, condensers, and other familiar laboratory apparatus. Physicians, herbalists, healers, and apothecaries adopted these methods to prepare a new generation of medicines. Jabir also revised the classical "elements" of antiquity. He proposed three categories of elements — "spirits" such as mercury or sulphur, which would vaporise when heated; metals, such as gold or silver; and non-malleable substances such as stones, which could be ground into powders. These systems of elements would persist in alchemy for several centuries, as would the medicinal use of compounds containing mercury and sulphur.

Mercury has a long and double-edged medical history. During Jabir's time, mercury-containing balms and ointments, usually prepared from the metal's main ore, cinnabar (mercury sulphide), were in common use for skin problems. Later, calomel (mercurous chloride) was prescribed as a laxative, purgative, diuretic, and as a treatment for syphilis. Sulphur compounds were also common on the alchemist's workbench and in the apothecary's jars. Sulphur-rich waters were said to ease skin conditions, joint problems, and parasitic infestations. Sulphurous mixtures acted as disinfectants and fumigants. Before the penicillin class of antibiotics, sulphonamides or "sulfa drugs" were widely prescribed for bacterial infections.

During the time of the Crusades, in the late 11th and 12th centuries, Arabic works on alchemy were brought back to Europe and translated into Latin, the language of scholars. Pivotal was Jabir's *Kitab al-Kimya* (*Book of Composition of Alchemy*), translated and made available in 1144 by Robert of Chester. In addition to early Egyptian mysticism and the philosophy of Aristotle, Arab practitioners

MASTER ALCHEMIST
Arab chemist, physician, and engineer Jabir ibn Hayyan wrote numerous pioneering alchemical and metallurgical works.

TOAD, SERPENT, EAGLE
In alchemical symbolism, the toad and serpent represent fixity and volatility, while the eagle stands for sublimation.

such as Jabir added great amounts of practical information about preparing medicines according to alchemical methods. In turn, Europeans wove Christian beliefs such as religious purification, confessions to cleanse the soul, and ascent into heavenly afterlife into the new translations. European alchemy grew in stature and many prominent religious dignitaries, from humble monks to the highest clergy, began to practise it.

Among such practitioners were Albertus Magnus and Roger Bacon. Albertus Magnus (c.1193–1280) was a German cleric who had vast knowledge of the natural world in the tradition of Aristotle. He was also a practical experimenter, and in around 1250 may have isolated the chemical element arsenic. Like mercury and sulphur, arsenic became a mainstay of alchemy, its mineral- or plant-extracted compounds being stimulants in very small amounts, but disabling or deadly in fractionally higher doses. Accounts, which were probably written and embroidered after Albertus' death, describe how he discovered the Philosopher's Stone and passed its formulation to his pupil, Thomas Aquinas – who then destroyed it, fearing it had come from Satan.

Roger Bacon (c.1214–94) was also a cleric – in his case a Franciscan friar. As a student and teacher, he followed his Order's approach to investigation and experimentation: "Of the three ways in which men think they acquire knowledge of things: authority, reasoning, and experience; only the last is effective and able to bring peace to the intellect". Bacon attempted both to transmute base metals to gold and to divine the elixir for everlasting life. He saw these as related endeavours: "That medicine which will remove all impurities and corruptibility from the lesser metals will also, in the opinion of the wise, take off so much of the corruptibility of the body that human life may be prolonged for many centuries". Bacon's many texts rejected magic spells and incantations, but reinforced the influence of the Church and the authority of the Bible. His works were widely circulated, and inspired many to explore alchemy further, especially as applied to medicine. Bacon also studied optics, engineering, astronomy, and astrology, and – most importantly to him – mathematics. In 1267, he produced his 840-page *Opus Majus* (*Greater Work*), one of the foremost encyclopaedic works of the age.

European alchemy continued to flourish during the Renaissance. A famous proponent of the early 1500s was Paracelsus (see pp.110–15). His contemporary and fellow wanderer around Europe was Heinrich Cornelius Agrippa von Nettesheim, usually known as Cornelius Agrippa. German-born, he wrote widely on matters of magic, religion, the occult, and medicine, including alchemy. His major work was the *De Occulta Philosophia Libri Tres* (*Three Books Concerning Occult Philosophy*). In his medical opinions and prescriptions, Agrippa often mixed remarkable common sense with magic and superstition. He recommended the herb creeping cinquefoil (*Potentilla reptans*) to ease fever, but he attributed this ability to the number five, in line with the doctrine of numerology – cinquefoil meaning "five leaves". He wrote: "It resists poysons by vertue of the number of five; also drives away divells…" Later in the century, German physician Andreas Libavius produced a chemistry-based manual, *Alchemia* (1597). Like Paracelsus and Agrippa, he was keen on the use of minerals and extracts as drugs, but less enthusiastic about the mysticism and Hermetic traditions of alchemy. In this respect, Libavius was moving closer to a more practical, evidence-based use of alchemical remedies.

By the 1700s, alchemy in Europe was fading in the face of its rising successor, chemistry. The latter adopted a much stricter, more rigorous, no-nonsense approach that shunned notions such as divine intervention, ancient mystical traditions, and esoteric soul-cleansing. But in relation to medicine, chemistry continued one of alchemy's practical functions – to provide raw materials, elements, compounds, and ingredients from which physicians, apothecaries, pharmacists, druggists, and dispensers could concoct medicines that would heal and cure.

THE DAWN OF CHEMISTRY
By the 19th century, alchemy had given way to
chemistry, a subject based on purely empirical
principles. The quests for immortality and the
universal cure-all gave way to the microscopic
study of the flesh in all its forms.

Traditional Eastern Medicine

TRADITIONAL CHINESE MEDICINE HAS A RECORD as long and distinguished as anything in the West. As Hippocrates lectured in Ancient Greece (see pp.30–39), Chinese physicians were compiling medical texts that would likewise persist for millennia, in the form of works such as the *Huang-di Nei'Jing* (*The Yellow Emperor's Inner Canon*). And as Claudius Galen held sway in Rome (see pp.40–45), foremost Chinese physician Zhang Zhongjing was founding medical institutions that would endure for centuries, in some cases to the present day. Like the Hippocratic Corpus and Galen's multitudinous writings, the *Huang-di Nei'Jing* has been revised and translated many times, making its authenticity and original content difficult to pin down. In general, it recounts discussions between the Yellow (or Golden) Emperor, Huang-di, and his associates and advisors, including First Minister Ch'i Po. The semi-mythical figure of Huang-di is credited with establishing China as a great civilization more than 4,500 years ago. In the text of the *Huang-di Nei'Jing*, produced some 2,000 years ago, the proponents ask and answer questions, and in the process set out an encyclopaedic store of Chinese medical knowledge and practices of the time. The work deals extensively

with fundamentals such as feeling the pulse, examining bowel products, observing the tongue, acupuncture, moxibustion, and concepts such as the flow of qi (energy), yin-yang, zang-fu, and the five phases.

Feeling the pulse was central to diagnosis and formulating treatment. It sometimes took more than an hour, and was best done soon after waking. The focus was on the wrists, which had six

YIN-YANG DUALITY
The tension between opposites (yin and yang) is central to Chinese philosophy. Yin and yang are here represented by a snake and a dragon respectively.

pulse sites each. The nature or quality of the pulse had many aspects, described in the *Huang-di Nei'Jing* in poetic terms: "like water dripping through a roof", "smooth as a flowing stream", or, more worryingly, "dead as a rock". Urine and bowel motions were studied intensively, not only by physicians, but also by relatives, soothsayers, fortune-tellers, political colleagues, and even financial advisers. Frequency, volume, density, colour, consistency, smell, undigested contents, and other features were analysed to discover the cause of an illness and how it might be relieved. The tongue was another important indicator of health and diagnosis: the size, shape, colour, coating, and flexibility were all regarded as pointers to the body's well-being. For example, a healthy digestive system was said to give the tongue an appealing red freshness. This was especially true for the middle of the tongue, which was intimately linked to the stomach, intestines, and spleen. The tongue's tip related to the heart, lungs, and chest area, while the back of the tongue was associated with the kidneys and the urinary bladder.

The concept of yin-yang, pervasive in Chinese philosophy and culture for thousands of years, represents the complementary duality inherent in all aspects of the universe. Derived from "shady place" and "sunny place" (referring to a hill), one cannot exist without the other. Yin tends to be dark, watery, cool, passive, and feminine, while yang is bright, dry, hot, active, and masculine. The allied distinction of zang-fu characterizes the lungs, heart, liver, spleen, and kidneys as zang, or yin, and the stomach, intestines, gall bladder, and urinary bladder as fu, or yang. In turn, yin-yang and zang-fu were incorporated into the concept of the five phases, or wu-xing – namely earth, water, fire, wood, and metal. These phases were so-called because they were energy states, rather than elements, and were in a constant state of flux. As the *Huang-di Nei'Jing* states: "The five elemental energies... encompass all the myriad phenomena of nature. It is a pattern that applies equally to humans". So, the liver was characterized as a yin, zang, and wood organ, while the stomach was yang, fu, and earth, and so on.

Additionally, the five phases concept embraces four main ways or cycles in which these energies interact. In the sheng (generating) cycle, each phase is in effect a "mother" that nurtures the development of the following "child" phase. So the fire phase supplies a generating force, or foundation, for the earth phase, which spawns and develops the metal phase, and so on. The ke (controlling) cycle holds that each phase affects and is affected by another – for instance, water controls fire, but is itself kept in check by earth to maintain equilibrium. The cheng (overactive) cycle involves one phase becoming too dynamic and having too much control over its associated subordinate phases, leading to imbalance and illness. In the wu (contradictory) cycle, a reversal of forces involves a subordinate phase taking control of the phase that would normally dominate it. For instance, water, instead of smothering fire in the balanced way, would control and burn fire. Again, this imbalance leads to disease.

The *Suwen* – the first part of the *Huang-di Nei'Jing* – takes account of all these aspects and their effects on the body's health and wellbeing, explaining their role in qi energy disturbances that underlie illness. For example, the pulse should be felt at daybreak: "The yang qi has not yet stirred, the yin qi has not been dispersed". The *Ling Shu* – the second part of the *Huang-di Nei'Jing* – contains some of the earliest descriptions of acupuncture. This therapeutic system probably evolved as far back as 4,000 years ago, and even perhaps has its origins or parallels in ancient Europe (see p.19).

Acupuncture aims to correct problems in the flow of qi energy around the body. The term "qi" has various literal interpretations, such as gas, vapour, or flowing breath. The four or five forms of qi are likened to "life energy" or "vital force" and move along channels known as meridians around and within the body, numbering some 20 main ones with subsidiary branches. The healthy, harmonious flow of qi can be disrupted by malfunctioning organs – or vice versa, with yin or zang organs having different effects to yang or fu organs. To address imbalance, the acupuncturists of Ancient China consulted patients and carried out examinations, looking especially at the pulse and tongue, as mentioned above. Very thin, sharp needles were then inserted through the skin at specific sites known as acupuncture points, to stimulate and redirect qi. Most acupoints were located on meridians and chosen for their energy links to body organs. The *Huang-di Nei'Jing* identifies or implies the presence of nearly 300 acupuncture points. (Some modern acupuncturists recognize more than double this number.) The needles might be left in position for a set time, or rotated, vibrated, or otherwise manipulated.

POWER LINES OF THE BODY
Traditional Chinese medicine sees disease as a disturbance of the flow of qi (energy) in the body. This energy moves along channels that can be stimulated by acupuncture.

"The superior doctor prevents sickness; the mediocre doctor attends to impending sickness; the inferior doctor treats actual sickness"

CHINESE PROVERB

Traditional Ancient Chinese medicine also incorporated many other ways to promote health and prevent illness. They included extensive use of herbs, special diets, bathing, massage, meditation, and physical exercise ranging from the simple moves and postures of calisthenics to strenuous martial arts.

For four centuries, until the year 220 CE, the Han Dynasty ruled Ancient China. Its foremost physician was Zhang Zhongjing (c.150–c.219 CE), by whose time medicine had moved on from the *Huang-di Nei'Jing*, though it still relied on central concepts such as zang-fu and the five phases. Zhang practised at the end of Han rule, when conflict between rebel armies and the Han overlords was causing poverty and chaos. The desperate situation led to malnutrition and epidemic infections, giving Zhang and his contemporaries plenty of patients. Zhang produced works that introduced many pharmaceuticals to the body of Chinese traditional medicine. The general name for this work is *Shanghan Han Za Bing Lun*, often translated as *Treatise on Febrile Diseases Caused by Cold and Miscellaneous Causes*. As usual, the original knowledge has been revised and muddied by later editors. The first section, "Shang Han Lun" (On Cold-Induced Damage), covers infectious diseases common at the time, which caused symptoms such as the fevers of yang, and the chills and shivering of yin. It describes more than 100 herb-based remedies. For instance, certain fevers could be reduced with preparations containing mahuang (ephedra), guizhi (cinnamon wood), zhigancao (liquorice root), and xingren (bitter apricot stone). The second section, "Jin-Kui Yao Lue", is known in English as Synopsis of the Golden Chamber or Vital Prescriptions of the Golden Coffer. Zhang states that there are thousands of diseases, but people

THE AGONY OF MOXIBUSTION
This 19th-century statuette shows a patient
in agony during moxibustion therapy.
A burn mark is visible on his shin.

die from three main causes: external causes,
meaning outside forces (spirits or disease
"nuclei") that enter through the skin and
invade the body's interior; internal causes,
meaning harmful forces or particles that
spread along the qi meridians to the zang
and fu body parts; or neither of the above
– a diverse category that encompasses
insect stings, animal bites, wounds from
weapons, and sexual abuse.

Jin-Kui Yao Lue concentrates mainly on the internal conditions
and lists more than 250 recipes and preparations predominantly
using plants. Kidney yang deficiency could bring on back pain and
leg cramps, so the advised remedy was jingui shen qi'wan, the kidney
qi remedy – containing, among other herbs, fu zi (aconite root),
mudan pi (peony root), fu ling (China root), and sheng di-huang
(rehmannia or Chinese foxglove).

Animal products were also used in traditional Chinese medicine.
These included snake flesh for eye problems, pulverized seahorse for
goitre (swollen thyroid), and syrup of elephant skin for skin ulcers
and sores. Information on surgery in Ancient China is scant. One of
the few surgeons mentioned by name was Hua T'o (c.143–208 CE),
who was also proficient in acupuncture and other healing arts.
Apparently, he invented an all-purpose anaesthetic, known as
mafeisan, based on wine with added secret ingredients – extracts of
cannabis, opium poppies, datura (a type of nightshade), mandrake,
and even mixtures of these.

The herb mugwort (wormwood) of the genus *Artemisia* was – and,
like many ancient Eastern practices, continues to be – the chief plant
used in a therapy called moxibustion. This was often employed
in conjunction with acupuncture. There are several species of mugwort
with various names, such as yomoge and gaiyou in Japan, ssuk in Korea,
and mogusa, ai-ye, and huang hua'ai in China. Dried mugwort might be
heaped onto a skin acupoint and left to smoulder there, being removed
before it burned the surface – or, if the practitioner advised, left to singe

MOXIBUSTION
This 10th-century illustration shows a Chinese country doctor applying burning mugwort to a patient's back. This painful treatment, called moxibustion, stimulates acupuncture points to enhance the flow of qi (energy) in the body.

(which could cause blisters and scarring). This was the direct form of moxibustion. In the indirect method, the processed herb was pressed into a moxa stick, lit, and held near the skin to subject the site to heat and vapours. Alternatively, the moxa substance was piled around or on top of an inserted acupuncture needle and ignited, and left until the physician deemed it had taken effect. Moxibustion was mainly used for illnesses characterized by damp, cold, sluggishness, and stagnation. It aimed to banish cold, to warm the meridians, and to stimulate qi energy to flow again. Muscle pains, joint stiffness, headaches, stomach and intestinal complaints, painful or irregular periods, and even infertility were all treated in this way.

In ancient times, moxibustion made its way from China to nearby regions, including Korea, where it became associated with the legendary ruler Tangun (Dangun), who founded Korea more than 4,000 years ago. The legend describes how Tangun's mother, Ungnyeo, was initially a bear who wished to become a human. She was challenged to stay out of sunlight in a cave for 100 days, eating nothing but garlic and mugwort. Ungnyeo persisted, her wish was granted, and she later gave birth to Tangun – and the herbs mugwort and garlic have enjoyed importance in traditional Korean medicine ever since.

Korean medical traditions inherited many theories and practices from China. However, the former tended to place more emphasis on the inner causes of disease, including eating habits, lifestyle, personality, and behavioural traits. The concepts of yin-yang and the five phases were followed, and also yuk-gi, the six atmospheric natural influences: han (cold), yeol (heat), hwa (fire), pung (wind), jo (dryness), and seup (moisture). When these influences become unbalanced, people fall ill. In about 1614, during Korea's Joseon Dynasty, the eminent royal physician Heo Jun (c.1540–1616) produced *Dongui Bogam* (*Mirror of Eastern Medicine*). Its five main sections cover "internal" disorders, especially those of the heart, lungs, liver, spleen, and kidneys; "external" disorders, such as those of the bones, muscles, blood, and skin; varied conditions ranging from excessive worry to jaundice and gynaecological problems; herbal remedies; and acupuncture. This work established Korean medicine as distinct and independent from its Chinese-influenced background.

As far back as the 5th century CE, the classical medicine of China also greatly influenced developing medical practices in Japan – much of the knowledge arriving by way of Korea. Japanese practitioners incorporated elements of Chinese medicine into their own therapeutic system, which is known as kampo medicine. Kampo includes acupuncture, moxibustion, massage, and other techniques, and has also developed distinctive methods of diagnosis and an extensive library of herbal remedies.

One of the earliest written works on Japanese medicine was the 100-volume *Dido Rui Ju Ho*, compiled by the year 808 at the request of Emperor Kanmu. Its vast contents cover medical knowledge of the time, as well as folk remedies and those based on religion and worship. In 984, the *Ishimpo (Essence of Medicine and Therapeutic Methods)* was published, written by Japanese physician Yasuyori Tamba. Again, this is based on ancient Chinese texts with Japanese input. In the 15th century, Japan's medical traditions, still fundamentally adopted from China, were "Japanized" by Dosan Manase (c.1507–94). Raised as a Zen Buddhist in Kyoto, he studied medicine at the Ashikaga School, one of Japan's earliest institutes of learning, in Ashikaga, north of present-day Tokyo. It was a time of great communication between Japan and the Ming Dynasty of China, and both cultures benefited from the exchange of medical ideas and practices. Dosan accumulated huge amounts of information, both traditional Chinese methods, and from local and academic knowledge in Japan. This fairly amorphous mass was synthesized into his great work, *Keiteki Shu (Textbook of Internal Medicine)*. It emphasized the logic of treating particular symptoms with specific herbs and became central to the further development and autonomy of Japanese medicine.

Kampo medicine emphasizes herbal treatments and is controlled and regulated as part of the national health care system in Japan. Like many of East Asia's classical medical systems, it has endured to the present day, adapting to the modern world.

KOREAN MASTER OF MEDICINE
Eminent physician Heo Jun wrote the defining text of traditional Korean medicine, *Dongui Bogam*.

Ayurveda

MOST MAJOR CIVILIZATIONS around the world have a so-called "Father of Medicine" – a real-life or perhaps mythical individual, who laid the foundations of an enduring system of medicine and healing – and who, ancient societies being what they were, was usually male. In India, this position is held by Charaka. Some 2,300 years ago, he compiled, wrote, and refined one of the classic texts that established India's primary form of traditional medicine – Ayurveda. This was the *Charaka Samhita*.

Samhitas are collections or compendia, usually written in the form of verses, hymns, or mantras. The term initially referred to India's most ancient religious texts or scriptures, the four *Vedas*, which date back at least 3,000 years, and were based on even more ancient texts. The Vedic traditions gave rise to Ayurveda (from "ayur", meaning life, and "veda", meaning knowledge) – a medical system that has parallels with other traditional systems, including those of Ancient Greece (see pp.30–39) and Ancient Rome (see pp.40–47). Central to the concept of Ayurveda are the five elements – namely jala or ap (water), tejas or agni (fire), privthi or bhumi (earth), pavana or vayu (air), and akasha (ether or space). These elements combine or compete in various proportions, and contribute to the three main doshas – which roughly correspond to the fluid-like bodily constituents that the Europeans called humours (see pp.106–107). The three Indian doshas are vata (wind), pitta (bile), and kapha (phlegm). As with the four humours theory, a serene balance of the doshas leads to health, whereas an imbalance causes illness. Each dosha

BRAHMA, GOD OF CREATION
According to tradition, Ayurveda was given to humankind by Brahma, the Hindu god of creation, as a way of reducing our suffering.

has qualities linked to a particular type of illness. If vata, named after the Hindu god of wind, becomes excessive, it can cause digestive problems such as abdominal cramps, constipation, and flatulence. Kapha, which is linked to phlegm and mucus, is slow, oily, and has protective qualities – as do the mucous membranes lining the body's inner passageways such as the airways and digestive tract. Since kapha controls these moist tissues, an imbalance can lead to colds, coughs, and asthma. The doshas move and flow around the body along channels, or through pores called srotas. In some forms of Ayurveda, the srotas also carry nutrients and waste, and even knowledge or information.

The *Charaka Samhita* described 13 of these srotas. Three are interfaces between the body and the environment, forming conduits for incoming air, food, and water. Seven are associated with the seven bodily tissues, or dhatus (see below), and the final three carry away waste. Other classical Ayurvedic writers added three more srotas – the flow of thoughts in the mind, the flows of blood in menstruation, and of milk during lactation. These 16 srotas are largely accepted in Ayurveda today.

Two further concepts central to Ayurveda are the dhatus and agni. The dhatus are structural components, analogous to tissues. The seven dhatus are blood, lymph, muscles, bones, bone marrow, fat, and reproductive products (semen and eggs), and each dhatu has corresponding dosha channels. So the mamsa or muscle dhatu is accompanied by mamsavaha srotas carrying muscle nutrients and waste; while the majja or bone marrow dhatu corresponds with the majjavaha srotas supplying the bone marrow nutrients – plus, in this case, the nutrients for the nerves and nervous tissues, including the brain. Agni, which roughly means "digestive fire", is the final principle in Ayurveda. Agni is the Hindu god of fire, and in this context refers to the body's ability to assimilate and process many aspects of life, from food to the general mass of biochemical reactions known as metabolism, even to experiences and memories, while igniting or burning waste for removal.

Little is known about Charaka himself. He was probably born between 300 and 200 BCE and may have been a court physician. According to one legend, knowledge was handed by Lord Brahma (the Hindu god of creation), who wished to ease human suffering, to another deity,

Dhanvantari. He then transmitted it to humans, passing it from a series of teachers to their pupils, including Atreya and Agnivesa, and eventually to Charaka, who turned it into the seminal *Charaka Samhita*. His text has been revised and re-collated over the centuries. This encyclopaedic work is written in a poetic style and has eight main sections, more than 120 chapters, and some 8,400 verses (a mode of expression that helps students to memorize the content). It deals mainly with the area of Ayurvedic medicine called kaya-chikitsa – "body treatment", or internal medicine. Like the teachings of Hippocrates, the *Charaka Samhita* describes the qualities needed by a physician, and instructs how he should go about examining a patient to find the root cause of a disease, and how to make a prognosis and prescribe treatments. These treatments are minimally invasive, and involve specific diets and exercises, and more than 2,000 plant-based remedies. The emphasis throughout the *Charaka Samhita* is on preventing illness by maintaining good hygiene and a healthy diet.

The other great founding work of Ayurveda, the *Susruta Samhita*, was probably compiled a few centuries earlier than the *Charaka Samhita*. It deals chiefly with the field of Ayurvedic surgery, shalya-chikitsa, and is credited to Susruta, who, like Charaka, was a somewhat shadowy figure, and who dates to around 2,500 years ago. This text was also revised and expanded over the centuries, and given the content relating to traumatic injuries, parts of the book were probably written during times of conflict and warfare.

The *Susruta Samhita* is massive in scope and describes many surgical techniques that are sophisticated and daring, both in theory and practice, along with equipment and medications. Details vary among the later editions, but the procedures include extracting teeth, draining fluids using trocars (a kind of syringe), repairing hernias and broken bones, venesection (see p.132), eye surgery (including cataract excision), widening tubes such as the oesophagus or urethra with strictures, cauterizing haemorrhoids with powerful acids, alkalis, or hot irons, and caesarian section. Surgical training is described, including knifework practice on dead animals and vegetables, and there is advice

AYURVEDIC PHARMACY
This 19th-century painting shows an Indian pharmacist preparing Ayurvedic remedies. The principles of Ayurveda were laid down between 500 and 300 BCE and are still relevant in the 21st century.

on how to deal with complications such as sudden bleeding, diarrhoea, vomiting, cough, impotence, and infertility. More than 1,000 medical conditions and 800 remedies, mostly herbal, are described altogether. The *Susruta Samhita* departs from mainstream Ayurveda's three doshas by suggesting a fourth – rakta, or blood – which is a dhatu or tissue in the standard system. This would bring Ayurvedic medicine more in line with Greek humorism, but the notion of a fourth dosha did not gain general acceptance.

After the *Susruta Samhita* and *Charaka Samhita*, and probably written between the 4th and 6th centuries, came the *Ashtanga Hridayam* and the *Ashtanga Sangraha*. These were probably the work of Vagbhata, a Buddhist healer and medical authority who may have lived in what is now Pakistan. Vagbhata organizes the *Ashtanga Hridayam* content into eight (ashta) sections: internal medicine; gynaecology and paediatrics; problems of the mind and spirit (what we might call psychiatry); head, eye, ear, and nose conditions; general surgery; toxicology (such as treating swallowed poisons and snake venom); rejuvenation; and sexual medicine, including aphrodisiac therapy. The author quotes or draws material from the two earlier works, but focuses more on the body's anatomy and physiology, and adds updated knowledge of surgery and drugs.

A fourth revered source for Ayurveda is the Bower Manuscript, named after the British military intelligence officer Sir Hamilton Bower, who obtained it while working in northwestern China in 1890. Dating from the 6th century, or even the 4th – roughly the same era as the *Ashtanga Hridayam* – the manuscript contains a great deal of information about medicine, particularly Ayurvedic medicine, and includes many recipes for remedies. One of the herbs cited at length at the start of the Bower Manuscript is garlic, *Allium sativum* (known as lahsun in Hindi, or lasuna in Sanskrit). This most revered of plants originally came from Central Asia, probably the Hindu Kush in the

"The person whose vata is unimpeded… lives for 100 years without sickness"

CHARAKA SAMHITA

western Himalayas. Its recorded medicinal uses go back at least 5,000 years, and it remains one of Ayurveda's most commonly advised plant remedies. Another founding treatise of Ayurvedic medicine, *Kashyap Samhita*, explains: "The taste of its seed is pungent, its stem salty and bitter, its leaves astringent and its vipaka [Ayurvedic term for post-digestive effects] is sweet". Vagbhata suggested that garlic is helpful for rejuvenation, for "smoothing" the digestion, and as a general stimulant, although it is also recommended as a decongestant and expectorant for coughs and colds, and (due to what we would now call its antimicrobial

INDIAN SAGE
Susruta, the author of the Ayurvedic classic the *Susruta Samhita*, lived in Varanasi, India, in the 6th century BCE.

properties) for alleviating skin problems. These range from plague sores, scrofula (a form of tuberculosis) ulcers, smallpox eruptions, and leprosy lesions to rabid dog bites, and oral and vaginal thrush.

Two popular spices in Ayurvedic medicine are cinnamon and cardamom. Cinnamon bark, from *Cinnamomum verum* and related trees, is reputed to have powerful effects on the kapha (phlegm) dosha, which makes it good for respiratory disorders such as colds, coughs, blocked nose, sore throat, and chest infections, as well as digestive complaints such as heartburn, indigestion, abdominal pains, and diarrhoea. Cardamom, from *Elletaria* and *Amomum* herbs, is regarded as "warm", and balances the vata and kapha doshas. Again, it is commonly used for problems with the stomach and intestines, such as nausea, stomach cramps, and flatulence, and problems in the lungs and airways, including allergies such as rhinitis. It is also reputed to stimulate the appetite and the general constitution.

Like many traditional medicines, the various forms of Ayurveda are still widely practised in its home region. It has also spread to other lands in recent times, taking its place as a contemporary form of complementary medicine (see pp.320–27).

PULSE DIAGNOSIS
According to Ayurveda, disease results from an imbalance in a person's doshas. For this reason, an Ayurvedic doctor spends considerable time feeling a patient's pulse – a practice that leads to diagnosis and treatment.

Native American Medicine

WHEN EUROPEANS FIRST EXPLORED the Americas, from the 1490s, they found a huge variety of native peoples with distinctive cultures, languages, customs, clothing, ceremonies – and systems of medicine. The number of main tribes in North America certainly exceeded 500, and with smaller groupings probably totalled over 1,000. Each followed its own beliefs and ways of dealing with disease and healing the sick, but they all had much in common. Many native North Americans viewed health as a balance between mind, body, and spirit, and healing involved addressing imbalances in a person's life, either by making offerings to the spirits, repairing personal thoughts and emotions, or receiving practical care such as a massage or herbal remedy. The key figures in this process, variously known as tribal healers, medicine men and women, or shamans (see pp.88–89) were regarded as mediators between the human world and the unseen realm of spirits and gods. Most medicine people underwent exhaustive training, including being apprenticed to a senior. They gained knowledge and experience to assess not just the symptoms of health problems but also the intricacies of the people who suffered them. These practitioners learned to select and prepare herbs, carry out ceremonies, employ tokens, charms, and offerings, make intimate contact with nature, and read signs and symbols from the spirits. Much of this was kept secret, since discussing matters with others might anger the spirits.

Many medicine people had bundles or bags containing treasured items and tokens known as medicine tools. These were often natural objects such as bones, feathers, crystals, and furs. One item usually included in the medicine bundle was a medicine pipe. Smoking herbs and other natural substances was a central part of healing ceremonies. The most sacred plant was tobacco. Exhaling its smoke made visible the body's breath, which was considered the most vital component of

RUNS MEDICINE
This picture, dating from around 1899, shows Runs Medicine, an Arapaho medicine man, in traditional dress.

SHAMAN'S DRUM
Shamans all over the world use a variety of
instruments – such as this Native American
drum – to summon spirits to effect healing.

life. Tobacco was also a gift that was
offered to the spirits when they were
being petitioned for help. During
treatment, the medicine person
might blow tobacco smoke at the
patient to drive away evil – and the
smoke then rose to carry messages to
the spirits above. Drumming and
chanting were also important for summoning
spirits to ask them what was needed. Medicine people were rarely
paid for their help, but they accepted gifts – tobacco was especially
valued. Each patient was unique, so a medicine person's actions and
treatments had to be carefully tailored. However, there was no
automatic right for a sick person to demand help. The medicine man
or woman could choose whom to treat, how, and when.

North American peoples used a multitude of herbs and other
plants for medicine, some of which have been taken up by modern
doctors. The bark or leaves of willow trees were chewed, or perhaps
boiled to make teas, for all manner of aches and pains, from headaches
to stiff joints. Willow bark contains acetylsalicylic acid (ASA) or
salicylate – the pain-relieving, anti-inflammatory, fever-reducing
active ingredient in one of the world's most widespread and
useful drugs today, aspirin. Willow was especially effective in
relieving the pain of dental caries and abscesses, earning it the
nickname of the "toothache tree".

The most widespread and revered medicinal herb for many Native
Americans was sage. Regarded as a powerful cleansing agent for body
and soul, it was believed to transport prayers to the spirits and purify
the air. Its traditional medical uses were legion – as a remedy for
internal problems of the stomach, bowel, lungs, and liver, as an
antiseptic salve for wounds, burns, and rashes, and as a soothing
relaxant either inhaled as smoke or drunk as a tea. Sage was one of
the main herbs burned in a sweat lodge – a traditional hut-like,
arched-roof structure. The design and building materials of a sweat

lodge varied greatly, but it was often fashioned from flexible saplings and covered by animal skins. It created a small, dark, calm space in which water poured onto hot rocks created steam that mixed with smoke from smouldering herbs. Rocks were usually heated by a fire near the lodge, passed inside (using deer antlers as carriers), and arranged in a pit within. The medicine person might waft or blow smoke at recipients as part of the healing ritual.

Hundreds of herbs and other plants were used by Native American healers: the boiled leaves of the creosote bush made a tea that was used for easing respiratory problems such as bronchitis, pneumonia, and tuberculosis; an infusion of broom snakeweed was prescribed to help women during childbirth; pleurisy root was given for many kinds of breathing problems and was especially good as an expectorant; the boiled, cooled extract from the inner bark of dogwood was employed to aid colonic irrigation; horsemint (bergamot, bee balm) was used variously as a cold or warm infusion for back and head pains, as an ointment to ward off infection, and as a mouthwash for toothache and painful gums; the boiled, reduced extract of the flowers of yellow-spined thistle was applied to the skin for burns, scalds, sores, and other lesions; the buds and leaves of the cedar tree were boiled and sipped to ease sore throats and coughs.

From the 14th century, the Aztecs rose to power in what is now central-southern Mexico. They too commanded a huge herbal medicine chest, and believed that many forms of ill health were handed down from gods and spirits. Other origins for disease included natural disasters such as plagues, earthquakes, floods, and erupting volcanoes. Aztec priests also believed that illnesses were sometimes visited on humans purely for the gods' fun or amusement, rather than as a punishment for forgetting to worship

HEALING SAGE
Sage is the most powerful herb in Native American medicine, providing relief from numerous ills and serving as a means for communicating with spirits.

or for some other sin. To appease the gods and have the sickness taken away, the patient might be rebuked by whipping or by having thorns and spines jabbed through their flesh, possibly accompanied by animal or even human sacrifices. One of the commonest Aztec "medications" was pulque or octli, a form of alcoholic beer fermented from a species of agave known as maguey (American aloe). It was usually drunk by rulers or priests, but could be offered to any sick person, especially when spiced up with other herbs, tree bark, and roots to help dull pain and reduce the symptoms of all manner of ailments. Another Aztec speciality was the black, glassy, volcanic rock obsidian, which was ground by healers into a powder and rubbed into the skin to treat ulcers, rashes, and injuries. Far more specialized was a mixture of squash plant, ayonel-huatl flesh, and eagle dung, which was used to bring on labour in heavily pregnant women.

During the first millennium, in the Yucatan Peninsula and northern Central America, before the glory days of the Aztec Empire, the Mayan people developed a sophisticated civilization with a complex medical system. They too regarded body, mind, and spirit as equally responsible for illness. In particular, they thought disease was due to misbehaviour or wrongdoing on the part of the sufferer. Cure demanded a mix of ritual, ceremony, worship of idols, and offerings of tokens to the angered gods, to pacify them and resolve the sin. The Mayans' written language recorded parts of their history and practices. Their treatments were extensive: herbal emetics (vomit-inducers) and purgatives (bowel-emptiers) to clean out the body's interior; massage; and sauna sessions in sweat baths akin to the North American sweat lodges. Also, like North American cultures, the Mayans had specialist healers or medicine men, known as ah'men – the equivalent of a modern-day doctor, herbalist, psychotherapist, and counsellor. An Ah'man spent time with the patient, asking details about his or her life, habits, and behaviour, and would gradually home in on worries and problems, such as an unhappy relationship, depression, or self-

"Before eating, always take time to thank the food"

ARAPAHO SAYING

MAYAN HERB JAR
This ceramic jar, dating from around 700,
was used by a Mayan ah'man to store
medicinal herbs, including tobacco.

doubt, which might contribute to the illness.
Ah'men used plants such as turbina, cacti-like
peyotes, and mushrooms – all with known
hallucinogenic properties – to induce trance-
like states that brought them closer to the
gods. One of their main plants was a bush-like
species of mimosa known as tepezcohuite,
jurema preta, or vinho de jurema (*Mimosa
tenuiflora*). The leaves, seeds, and especially
the root bark were infused, boiled, roasted, or
fermented to make treatments for a wide range of problems, from skin
rashes to coughs and backache. Plant extracts were often mixed with
animal body parts (especially from reptiles), birds' eggs, and guano.

The rainforests of South America's Amazon region are globally
acclaimed as a treasure store of medicinal plants. Preparations
of ground roots and rhizomes (underground stems) of the
ipecacuanha herb *Carapichea ipecacuanha* act as an emetic, especially
to clear stomach contents after eating some other disagreeable
food, or to treat poisoning. To kill animals for food, native Amazonian
hunters fired blow darts and arrows tipped with curare or ampi – the
extract of plants such as the trailing vine *Chondrodendron tomentosum*. The
active ingredient, an alkaloid called D-tubocurarine, works as a
muscle relaxant, which can still help as an addition to anaesthesia
during surgery. Native South Americans also made extensive use of
coca bushes (*Erythroxylum coca* or *E. novogranatense*). They chewed the
leaves of these as a pick-me-up to ward off fatigue, thirst, and
hunger. Its active substance, cocaine, a powerful stimulant, made
its way into Western medicine chiefly as a local anaesthetic, before
being replaced by safer and more effective compounds. However,
illegal use of cocaine as a highly addictive stimulant – "coke" and
its freebase form "crack-cocaine" – continue to cause massive
problems worldwide.

Shamanism

The shaman, or "medicine man", is a combination of priest, healer, and teacher found in many traditional or tribal societies. Shamans are believed to be in contact with the spirit world, and use rituals and amulets that are said to heal the sick and prevent disease.

MASK (1497)
Iroquois shamans wore a mask with a broken nose, representing a legendary healer named Hado'ih. Hado'ih had injured his nose on a mountain during a display of spiritual power between himself and the creator deity.

MEDICINE JAR (c.100–1550)
This Mexican ceramic jar bearing the image of a deity probably belonged to a shaman and may have contained hallucinogenic drugs used in healing rituals.

SHAMAN'S CROWN (19TH CENTURY)
This crown was worn by a shaman of the Tsimshian people of Alaska. Made of mountain goat horns, it indicates the shaman's belief that he could transform himself into the spirit of this powerful animal.

NECKLACE (1801–1900)
The human teeth and glass beads
threaded onto this Apache medicine
man's necklace were believed to
protect the wearer from evil or illness.

HEALER'S CIRCLET (1880–1920)
Worn by a west African healer, this circlet
is decorated with cowrie shells and beads.
Used in Africa as money, cowrie shells
were not only valuable but also had
spiritual significance.

SOULCATCHER (c.19TH CENTURY)
Shamans believed that a person's soul could
be drawn from their body, leading to disease.
Amulets such as this were used to restore souls,
and to draw out and trap evil spirits.

RATTLE (1884)
Shamans from the Haida people of British
Columbia sang songs accompanied by rattles
like these. Knowledge of songs and stories is a
crucial part of a shaman's place in a tribe.

DIVINATION BONES (1880–1930)
One of the shaman's tasks was to make
spiritual journeys to find the answers to
important questions. An African shaman
used tools such as animal vertebrae, pebbles,
and similar objects in these divination rituals.

HAND DRUM (c.19TH CENTURY)
Shamans use percussion instruments, especially
drums, to beat out a rhythm. The effect of the
continuous drum beats helps the shaman to
enter an altered state of consciousness, in which
he or she can contact the spirit world.

African and West Asian Traditions

TRADITIONAL MEDICAL SYSTEMS in Africa have certain similarities with those of native America (see pp.82–89). In general, the root causes of ill health are viewed primarily as spiritual or supernatural, emanating from gods and the spirit world, rather than having natural origins within the body or the immediate environment. The usual reason for visiting disease on a person is some kind of misdemeanour or sin against the gods, the memories of ancestors or the local community, or perhaps disturbing harmony in the natural world's plants, animals, soil, rocks, and water. To effect healing, the spirits are appeased by offerings, chanting, ceremonies, and sacrifices, while the patient tries to feel remorse and repent. The spirits may also advise on practical remedies, often herb-based, but perhaps also massage, special diets, fasting, purging, and other treatments. They do so through traditional medical practitioners with special knowledge and powers who act as intermediaries between the human world and the dominion of the spirits. These individuals are known variously as healers, curers, witch doctors, diviners, shamans (see pp.88–89), and hundreds of local names.

Many traditional African practitioners do not identify an illness in the way that modern science-based medicine does – that is, by selecting the most likely condition from a range of related options, such as differentiating between pleurisy, bronchitis, and pneumonia. Rather, the traditional healer seeks the ultimate cause – the original reason for angering the spirits or displeasing the gods.

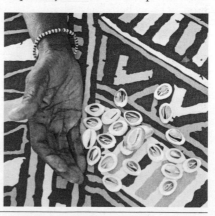

READING GOD'S WILL
Cleromancy is a form of divination in which stones or shells are cast onto the ground to form patterns. These reveal information about a person's past, present, and future.

Finding the cause then determines the spiritual aspects of the treatment, such as which incantations and offerings to employ. At the same time, practical remedies such as herbs are advised, and these can be selected as much for the symbolism attached to each remedy as for its known effects on symptoms.

Some patients may need the skills of a diviner. Common across Africa, divination takes many forms, and seeks to explain the past as well as predict the future. Divination by fire (pyromancy) may involve reading signs in flames or sparks, or throwing objects into the blaze to see how they burn. In water-based divining (hydromancy), the diviner studies ripples, splashes, or reflections in water, or watches the behaviour of objects such as floating twigs or leaves. This provides clues to the cause of an illness and how it can be addressed. The casting of lots (cleromancy) attaches mystical powers to special objects, which are thrown or cast onto the ground. A medical opinion is then divined from the arrangement or pattern in which they fall. Objects read in this way range from stones, seeds, and twigs to animal parts, such as bones, teeth, shells, skin, dried eyeballs, and fresh entrails. Each diviner has his or her own sacred groups of objects and chooses those that are relevant to each situation. Geomancy is a related technique, in which objects are cast onto patterns drawn on the ground.

For medical purposes, some diviners work in silence – others recite incantations, verses, or spells. They may talk to the patient and ask probing questions, which help to determine a course of action. Some diviners use no physical objects, but enter a trance and receive awareness of the spirit world intuitively, from within themselves. Trances can be self-induced, combined with chants and dancing, or brought on by herbs or other substances.

Among the Lobi people of Burkina Faso and the Côte d'Ivoire, diviners, known as buor, use idols or statues called batebas on which patterns are engraved that link them to the spiritual world. A medical diviner sits in front of the appropriate statue and holds the patient's hand. As the diviner questions the spirits, he also feels the way the patient's hand moves, perhaps tightening or loosening its grip. These changes indicate the basis of the sickness and offer ideas for treatment.

To heal the sick, traditional African medicine usually treats both the spiritual or religious realm and the physical body of the patient. Some healing focuses on restoring harmony between the patient and the gods. This can involve spells and ritual offerings such as money,

LOBI STATUETTE
The Lobi people of Burkino Faso
and the Côte d'Ivoire use statuettes
to call on the gods for spiritual aid.

food, drink, clothing, or jewellery. Through the healer,
a god can demand an animal sacrifice – perhaps a
wild creature like a monkey or a snake, or domestic
beasts such as chickens, goats, or even cattle. This might
be preceded by bleeding the animal and perhaps
drinking its blood.

Many African practitioners are expert herbalists
and have an encyclopedic knowledge of the plants,
mushrooms, toadstools, and other fungi of their region.
The violet tree *Securidaca longepedunculata* is known by local
names such as uwar maganigunar, ezeogwu, mpesu,
chipvufana, mufufu, umfufu, and maba. The main
medicinal parts are the roots and bark, which are – like
numerous medicinal substances – harmful in high
quantities. In smaller amounts, usually taken orally as an
infusion or soup, these serve as remedies for a huge array
of ailments, ranging from headaches and toothache to
coughs and chest infections, sexually transmitted diseases, and
constipation. Boiled root or leaf infusions of the violet tree can also be
applied topically (to the body's surface), such as by rubbing on the scalp
(for headaches), bandaged onto swollen joints (for arthritis), or as a
cleansing wash (for skin sores, insect stings, snake bites, and ulcers).
The Venda people of South Africa make a drink of the powdered root
with sorghum and maize to treat men who are "deficient below".

African pumpkin or balsam pear *Momordica balsamina* (mohodu,
nkaka, intshungu) is another widespread plant remedy. The bark,
leaves, fruits, and seeds have all been utilized. In the Okavango region
of southwest Africa, watery or plant-oil infusions of its fruits are
incorporated into poultices, balms, and liniments for skin sores, cuts,
boils, bruises, burns, and blisters – and also for haemorrhoids.

Another widely used traditional plant is the African stinkwood
tree *Prunus africana*. It too has many local names, such as entasesa in
Uganda, tikuur-inchet in Ethiopia, m'konde-konde in Tanzania,
muu'iri in Kenya, and inja'zangoma-ilimn'ama in southern Africa.

Traditional healers advise using its bark in preparations for stomach pains and bowel complaints, fevers, cuts, and abrasions, low fertility in men, and urinary difficulties.

With regard to urinary problems, the rainforests of West and Central Africa are busy with modern bioprospectors looking for native medicines to convert into the latest "wonder drugs". The bark extract from the stinkwood *Prunus africana* is processed in commercial quantities as the remedy pygeum. It is marketed worldwide for urinary problems in men with an enlarged prostate (benign prostatic hyperplasia). Harvesting the bark has made wild trees rare in many areas, so to make harvesting more sustainable, plantations are being established.

Traditional forms of medicine in North and East Africa have long cross-pollinated with those from the eastern Mediterranean and West Asia. Camel caravans and seagoing vessels transported herbal products for trade as well as the plants themselves. One example is the frankincense tree *Boswellia sacra*, producer of the legendary fragrance for perfumes, aromatherapy (see p.324), and herbal medicine. This small tree grows in dry, rocky regions of north-west Africa and Arabia. Its gum or sap is tapped and harvested to make frankincense. Its aroma was said to purify the "stale air" historically blamed for causing infections such as malaria and the dreaded Black Death (see pp.54–55). As a medicine, frankincense has been used across North Africa and Asia for several sets of conditions. Taken by mouth, it is said to ease digestive complaints, from stomach pains to ulcerative colitis. Local healers advise breathing it as a vapour or steamy inhalation for chest infections and tight, wheezy respiration. To help skin conditions such as rashes, eczema, and cuts, it is incorporated into salves and creams.

Frankincense has been known since antiquity. In the Bible it was offered to the infant Jesus by the Three Wise Men. It was mentioned by Hippocrates of Greece (see pp.30–39) and Galen of Rome (see pp.40–45), and the eminent Islamic

FRANKINCENSE GRAINS
Made from the gum or sap extruded from *Boswellia* trees, frankincense has long been used in treatments for chest infections, stomach complaints, and skin conditions.

AFRICAN MEDICINE MAN
A group of Bonda women stand with their
medicine man and his assistant in Freetown,
Sierra Leone, in 1900. A mask helps to
depersonalize the medicine man during
healing rituals in which he invokes the gods.

"The way a man dies is determined by his occupation"

AFRICAN PROVERB

physician of the Middle Ages, Ibn Sina (see pp.100–105) valued it for controlling fevers, vomiting, and diarrhoea: "If you give a drink of white flowers in wine, it helps [recovery] from dysentery... If you make a drug patch made from fresh flowers... it prevents conception".

Another tree product famous for thousands of years and still around today is mastic or arabic gum, from the mastic tree *Pistacia lentiscus*. It was chewed as a medication for halitosis (bad breath), toothache, inflamed gums, and mouth ulcers, and swallowed to combat digestive disorders such as gastric ulcers or an irritable bowel. Mixed with plant oils such as olive oil, it could be soaked into a pad of moss and tied onto snake bites and insect stings.

Not to be confused with arabic gum is gum arabic (meskar, awerwar, or chaar-gund) which comes from certain types of acacia trees, especially *Acacia senegal*. Aside from its many industrial uses as a binding and gumming agent in products ranging from confectionery to paints, gum arabic has a long history in traditional African and Asian medicine. Its soothing physical properties are believed to ease irritation, reduce inflammation, and promote the healing of body membranes and surfaces. Topically, it is advocated for swollen, painful areas and for sore nipples.

Yet another sap or gum highly prized by traditional Asian healers is asafoetida, obtained from species of the giant fennel *Ferula*. Native to Iran and Afghanistan, it is named from its foul or "foetid" smell and bitter taste. Its medicinal preparations come mostly from the underground stems or main roots. Popular through the ages in the Arab world, it is given for digestive upsets, to relieve pain, for colds and coughs, and – depending on mood – as a relaxant and aphrodisiac. It also embodies the popular global belief that if a medicine smells and tastes bad, it must be good.

Asafoetida was exploited in another way in both African and West Asian classic medicine – as an aid to exorcism. Combined with garlic for extra kick, it was worn around the neck during rituals to drive evil spirits from a sufferer's body and mind. More than 3,000 years ago, in Babylonia, royal physician Esagil-kin-apli compiled what has

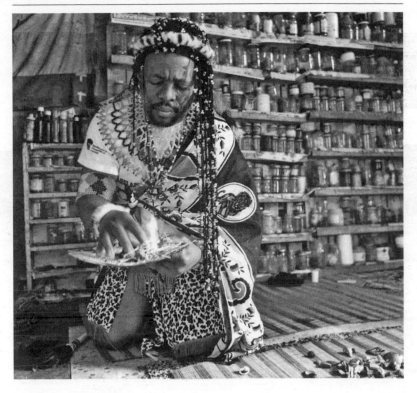

READING THE FLAMES
Pyromancy is the ancient art of reading flames for signs
that shed light on the past and the future. A doctor
may use it to understand a patient's condition.

become known as *The Manual of the Exorcist*. It instructs training and
practice for exorcisms, with details on rituals, spells, omens, and
tokens. Esagil-kin-apli also produced *Sakikku* (usually translated as
Diagnostic Handbook). It was a huge compendium of symptoms and their
underlying conditions, and included many methods for divining the
deity responsible for each disease.

The Rise
of Scientific
Medicine

900–1820

While Europe was in its Dark Ages, Islam expanded in West Asia and enjoyed a golden age. Its most famous physicians included al-Rhazi and the polymath Ibn Sina, who wrote more than 40 works on health, medicine, and well-being. Taking leads from Greece and Rome, Islamic scholars kept both the art and science of medicine alive and moving forward.

Early in the Renaissance, Western medicine emerged from stagnation and became more formalized. Universities opened medical schools and set up recognized qualifications, soon creating a medical elite. There was still room for a rebel. In the Italian city of Padua in 1543, against the trends of the time, Andreas Vesalius produced *De Humani Corporis Fabrica* (*On the Structure of the Human Body*). This magnificent book helped to break Galen's spell and usher in a new age when doctors trusted their own eyes, ears, and hands, and examined and talked to their patients. Another unorthodox figure was Ambroise Paré, a French "barber-surgeon", whose harrowing battlefield experiences led him to raise surgery from a menial trade to a respected profession.

The roles of the heart and blood had been subjects of speculation since ancient times. In 1628, English doctor William Harvey grafted his own research on to earlier ideas to explain the workings of the cardiovascular system. Similarly, in 1798, another English physician, Edward Jenner, built on pioneering work with his own experiments to establish smallpox vaccination. The light microscope, invented around 1590, took a couple of centuries to permeate medicine but, in the 19th century, the ground-breaking work by German physician Rudolf Virchow became the foundation of that essential branch of modern medicine, cellular pathology.

Al-Rhazi, Ibn Sina, and the Arab Revival

DURING THE 5TH CENTURY CE, the Western Roman Empire was in decay. Roman military dominance, social order, public health, and medical services fragmented in the face of Visigoths, Vandals, and a host of other invaders. Societies became more varied and disorganized, and written works, including historical records, became scarcer and more sporadic. Europe was drifting into the so-called "Dark Ages". In contrast, from about the 8th century in the Middle East and western Asia, the spread of Islam ushered in a golden age. Centred on Baghdad, in what is now Iraq, pursuits such as philosophy, literature, art, architecture, and science flourished in an age of intellectual progress. Knowledge was gathered, recorded, expanded upon, and disseminated. Dominating the fields of health and medicine through the following centuries were two great figures whose works would hold sway for 500 years and more: al-Rhazi (or Rhazes) and Ibn Sina (or Avicenna).

Al-Rhazi (c.866–925) came from the Persian (now Iranian) historic city of Rey (Rayy), now subsumed into Tehran. He was educated, became a physician, and held senior positions at hospitals both in Rey and in Baghdad. Like many great minds of those times, al-Rhazi was widely versed and active not only in medicine, alchemy, and chemistry, but also in philosophy, Islam and allied faiths, and other intellectual pursuits. He wrote widely and prolifically, producing more than 50 major works and more than 200 articles and smaller publications. In the area of medicine, he took his lead from many noted works of classical history, including those by Hippocrates of Greece (see pp.30–39) and Galen of Rome (see pp.40–45), the traditions of his own Persia, the Indian

MUHUMMAD AL-RHAZI
One of the greatest figures of the Arab revival, al-Rhazi made contributions to numerous fields of medicine, particularly pediatrics and ophthalmology.

Ayurvedic approach (see pp.74–81), and Chinese concepts such as yin-yang and qi (see pp.64–73). He drew upon these works and synthesized them, modernized them with the latest knowledge of his time, and added his own experiences from in-depth observation and sympathetic treatment as a practising physician.

Al-Rhazi championed a strict ethical code and a humane approach to patients that echoed those of Hippocrates. He recognized that some diseases were incurable, that physicians should not be blamed for such cases, and that they should not subject sufferers to supposed "cures" that were likely to worsen their quality of life. Physicians also had a duty to research and assimilate the latest medical knowledge and practices, and to treat each and every patient with equal courtesy and attention. Al-Rhazi was an acknowledged expert on ophthalmology, one of the great specialisms of the time, although he himself suffered cataracts and gradually lost his eyesight.

Clinically, al-Rhazi was probably the first physician to record the distinction between the terrible scourge of smallpox and the less deadly but still debilitating measles. He espoused a "fermentation theory" of disease, whereby the blood bubbles and boils in the manner of a fermenting alcoholic drink, giving off morbid vapours through the skin – manifested by the blisters and sores of the pox and measles. His work *al-Judari wa al-Hasbah* (*Concerning Smallpox and Measles*) advises: "Restlessness, nausea and anxiety occur more frequently with measles... pain in the back is more apparent with smallpox".

Therapeutically, al-Rhazi described many medicinal herbs and minerals, and introduced several drugs that contained mercury. He also improved medical equipment. Based on his work in alchemy and chemistry, he introduced new versions of utensils and tools that would persist for centuries, including the pestle and mortar for grinding, flasks for mixing, and phials for storage. He was also an early proponent of animal gut for sutures and a material similar to plaster of Paris for casts to immobilize and protect the patient.

Al-Rhazi's numerous writings include two massive encyclopedic works encompassing medical theory and practice, medical philosophy, and life in general. *Kitab al-Mansouri fi al-Tibb* (*The Book on Medicine Dedicated to al-Mansur*), known as *Liber almansoris* in Latin, was named in honour of Mansur ibn Ishaq ibn Ahmad ibn Asad, the governor of his home city of Rey. Its ten chapters cover diet, hygiene, anatomy, physiology, pathology theory, and aspects of medical practice such as diagnosis, therapy, and surgery. The second work was *Kitab al-Hawi fi al-tibb* (*The Comprehensive Book on Medicine*), Latinized to *Continens Liber* (and morphed to *Virtuous Life* in English), which comprises a multi-volume compendium of al-Rhazi's clinical observations, notes, and records, and views on previous medical works going back to Ancient Greece, Rome, and India. Parts of this volume were his own work, and others were assembled after his death.

Both books were soon established throughout the Islamic world. They were translated into other languages (including Latin for Europe), and became recommended reading for physicians and their students for several centuries. Al-Rhazi also produced numerous smaller books, articles, and commentaries, ranging from *Misconceptions of the Abilities of the Physician* to *Fruits Before and After Lunch*.

A century after al-Rhazi, Ibn Sina (c.980–1037) gained fame in western Europe under the Latin version of his name, Avicenna. His interests were even more extensive than those of al-Rhazi, and his written output greater. He was born near the historic Silk Road city of Bukhara (now in Uzbekistan), and apparently qualified as a physician by the age of 18, after which he set off on extensive travels around the Persian lands of West Asia. During these, he assimilated vast amounts of knowledge, treated patients, lectured on a variety of topics, penned over 40 works on physical and spiritual well-being, and managed to gain the patronage of rulers. These included Abu Ja-far Ala Adduala, the ruler of Hamedan (in northeastern Iran), with whom he spent his last decade as a physician and scholarly companion. His two most celebrated works are *Kitab al-Shifa* (*The Book of Healing*) and *Al-Qanun fi al-Tibb* (*The Canon of Medicine*), the latter being his masterpiece. Published in about 1025, *Al-Qanun* rapidly gained prominence throughout the Islamic world, and was translated from Arabic into Persian, Latin, most major European languages, and even Chinese. It influenced

"That whose existence is necessary must necessarily be one essence"

IBN SINA

TREATING SMALLPOX
A miniature from a Turkish edition of Ibn Sina's
Al-Qanun shows a remedy being prepared for a
smallpox victim.

physicians and medical students for the next five centuries, in Europe
and beyond, and is still regarded as one of the greatest works in the
history of medicine.

Among the attractions of *Al-Qanun* were its methodical and orderly
organization, and its vast scope as a self-contained work of reference
for both trainee and practising physicians. It selected, summarized,
and extended the medical knowledge of the ancients, and interwove
progressive contemporary ideas about diagnosis and treatments,
especially regarding transmissible diseases and drug therapies.

To modern eyes, some of the content of *Al-Qanun* is difficult to
appreciate. In first part of the work, Ibn Sina discusses the aims and
methods of medicine as "a science from which one learns the
conditions and states of the human body with regard to health and
the absence of health... the aim being to guard health when it exists
and restore it when it is lost". Following the medical philosophies of
his age, he invokes and describes many causes of illness – elements,
humours, temperaments, formal and efficient and accidental causes,
vital force, vital faculties and abilities, and much more that is

أراكَ قَدْ أبرزتَ لي رأسكَ قَبل أنْ تُبرِزَ قرطَاسكَ ولَيتني قدَ أكل ذ الكَ ولم أقرأ ذ الكَ ولستُ
ممن يبيع نقدًا بدين ولا يطلب أثرًا بعد عين فإن أنت رضختَ بالعين جمتُ في

PUBLIC VENESECTION
Surrounded by spectators, an
Arab physician draws blood from
a patient. The procedure was
believed to bring balance to the
patient's humours.

خلفَ عينٍ وإن كثُ تراً الشيخ أولى وخرتَ اَ لفلَس
غرب غيَّ والأ قفالَ الفتَى والَّذي حرمَ مصنوع ا

unfamiliar today. Some of these concepts derive from earlier ages, such as the four humours and four temperaments as described by Hippocrates, some are adapted from the ideas of al-Rhazi and others, while some were added by Ibn Sina himself.

Al-Qanun has five main parts. The first section covers the origins of health and illness, and various aspects of the body's structure and function. Ibn Sina regards the body as amenable to observation and dissection – however, the cause of disease and methods of treatment should be arrived at by reason and deduction. There are detailed descriptions of the brain and eyes, general therapeutic procedures, and the best ways to maintain health, namely through attention to exercise, food, and sleep. The second part of the book is a *materia medica* – lists and assembled information for more than 700 mineral preparations, herbal extracts, compound remedies, and other drugs and medicines. The third part concerns the diagnosis and treatment of diseases specific to certain parts of the body, following a pathway from the brain and nerves, eyes, and ears, down to the feet and toes, and including swellings and joint pains. Next come conditions that affect the whole body, such as fevers, poison bites, various fractures, broken bones, and even obesity. The fifth part lists compound remedies and their uses.

Scattered throughout *Al-Qanun* are Ibn Sina's personal experiences, anecdotes, advice, and pronouncements. He muses on the contagious or transmissible nature of phthisis or consumption (pulmonary tuberculosis); on how some diseases seem to be spread by water or in soil; and on sexual activities such as masturbation in men and women: "Women [with hysteria] should not resort to rubbing… this is suitable only for husbands and doctors".

Al-Rhazi and Ibn Sina kept alive and advanced much medical knowledge that had largely vanished from Europe – knowledge that had originated in Ancient Greece and Rome, and then spread through Constantinople and Gundeshapur to Baghdad and Bukhara, where it was combined with learnings from India and China, and was eventually translated back into European languages to form a basis for the flowering of the Renaissance. This reawakening of Classical thought inaugurated the age of the university, when medical schools were established throughout Europe, the Middle East, and beyond.

The Four Humours

The Ancient Greeks believed that the body contained four fluids, called humours – blood, yellow bile, black bile, and phlegm. To be healthy, they had to be kept in balance; their proportions could be changed by diet, activity, the season, or a person's age. Physicians from the time of Galen in the 1st century CE (see pp.40–45) to the 19th century believed that bloodletting (see pp.132–33) removed excess humours from the body and restored its natural balance.

ZODIAC LUNAR SCHEME FOR BLOODLETTING
ENGLAND, 1486
This device, from the guild of barber surgeons of York, England, calculated times for bloodletting. It had two movable discs: the "index of the sun" pointed to the day of treatment; the "index of the moon" (now missing) pointed to the cycle of the moon and a corresponding zodiac sign. Each sign related to one of the four elements, and to one of the humours – bloodletting of the relevant body part (see below) was to be avoided in that lunar phase.

The four elements

One of the oldest theories of matter, going back to Ancient Greece but also influencing Christian physicians in the Middle Ages, stated that everything in the world is made up of four elements – air, fire, earth, and water. Each of these elements was associated with one of the humours: air with blood, fire with yellow bile, earth with black bile, and phlegm with water. Ancient writers also linked parts of the body with the elements, for example, the lungs with air and the digestive system with fire.

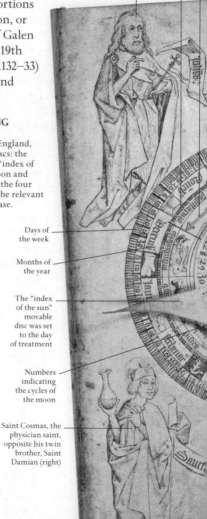

15TH-CENTURY ILLUSTRATION SHOWING CHRIST BINDING THE FOUR ELEMENTS

Signs of the zodiac, each linked to one of the four elements

Each sign occupied thirty degrees

John the Baptist, one of the patron saints of the guild.

Days of the week

Months of the year

The "index of the sun" movable disc was set to the day of treatment

Numbers indicating the cycles of the moon

Saint Cosmas, the physician saint, opposite his twin brother, Saint Damian (right)

John the Evangelist, the guild's other patron saint

The four temperaments

According to the theory of humorism, physicians believed that the humours influenced a person's character, emotions, appearance, and mental health. Galen named four personality types, each corresponding to, and influenced by, a specific humour.

SANGUINE
Men and women with a sanguine (blood-influenced) temperament were said to be impulsive, sociable, and good with people. Other character traits associated with this type included courage, optimism, and pleasure-seeking.

CHOLERIC
People believed that yellow bile made choleric individuals ambitious and disposed them to be good leaders. The downside was that they were inclined to lose their temper easily.

PHLEGMATIC
Phlegmatic people were generally relaxed, made loyal friends, and were able to keep calm in a crisis. However, they also tended to be rather unemotional.

MELANCHOLIC
Those with a melancholic disposition, influenced by black bile, were thought to be pessimistic and often suffered from insomnia. They were also said to be thoughtful, inventive, and artistic.

Schools of Medicine
and Life

MOST BIG TOWNS AND CITIES have medical schools and teaching hospitals. Indeed, where people's lives are at stake, it seems vital to have highly trained professionals gaining qualifications from officially recognized organizations. In the early Middle Ages in Europe, however, this was far from the case. Almost anyone could set up as a medical practitioner, and almost anyone did. Religion and medicine were intricately entwined, and many diseases were viewed as punishments for sins in this life or a previous one. Priests, monks, and nuns practised their cures in infirmaries and sickhouses attached to churches and monasteries, and wandering healers preached the wonders of their magical potions to anyone who cared to listen and pay. All this began to change towards the end of the First Millennium, as the achievements of Islam's golden age gradually spread through Europe.

The first generally recognized European school of medicine was the Schola Medica Salernitana in Salerno, southwest Italy. Here, great medical works by Arabic practitioners and communicators such as al-Rhazi (see pp.100–102) and Ibn Sina (see pp.102–105), carrying knowledge from Ancient Greece and Rome and augmented by their own advances, were translated into Latin, the language of Europe's scholars. Many of these works came from the library at Monte Cassino – the great Benedictine centre of religion and learning that stood 120km (75 miles) northwest of Salerno on the road to Rome.

One of the Schola Medica's inspirations was Alfanus I, who was Archbishop of Salerno for almost 30 years from 1057. A multilingual physician, he worked to establish the school and translated many of the Arabic texts, then used his position as Archbishop to increase the school's funding and powers. Another major figure of this time was Constantine the African, who first arrived in Salerno in around 1065. A scholar and trader from Tunisia, Constantine had travelled widely through Islamic regions and gathered a marvellous collection of books. Able to translate between Arabic and Latin, he also had knowledge of West Asian and Indian medicine. Alfanus welcomed Constantine and encouraged him, after several visits, to settle in

Salerno and to continue his studies. As a result, Constantine produced many lengthy translations that became staples in medical libraries around Europe for the next five centuries. He also lectured and demonstrated at the Schola Medica, before becoming a Christian convert in his final years at Monte Cassino.

During the late 11th and 12th centuries, the reputation of the Schola Medica spread and Salerno became known as Hippocratica Civitas (the Town of Hippocrates). Aspiring physicians, healers, surgeons, and apothecaries arrived to learn their craft and to gain certificates. The sick and ill also flocked in with the hope of a cure, or at the least of redemption. Arabic and also Jewish medical influences continued to spread across the Mediterranean, and Greek and Roman learning was integrated into the literature. Salerno became a gateway for medical knowledge entering Europe.

Training courses were highly organized at Salerno, with students passing from one level to the next only upon achieving the required passes. There could be three years of initial study, then four years of medical training, including practice with specialist physicians, surgeons, medical herbalists, and others. High standards were upheld in all fields, from hygiene to ethics, and (almost unheard of at the time) women were admitted and given licenses, not just for gynaecology, obstetrics, midwifery, and pre- and postnatal care, but also for general practice on both women and men. The physician's behaviour and bearing were also taught. *The Coming of a Physician to His Patient* advises the doctor on bedside manner: "When the doctor enters the dwelling of his patient, he should not appear haughty nor covetous, but should greet

CONSTANTINE THE AFRICAN
Benedictine monk Constantine the
African lectures on uroscopy – the art
of studying urine for signs of disease.

CAUTERIZING WOUNDS
A miniature from the 14th-century manuscript *The Surgery of Master Rogerius* shows a physician at Salerno's medical school cauterizing a wound.

with kindly, modest demeanour those who are present… Put the patient at his ease before the examination begins and the pulse should be felt deliberately and carefully… The friends standing round will be all the more impressed because of the delay and the physician's words will be received with just that much more attention".

Salerno became the model for other medical schools wishing to attract the most able physicians, papal approval, and royal patronage. One of these was the medical school at Montpellier, on France's Mediterranean coast. Another school was founded at the university of Bologna in northern Italy, around 1200, and it was here that the controversial practice of dissection appeared on the curriculum, from where it spread to other universities. As Bologna University matured, however, its promise of freedom to learn became compromised, and many students moved to Padua, where a university had been founded around 1200. Padua's medical faculty remained a progressive institution, and appointed a series of free thinkers to professorships such as anatomy and surgery, most famously the Flemish anatomist Andreas Vesalius (see pp.116–25).

Gradually, during the 14th and 15th centuries, more and more organized medical schools were established around Europe, each insisting on high levels of scholarship, unblemished morality, and wide-ranging studies, from Hippocrates and Galen to the Islamic golden age advances. This was fine and good for the well-connected and the wealthy. But for peasants in the countryside, healthcare remained entrenched in the Dark Ages, rooted in superstition and religion.

Philippus Aureolus Theophrastus Bombastus von Hohenheim was not quite from peasant stock. Born in Switzerland, his father was a minor-league physician who encouraged Philippus Aureolus to study theology and medicine, first at Basel in Switzerland, then Vienna,

Austria, and then at Ferrara, Italy. But no mere college could hold the youngster for long. Driven by wanderlust, and the desire both to make a name for himself and to help humanity, Philippus Aureolus decided to call himself Paracelsus – meaning "Better than (or beyond) Celsus", in barbed honour of Aulus Cornelius Celsus of Ancient Rome, who compiled massive encyclopedic works, including *De Medicina*. Being "better than" Celsus was, of course, a manifesto – a statement that the Ancients should not be trusted, and that the best teachers might not be found at universities, but rather in nature herself.

Paracelsus spent most of his time on long journeys, not only around Europe, but north to Scandinavia and Russia, south to North Africa, and east to the Holy Land and Asia Minor – perhaps even as far as India and Tibet. All the time, he learned and lectured, treated the sick, devised new operations and drug-based cures, and argued with anyone who cared to offer a contrary view. Details of his life are sketchy, but it seems that he was opinionated and awkward, spiky of temperament, probably emotionally unstable, perhaps an alcoholic, forever keen to tilt at the establishment and rebel against tradition. However, he also possessed a sharp intellect, an enormous amount of knowledge, and an obsessive need to write about and publish his discoveries – his fields included alchemy, religion, astrology, the occult, philosophy, and numerous other disciplines.

At one juncture, in 1527, Paracelsus found himself back in Basel as town physician and medical professor at his old university, where his unconventional views and rejection of the old authorities (such as Hippocrates and Galen) soon created controversy. He advocated, for example, that a wound should be allowed to drain itself freely of pus and fluids, rather than be bound tightly or cauterized. There were also arguments over his finances and his appointment of like-minded insubordinate junior physicians without the knowledge of the city council or the university congress – but

"Medicine rests upon four pillars – philosophy, astronomy, alchemy, and ethics"

PARACELSUS

A LESSON IN LIFE
Physicians at the Montpellier medical school give students a lesson in human anatomy. Founded in the late 11th century, the school attracted numerous surgeons and teachers — and patients hoping for a cure.

real trouble came on Midsummer's Day, when, in a public demonstration of his contempt for tradition, he made a bonfire out of the revered works of Galen, Ibn Sina, and others – an act that outraged the city's establishment. In a now-familiar pattern, Paracelsus had settled down with high hopes, stirred up a hornet's nest, and within the year had moved on again.

The doctrines of Paracelsus seem mystifying to us today. He adhered to the time-honoured idea of the four humours (see pp.106–107), and to this he added a "holy trinity" of three minerals: salt, sulphur, and mercury. He claimed that these substances contributed certain qualities to objects and beings, from mountains to humans, in line with each mineral's chemical properties. Salt, for example, signified stability and solidity; mercury (or quicksilver) brought change and transformation; while sulphur mediated between the two, leading to a balance between change and permanence.

Paracelsus's overall view of medicine was based on four central pillars: philosophy, astronomy, and alchemy, coordinated by the fourth, the virtue of the physician. Later, he also described disease as emanating from the interaction of five entities – namely, the body's own constitution, astrological influences, toxins, spirits good and evil, and God. Another of Paracelsus's many guiding ideas was that the human body is a microcosm – a distillation and focused reflection of the whole of nature, which is the universe or macrocosm. He wrote: "Man is a microcosm, or miniature world, being an extract from all the stars and planets of the whole firmament, from the earth and the elements; and thereby he is their quintessence". Health followed when the microcosmic body was in balance and harmony with the macrocosmic universe. Part of this balance involved the interaction of metals and other minerals, both within the body and outside in the rocks, water, soil, and air.

PARACELSUS
German-Swiss physician Paracelsus is often called the "father of toxicology" for his work on the effects of poisons on the human body.

THE GOOD PHYSICIAN
A woodcut from Paracelsus's *The Great Surgery Book* shows a sick man being attended to by a serving woman and a physician. The book encourages doctors to observe and experiment with nature, rather than simply to rely on textbooks.

Such ideas indicate that minerals were among Paracelsus's abiding passions – and herein lies one of his main contributions to medicine. He is often cited as the founder of toxicology – the study of the harmful effects of certain substances (i.e. "toxins" or poisons) on living things, and especially the damage they cause in the human body, and how these injuries can be treated. Paracelsus gained expert chemical, alchemical, and mineralogical skills from his extensive travels. He gathered knowledge from all manner of sources, including gypsies, outlaws, "old wives", and farm workers. He extracted a vast range of substances, mainly from plants, but also from soil, rocks, and occasionally animal bodies. He believed that any material could be both poisonous and therapeutic, depending on the amount, or dose, absorbed by the body. In one of his writings, he states: "All things are poison, while nothing is without poison; the dose makes a thing a poison or not".

This approach led to Paracelsus recommending mercuric minerals to treat syphilis. He also championed improved ways to deal with wounds, devised several new surgical procedures, and wrote copiously, not only on mineral-based medications and their uses, but on a wide range of topics from magic to the stars and planets. Probably his major book, earning him fame and financial security, was *Die Grosse Wundarzney* (*The Great Surgery Book*) of 1536. But even during his final years in Salzberg he remained cussedly independent. As he claimed: "No man should belong to another, but answer only to himself".

Vesalius and the Anatomists

IT SEEMS SENSIBLE that the best way to understand the human body is to open one up – preferably a newly dead body, and a healthy one that has died by accident or execution, so that its innards are not distorted by disease. Sensible indeed, since anatomy (the study of the body's "fabric" or structure) is a cornerstone of medicine. In the early 16th century, however, an obstacle stood in the way of this idea – indeed, it had stood there for 13 centuries – in the person of Claudius Galen (see pp.40–45). Such was the status of this legendary Roman physician that his pronouncements on anatomy, physiology, and disease were not questioned by the academic medics of medieval Europe – even though his works had been handed down in various forms of Latin and cod-Latinized texts, had been translated into Arabic and back again, had been added to by all manner of do-gooders, and were full of illustrations that had been copied and re-copied with varying degrees of quality and accuracy. And if a physician opened a body and dared to see things that Galen had not described, then either his eyes were at fault, or the body was malformed, or someone had introduced an error into Galen's text – or indeed the human body had changed since Galen's time. On no account, however, could it be said that Galen was wrong.

Luckily for medical progress, Andreas Vesalius (1514–64) had never really fallen under Galen's spell. Often credited as the founder of modern scientific anatomy, Vesalius came from a family of eminent medical men based in what was then the Hapsburg Netherlands. His father, Anders van Wesel, was apothecary

ANDREAS VESALIUS
Flemish physician Andreas Vesalius overturned centuries of medical dogma through his pioneering anatomical work.

(pharmacist) to Archduchess Margaret of Austria, and to Holy Roman Emperor Maximilian I and his successor Charles V. His grandfather was the royal physician to Maximilian I, and his great-grandfather had been a physician and instructor at the University of Leuven (Louvain), in present-day Belgium. At the age of 15, despite his medical background, Vesalius began studying art at the University of Leuven, and developed a talent for illustration. Five years later, however, he switched to studying medicine in Paris, where he read and re-read the works of Galen and other ancients, which had recently become widely available due to advances in printing technology. It was here, under the eyes of tutors Johann Winter von Andernach and Jacobus Sylvius (Jacques Dubois), that he learned the science of anatomy – Sylvius particularly impressed him by allowing his students to see inside corpses. These lessons showed Vesalius that the wisdom of the ancients – and that of the 14th-century Bolognese professor Mondino de Liuzzi – might not agree with what he was uncovering on the autopsy slab himself.

In 1536, when war broke out between France and the Holy Roman Empire, Vesalius returned to Leuven. He obtained basic medical qualifications, quarrelled with his superiors, and spirited away the corpse of a criminal from the scaffold to further his dissecting skills. He then moved on via Venice to the famed University of Padua, Italy, where his talents were quickly recognized. In 1537, apparently the day after his graduation, Vesalius was offered the post of Professor of Anatomy and Surgery, which he accepted.

Vesalius's Paduan superiors knew little of his rebellious streak, but this soon became apparent when he began teaching. Extending Sylvius's lead, he wielded the knife and opened up the dissection bodies himself, allowing his students to peer inside. The standard practice of the day was to allow an assistant or lowly barber-surgeon (see pp.126–33) to do such work, and even then, this physical side of the lesson was usually just a supplement to the reading of the sacred works of Galen, de Liuzzi, and the rest. Another of Vesalius's innovations was to record what he saw with his own eyes in the form of detailed illustrations that were faithful to the specimens before him, rather than relying on older renderings. Using his drawing skills, and taking advice from professional artists, Vesalius built up a collection of accurate and skilfully executed illustrations. News soon spread of Vesalius and his fresh approach, and in 1538 this led him to publish six of his early works as *Tabulae Anatomicae Sex* (*Six Anatomical Plates*), the illustrations of which were possibly prepared from his originals by Jan van Calcar, a pupil of the painter Titian. Vesalius's work was soon "pirated", which rapidly spread his name and fame around Europe, but left him concerned about unauthorized replications of his work.

By 1540, Vesalius had edited one of Galen's works, *Institutiones Anatomicae*, and published "revisions" of some of the details. He also had an encounter during a public dissection at Bologna with one of Italy's top professors, Matteo Corti, about details of the liver and muscles. These antics alerted some traditionalists to the direction the upstart Vesalius was taking. Meanwhile, a local judge in Padua, fascinated by medicine, and by Vesalius's approach in particular, permitted him to use the corpses of executed criminals for autopsies. As a result, Vesalius soon had numerous corpses in various stages of dissection taking up space in his university rooms – including his personal quarters.

As part of his academic duties, Vesalius visited Pisa, Bologna, Venice, and other universities to lecture and lead teaching sessions. One such trip to Bologna in 1541 reminded him forcefully that much of Galen's anatomical work – especially dissection – had not been carried out on humans. Such work had been forbidden in Ancient Rome, so Galen had therefore opened and described the anatomy of animals (ranging from pigs to macaque monkeys) instead and assumed that their insides were similar to ours. Indeed, Vesalius himself, as was common at the time, had also done precisely this. He now came to realize that this was the origin of the "discrepancies" in Galen's work, and that, for the good of medical knowledge (and for patients), they had to be corrected.

ABDOMINAL CAVITY
This illustration from *De Humani* shows a man's abdominal cavity – minus its intestines.

"I am not accustomed to saying anything with certainty after only one or two observations"

VESALIUS

An emboldened Vesalius, equipped with fresh human corpses and a new slant on Galen, decided to produce his own great work on anatomy. Two years later, the immense seven-volume *De Humani Corporis Fabrica (On the Fabric of the Human Body)* was published, and was a great success. By the year's end, despite its immense size and breathtaking price, the book had sold out. Not only were *De Humani*'s originally woodcut images (probably prepared in Venice on pear wood) hugely detailed and beautifully executed, they were also accurately taken from life. They showed bodies in lifelike poses and familiar contexts, with many set against the Italian countryside. An illustrated aside showed a dog with one paw as a human foot, perhaps a reference to the fact that Galen's animal subjects included many dogs.

Aged just 30, Vesalius had masterminded the project himself, but others had almost certainly produced the illustrations. Some experts again suggest Jan van Calcar, who was an acknowledged expert copyist and mimic (and occasional forger) of great works. Other authorities consider the *De Humani* pictures to be by general studio artists familiar with the style of Titian. Nevertheless, Vesalius had attended to every detail of *De Humani*, and chose the renowned printer Joannis Oporini of Basel to produce it — which he did using the intaglio method, in which engraved copper plates are taken from woodcuts. The resulting detail and clarity astonished Vesalius's readers.

The 663 pages of *De Humani* were divided into seven "books", more akin to what we might today call chapters, that summarized Vesalius's extensive findings. The sheer size of the pages — 42cm (16½in) by 28cm (11in) — was daunting, as were the 400-plus individual images that they contained, which featured textures and contours in three dimensions, quite different from the "flat" style of the times. Then, of course, there were Vesalius's observations, which were born of his recognition that form reflects function. He understood that the positions, shapes, sizes, and connections between the body's organs, muscles, tubes, ducts, and other parts gave clues to what they did. His discoveries included that men and women have the same number of ribs; that the lower jaw, or mandible, is a single bone, not two (an error derived from dog anatomy); that the breastbone, or sternum, has three parts, not seven (an error derived from monkey anatomy); that nerves are solid, not hollow, and that they are involved in muscle control and sensation; that nerves either originate or end in the brain, and do not run between other organs, such as the heart, as had been believed since Aristotle's time; that the liver has two lobes and not five; that the heart rather than the liver is central to the vascular system; that there are no traces of connecting holes or pores in the septum between the heart's left and right sides, as had long been imagined – which had great implications for later investigators such as William Harvey (see pp.134–43). He also gave detailed descriptions of several complex abdominal parts, such as the omentum (a fold of tissue lining the abdomen), and suggested that the kidneys filter blood to produce urine, which travels along ureters to the bladder (previously it had been thought that the kidneys filter urine). By far the mainstay of the book, however, are the hundreds of pictures of muscles, showing the tendons and ligaments that connect them to the skeleton, and the manner in which they move.

As well as being an ingenious anatomist, Vesalius clearly had a flair for furthering his own career, which he surely did when he dedicated the first edition of De Humani to Holy Roman Emperor Charles V, whom his father had served. A special silk-bound, vellum-paged, hand-coloured copy was presented to the emperor – and indeed, Charles duly responded by appointing Vesalius court physician in 1545. Vesalius accepted the post and literally burned his bridges to medical academia, by burning many of his learned works and notes, including volume after volume of Galen. Then off he went, accompanying the emperor and his entourage to their various palaces and homes, and on forays to visit allies around much of Europe. In the early 1550s, Vesalius also established a lucrative practice as a private physician in Brussels,

FRONTISPIECE OF *DE HUMANI*
The frontispiece of *De Humani* shows the author conducting a dissection at the School of Medicine, Brussels.

ANDREAE VESALII
BRVXELLENSIS, SCHOLAE
medicorum Patauinæ professoris, de
Humani corporis fabrica
Libri septem

CVM CAESAREAE
Maiest. Galliarum Regis, ac Senatus Veneti gra

a job that came with a magnificent house, stables, and an orchard. In 1556, Charles abdicated as emperor, but Vesalius had perhaps knowingly covered this eventuality as well when he dedicated an abridged "digest" version of De Humani (published in 1543, less than three months after the original) to Charles' son, Philip. Usually known as Epitome (from De Humani Corporis Fabrica Librorum Epitome), this version of De Humani had more images and a shorter, simpler version of the text. In 1556, this same Philip, now Philip II of Spain, invited Vesalius to be his royal physician, which of course Vesalius accepted – along with the awards, titles, and wealth that also came his way.

During this time, there was a backlash against Vesalius, his methods, his disregard for long-held beliefs and ancient teachings, and the more radical elements of De Humani and his other works – particularly those contradicting Galen. Some critics were outraged at the immoral sacrilege of organized dissections, which desecrated "God's handiwork". Vesalius was also taunted as a "mere barber" by eminent court physicians, academic professors, and others of nobility and title – barber-surgeons being the main practitioners of the time, though they were generally regarded as uneducated inferiors by medicine's upper strata (see pp.126–31). Vesalius himself rarely responded, although criticism did lead to errors being recognized in a second edition of De Humani, which appeared in 1555. In this edition, he covered greater ground, removed more animal material and added a good deal more about female anatomy, including pregnancy.

In 1564, Vesalius arranged a pilgrimage and medicinal plant-hunting expedition to the Holy Land, perhaps to escape the confines of Philip's court and the pressures of the infamous Spanish Inquisition. His itinerary included Jerusalem and Jericho, where he wished to collect and study therapeutic herbs. However, the trip was allegedly curtailed when a message arrived in Jerusalem requesting that Vesalius return to take up his former professorship at Padua following the death of Gabriele Falloppio. Vesalius duly sailed back, but adverse weather shipwrecked him on the Ionian island of Zante (Zakynthos), where, far from the courts of Europe, he is said to have died in confused and lonely circumstances, perhaps of plague. His burial site is unknown.

The momentous De Humani echoed the spirit of the age. As in other areas of Renaissance science, literature, and art, it hastened a break with ancient traditions and long-established but unverified information. Through it, Vesalius pioneered the approach of relying on personal observations and investigations. He also set new scientific benchmarks and ethical standards that gradually permeated the whole of medical practice. In establishing the modern science of anatomy, Vesalius corrected long-held misbeliefs, introduced new discoveries, and inspired a fresh breed of anatomists, physicians, and surgeons.

Among Vesalius's pupils and contemporaries were Gabriele Falloppio and Bartolomeo Eustachi, both of whom contributed a deeper understanding of anatomy. Falloppio advanced anatomical studies of the head, especially the ear, describing the tiny organs of hearing such as the eardrum and cochlea that lie deep within the temporal bone of the skull. He also studied the reproductive organs, and his name lives on in this area. In the female body, ripe eggs released from the ovary travel to the womb along the oviduct – the fallopian tube.

Eustachi also furthered knowledge of the ear. The small air tube that equalizes pressure between the middle ear and the back of the throat (and thence to the general outside atmosphere) is called the eustachian tube. Nine years after Vesalius and *De Humani*, Eustachi completed his own epic anatomy work, *Tabulae Anatomicae* (*Anatomical Engravings*), but he forbade its publication in case he was prosecuted or excommunicated by the Catholic Church. To avoid confusion with Vesalius' earlier *Tabulae Anatomicae Sex*, this later work is sometimes known as *Tabulae Anatomicae Bartholomaei Eustachi*. It did not become generally available until 160 years later, in 1714.

A poignant reminder of Vesalius resides at the University of Basel, the city of *De Humani*'s launch. The "Basel Skeleton", as it is known, originally belonged to a notorious local villain by the name of Jakob Karrer von Gebweiler. While overseeing *De Humani*'s publication in 1543, Vesalius happened to visit Basel when von Gebweiler was being publicly beheaded. Since he was known for his great skill with the knife, Vesalius was invited to carry out an autopsy on von Gebweiler – also in public. After the autopsy, the bones were reassembled into a preparation or specimen that Vesalius presented to the city. The Basel Skeleton still resides at the University's Museum of Anatomy. For a man who gave the medical world such an epochal publication, and a springboard to a new era of progress, the skeleton remains the only known well-preserved specimen prepared by Vesalius himself.

VESALIUS IN PADUA
Vesalius conducts an anatomy lesson in the
world's first dedicated anatomical theatre, at the
University of Padua. It was here that it became
normal to study anatomy by dissecting human
corpses, rather than by studying ancient texts.

Paré and the Barber-Surgeons

THE BARBER-SURGEONS of medieval Europe practised a curious mix of trades: haircutting and shaving, with lice and flea removal often thrown in for free; also removal of warts and similar skin blemishes; perhaps a few tooth-pullings; the always-popular bloodletting by leech (see p.132–33); and cauterizing open wounds by pouring on boiling oil – plus emergency limb amputation, usually in hellish battlefield conditions. Ambroise Paré was schooled in all of these procedures, but he was also a pioneer who led a revolution in surgery – one that greatly eased pain and suffering, promoted healing, and vastly improved prospects for the seriously wounded.

Paré was brought up in an unremarkable artisan family in Laval, northwest France. From 1532, he trained at the Hôtel Dieu, Paris's leading hospital and seat of medical learning. As in much of Europe, its approach was rooted in the teachings of Ancient Rome's Claudius Galen (see pp.40–47), whose colossal reputation meant that even 13 centuries later, physicians almost blindly followed his doctrines. They refused to accept the evidence of their eyes and acknowledge Galen's mistakes in human anatomy, even when confronted time and again with dissected corpses whose body parts were not where Galen said they should be (see p.116). These physicians were highly educated, principled men, usually from privileged, well-connected backgrounds. They haughtily held court to diagnose patients' ills, recommend treatments, and perhaps even administer an occasional tincture or potion, but they rarely got their hands dirty. Practical treatment was left to barber-surgeons, who were generally from middle-class or perhaps peasant stock, less educated, or even

AMBROISE PARÉ
French barber-surgeon Ambroise Paré is one of the fathers of modern surgery. His revolutionary techniques were tested on wounded soldiers.

illiterate, aware of their status, but with hands-on skills, and tolerant of pus, blood, urine, excreta, and gangrenous flesh. Indeed, by the time Paré attended the Hôtel Dieu, the reputation of barber-surgeons was growing. The Hôtel Dieu was affiliated to the Faculty of Medicine at the University of Paris, so trainees could attend university lectures on surgery and anatomy.

A fast learner, Paré progressed rapidly through his barber-surgeon apprenticeship, and was appointed army regimental surgeon in 1536. At the time, France was embroiled in several military campaigns, so Paré was kept busy treating war wounded in extremely primitive field hospitals; a common duty was running hopelessly mutilated soldiers through with a sword, or cutting their throats, to end their suffering.

The traditional treatment for open wounds was to cauterize and seal them with boiling oil (elder oil was favoured) or red-hot irons. This reduced complications such as gangrene, but it also brought further agony and prolonged suffering. Such treatments were especially favoured for the relatively new phenomenon of gunshot or firearm wounds. Gunpowder itself, and the burns and penetrating damage its projectiles caused, were considered poisonous to flesh and so required detoxifying with scalding oil.

Intense pain and dreadful suffering were common at the time. Indeed, they were viewed as essential components of surgical treatment and recovery. Pain relief was limited, with no anaesthetics as we know them available, only roughly prepared potions containing worryingly approximate amounts of potentially deadly opium, henbane, mandrake, or alcohol. This was also the pre-antibiotic era, and an agonizing but swift treatment such as boiling oil or red-hot iron reduced the risk of infection, and improved chances of eventual survival, albeit with the legacy of disfiguring scars, missing limbs, and long-term discomfort.

Paré was appalled at such barbarous procedures and vowed to do better – and his chance came in 1536, when King François I declared war on the Duke of Savoy, leading to a siege of Turin. In the ensuing bloodbath, the fighting was so destructive of the army ranks that Paré ran out of boiling oil. Freed from the stricture of his army orders to use the treatment, he jumped at the opportunity to try an alternative. This was a soothing balm made from turpentine, egg yolk, and oil of roses. Paré had confiscated supplies to mix the balm, which he developed from a combination of folk remedies. The following day, Paré checked and compared his patients. Those who suffered boiling oil or hot irons were in great pain, feverish, even delirious, with wounds and surrounding tissues swollen, red, and raw. Those who had been treated with the balm had less pain and were healing faster. In 1545, Paré publicized this new approach in his *Method of Treating Wounds*. Following his convictions, and eager for his fellow barber-surgeons to benefit from his discoveries, he wrote this not in the Latin used by qualified physicians and learned scholars, but in vernacular French.

Paré trialed a further innovation at the Turin campaign in 1537, and went on to develop this as a reliable procedure. It concerned sucking chest wounds leading to collapsed lung – or pneumothorax, in modern terminology. Penetrating sword or lance wounds to the chest could allow air into the interface between the outer covering of the lung and the inner lining of the chest. Normally there is no air here and the lung adheres to the chest lining, so that as the ribs and chest expand on breathing in, the elastic lung tissues are stretched with it and increase in volume, sucking in air down through the windpipe. With a penetrating chest wound, air can take an easier route. On breathing in, air is sucked in through the wound and creates an air gap around the unstretched lung, which comes away from the chest lining and collapses. Breathing out pushes the air in the reverse direction, leaving the lung still collapsed. Fighting for breath, but with no air exchange inside the lung itself to provide oxygen for the blood, the patient in effect suffocates. The conventional emergency procedure was to suture (stitch) the wound closed, but this rarely helped, as most battlefield surgeons understood. As dreadfully injured victims lay dying all around, a surgeon would often pass by a soldier with a sucking chest wound to look for someone whose injuries were easier to treat successfully. Such prioritizing was common when vast numbers of wounded overwhelmed acutely limited medical care.

Paré described how he attended a soldier at Turin with a deep wound under the left breast. The wound had been sutured by another medic, trapping air and blood from internal bleeding around the lung. For the soldier, the end was near. Paré removed the stitching to reopen the gash, then he positioned the soldier with his legs elevated, and his head and chest low over the side of the bed. He advised the soldier to breathe in slowly to maximum, close his nose and mouth, and try to compress his chest as if breathing out hard. His hunch was that this should force out material from around the lung. Paré reported that this caused a fluid filled with congealed lumps of blood "to jet through the wound... I put my finger deep in the wound to break up the coagulated blood, and seven to eight ounces of fetid and corrupt blood drained". Paré then irrigated the wound with barley water containing rose oil, honey, and sugar candy, while placing the soldier at various angles and positions to encourage maximum drainage. "To conclude, this injury was so well handled that beyond my expectation, the patient recovered".

Following wound balms and sucking chests, Paré introduced another revolutionary technique. Many soldiers with gruesomely extensive limb damage underwent rapid amputation, but then

THE SURGEON AT WORK
A barber-surgeon removes a stone from a man's
head at a public fair. Other such stones hang in
the background as proof of the surgeon's skill.

bled profusely and died from medical shock brought on by blood loss. This could occur even after attempts to sear and seal the amputation wound using a red-hot iron. Acutely observant, Paré saw that most of the blood gushed from one or two severed arteries at the stump, rather than from general tissues such as muscle. He reasoned that if these arteries could somehow be compressed slightly nearer the heart, haemorrhaging would be reduced. So he tried tying ligatures or tight cords adjacent to the proposed amputation site. It worked: upon amputation, the restricted artery no longer spurted high-pressure blood from the stump. Survival rates climbed, and Paré used his anatomical knowledge to find the best ligature sites for various levels of amputation.

News of Paré's handiwork spread through the army ranks and other barber-surgeons took up his idea. He gained fame and promotion within the military, but few in the medical establishment, especially back at the Faculty of Medicine in Paris, were receptive to his ideas. However, despite such academic snubs, in 1552 he was appointed to a royal position, in the service of Henry II of France. It was the first of many royal appointments, which saw him employed for almost 40 years under four monarchs – Henry II, Francis II, Charles IX, and Henry III – holding the office of chief surgeon to the last two.

Rather than enjoying the luxuries of the royal court, Paré continued his pioneering

"WOUND MAN"
This 15th-century illustration from a barber-surgeon's manual indicates the various wounds a soldier could receive in battle.

"The art of medicine is to cure sometimes, to relieve often, to comfort always"

AMBROISE PARÉ

work on amputation. He designed and made a series of limb prostheses – artificial arms, legs, hands, and feet – as well as trusses, artificial eyes, and tooth implants.

Experimentation and rational deduction also continued to fascinate Paré. He had long been suspicious of so-called "bezoar stones" – masses of material extracted from the stomach or digestive tract of humans and animals. According to legend, the stones had medicinal properties, and were in particular an antidote to all manner of poisons. In 1567, an opportunity arose to test this notion. A thief at the royal court was sentenced to death by hanging, but he agreed to take poison instead, provided he could then take a bezoar preparation. If he survived, he would be freed. Paré recorded the proceedings and noted that the thief died from taking the poison after several hours of excruciating pain, thereby showing that a bezoar was ineffective in this case.

For all his achievements on the battlefield and elsewhere, perhaps Paré could be excused his occasional lapses. His book *On Monsters and Marvels* was an illustrated compendium of human and animal birth defects, fanciful beasts from hearsay and legend, and other weirdly wonderful phenomena. His causes of birth defects in human babies included "Wrath of God", "Corrupt seed", and "Indecent posture by the expectant mother". A two-headed child, for instance, resulted from "Too much seed". Nevertheless, despite initial scepticism and even rebuttal from the medical establishment, Paré's reputation grew over the centuries, and he is now regarded as a major innovator in battlefield surgery, and a humane and caring barber-surgeon. Devoutly religious throughout his long life and distinguished career, he retained the motto: "I treated him; God healed him".

Bloodletting

First-century Roman physician Galen believed that blood, as the strongest of the four humours (see pp.106–107), had a powerful influence on health. He theorized that blood was created by the heart and liver and consumed by other organs, and that it could stagnate in the extremities of the body, causing disease. Based on this idea, surgeons bled patients to remove stagnant blood, and to restore the balance of the humours. This practice, common since the time of the Ancient Greeks to treat a range of diseases, was such a popular procedure that it continued long after the 17th-century discovery of blood circulation.

LEECH JAR AND LANCETS
ENGLAND, c.18TH–19TH CENTURY
A popular method of bloodletting was to place medicinal leeches – bloodsucking freshwater worms – on a patient's skin. Leeches have triple jaws that pierce the skin so they can suck out blood. Surgeons stored them in special jars.

A cure for all

Bloodletting was recommended for all kinds of diseases, from headaches and indigestion to pneumonia and strokes. The treatment was often carried out by surgeons and barber-surgeons, who combined shaving and hair-cutting with basic surgical work (see pp.126–31). Surgeons also bled healthy people as a preventive measure. The most common method was venesection – applying a tourniquet to the patient's arm so that a vein would swell, cutting open the vein, and draining off the blood.

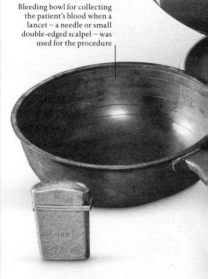

Bleeding bowl for collecting the patient's blood when a lancet – a needle or small double-edged scalpel – was used for the procedure

17TH-CENTURY ILLUSTRATION OF A MAN WEARING A TOURNIQUET BLEEDING INTO A BOWL.

Ventilation holes in the lid allowed the leeches to breathe

The jar held water, in which the leeches lived

A metal box holds two sharp lancets for opening a vein

The medicinal leech (*Hirudo medicinalis*) secretes an anticoagulant, to make the blood flow

Tools of the trade

The use of leeches was widespread in the 19th century – so much so that the high demand almost made the species extinct. This was one of the reasons surgeons resorted to other methods of bloodletting, including cupping and the use of mechanical devices to remove patients' blood.

BRONZE BLOOD CUP
This blood cup from Sicily dates back to between 400 and 100 BCE. Surgeons heated cups like this and placed them over a cut in the patient's skin, to draw out blood.

SCARIFICATOR
In the 18th and 19th centuries, instruments called scarificators, consisting of several blades mounted on a handle, were used to make multiple incisions in the skin, piercing numerous superficial blood vessels. Designed to be less painful and more efficient than a single lancet, scarificators were usually used in conjunction with cupping.

MECHANICAL LEECH
This syringe-like suction device enabled surgeons to control the amount of blood removed. It did not fall off the skin and reattach itself somewhere else as real leeches tended to do, and could be used on parts of the body on which it was not practical to use a live creature.

Harvey and Blood Circulation

SINCE ANCIENT TIMES, blood has been regarded as the very stuff of human existence – a red liquid that, as it leaked away, took life with it. Likewise, the heart has always been at the centre of our ideas about character – today, to "have a heart" means to be generous and forgiving. Perhaps no other parts of the body have been subject to so much myth and superstition, nor had their workings guessed at so many times – the simple fact that the heart pumps blood around the body took until the 17th century to be discovered. The breakthrough came in the 1620s, when English physician William Harvey performed experiments that overturned centuries of guesswork about veins, arteries, and the workings of the human heart.

About 2,000 years ago, the immense Chinese work *Huang-di Nei' Jing* (*The Yellow Emperor's Canon of Medicine* – see p.64–69) referred to a form of "circulation" by which blood, mixed with qi (life energy), was distributed around the body. In Ancient Greece, Hippocrates (see pp.30–39) also suggested that there might be a form of circulation in the body. The trouble was that in most dissected corpses the arteries seemed to be empty, while the veins were always engorged with blood. This led Hippocrates to think that arteries contained air, while only veins contained blood – the truth being that arteries (which move blood *away*

WILLIAM HARVEY
English physician William Harvey demonstrates the circulation of blood in a stag. His was the first complete account of the mechanics of the heart and the blood system.

from the heart) have thick, muscular walls, which contract after death, shifting along any contents, whereas veins (which *return* blood to the heart) have thin walls and tend to retain their contents. Another Greek physician, Erasistratus, studied the heart, blood vessels, and lungs, and suggested that a life-force called "pneuma" was breathed into the lungs (from the air) and passed into the heart, where it was converted into a form of "animal spirit" that spread like a vapour around the body – via the apparently empty, hollow arteries. For Erasistratus, then, veins were still the principal vessels of the blood system, and the fluid within them ebbed and flowed, to and fro, into the heart and out, with each heartbeat.

In Ancient Rome, Claudius Galen (see pp.40–47) had given vent to copious opinions on the heart and the blood, and cleverly combined several existing beliefs into a complex theory that would, like many of his pronouncements, last for centuries. One advance he did make, based on experiments with live animals, was that arteries contained blood, rather than air, and that this blood was bright red and actively spurted – unlike venous blood, which was dark and slow. So Galen appreciated that there were two sets of blood vessels – arteries and veins – but he regarded them as distinct systems. With no microscope, he had no knowledge of the capillaries in the tissues that linked the two, but he did suggest another set of tiny connections – in the heart itself. He contended that digested food went from the gut to the liver, where it transformed into blood, and from here the sluggish venous blood ebbed and flowed to and from all the major parts of the body, distributing nutrition and also a variant of pneuma known as "natural spirit". The heart's job was to mix blood that came into its right side from the liver, with air from the lungs, which arrived along what we now call the pulmonary arteries. Blood impurities were removed in the heart and returned to the lungs, where they were breathed out, while the cleaned blood returned to the liver. On the issue of the connection between veins and arteries, Galen proposed that some of the blood in the heart's right side managed to seep through tiny pores in the dividing wall (known as the septum) into the left side. There was no visible evidence of these septal pores, but Galen was convinced that they existed. In the heart's left side, the formerly dull, oozing blood was energized by a version of pneuma called "vital spirit", from air conveyed along the vessels that we call the pulmonary veins. Now vivid and pulsing with "vital spirit", this blood then spread around the body and was consumed, especially in the brain.

The Galenic view of the heart and blood persisted through medieval times, with only minor modifications here and there. One such modification came in the 13th century, when Arab physician Ibn al-Nafis commented on the works of Ibn Sina (see pp.100–07), and challenged the latter's belief in Galen's septal pores. Instead, al-Nafis contended that blood flowed from the heart's right side to the lungs, where it mixed with air and then returned to the left side. He also conjectured on minute pores or networks between the arteries and veins in the lungs – which, four centuries later, were identified as capillaries. Al-Nafis' account thus describes the pulmonary part of the blood's circulation as we know it today.

It was during the Renaissance that Galen's view was finally overthrown. In the early 1500s, Leonardo da Vinci drew the heart's outer and inner structure with accuracy and elegance, distinguishing four chambers, as opposed to Galen's three (which came from his study of the three-chambered hearts of reptiles). Based upon his knowledge of mechanics, da Vinci also guessed at the function of valves as flow controllers – but he failed to make the leap to the idea of continuous circulation. Instead, he stuck with the ebb-and-flow model, and even illustrated Galen's tiny "pores" in the septum, though he never saw them.

In the 1540s, Amato Lusitano, a Portuguese-born physician and anatomist working in Italy, experimented with the membraneous, flap-like, one-way valves in the main veins. By blowing through the veins, he showed that air, and so presumably blood, could not stream past them away from the heart, according to the age-old conviction. In the 1550s, the celebrated Renaissance anatomist Andreas Vesalius (see pp.116–25) declared that he had failed to find Galen's septal pores – and in 1559, one of Vesalius's successors, Matteo Realdo Colombo, proposed that blood flowed between the lungs and the heart along the pulmonary vein. Colombo came to this conclusion by observing living animals, in which the pulmonary vein from the lungs to the heart always contained blood, not air. He also demonstrated that the blood vessels pulsated in time with those of the heart. Thus, he

DA VINCI SKETCHES
Leonardo da Vinci produced many accurate drawings of the heart and the blood system. He proved both that the heart is a muscle and that it does not warm the blood.

proposed that with each beat, the heart's muscle forcefully contracted to push blood out into the vessels – the phase of the heartbeat we know as "systole". This idea turned on its head the old view that the heart actively enlarged to suck in blood. In fact, that phase, known as "diastole", allows blood to flow in from the veins as the heart passively relaxes. Another Italian to pen ideas about the heart, and who used the concept of blood "circulation", was botanist-cum-doctor Andrea Cesalpino, who at one stage declared: "The movement of blood... is constant from the vena cava [great vein] through the lungs and through the heart to the aorta".

Such was the state of cardiovascular science at the turn of the 15th century. Strands of evidence had accumulated about the structures and workings of the heart and blood vessels, and there had been several accounts that used the concept of "circulation". But no one had yet fashioned them into an overall proposal and fully understood the idea of a circulatory system.

Enter English physician William Harvey. In 1599, after graduating from Cambridge, Harvey arrived at the University of Padua, Italy, where he studied under Hieronymus Fabricius, follower of famed anatomist Gabriele Falloppio (see p.123), himself successor to Realdo Colombo. The young Harvey read Colombo's works on the heart and blood, and also those of Fabricius, who had provided the first accurate descriptions of valves in major veins. Returning to England, Harvey worked his way through London's medical establishment to become Chief Physician at St Bartholomew's Hospital, a celebrated lecturer on anatomy, and eventually a physician to the rich and powerful, including King James I and his heir Charles I.

An enthusiastic demonstrator and experimentalist, Harvey reputedly dissected the bodies of both his father and his sister. After travelling around Europe in the 1630s, he accompanied Charles I to

"All we know is still infinitely less than all that remains unknown"

WILLIAM HARVEY

ROYAL PHYSICIAN
William Harvey gives
Charles I of England
a lesson in blood
circulation. During the
English Civil War, Harvey
treated many of the
wounded, and looked
after the king's children.

Oxford during the troubles of the English Civil War, settled there for a time, and spent his later years in retirement back in London. His historic publication — *Exercitatio Anatomica de Motu Cordis et Sanguinis in Animalibus* (*An Anatomical Exercise on the Motion of the Heart and Blood in Living Beings*), usually known as *On the Motion of the Heart and Blood*, or *De Motu Cordis* — appeared in 1628. A slim 72 pages, it was the result of more than 20 years of deliberate, detailed, step-by-step, occasionally obsessive dissections, observations, and experiments on over 60 different species of dead and living animal — ranging from tiny freshwater shrimps, snails, crabs, and fish to toads, frogs, birds, dogs, pigs, and, in particular, snakes. Cold-blooded creatures like frogs and reptiles were useful to Harvey because the motions of their hearts and pulsating vessels were generally slower and easier to follow than those of warm-blooded birds or mammals — and their bodies stayed fresh longer when they were opened up and subjected to various procedures. Harvey peered intently and recorded diligently as he prodded, twisted, nicked, sliced, injected with fluids, emptied by needle aspiration, tied off, and removed their hearts and vessels for detailed inner examination.

De Motu Cordis was the first well-rounded, scientific, evidence-supported description of the circulatory system and its function — how the heart pumped blood round and round the body. As we know today, there are in fact two "sub-circulations". One, as uncovered by several of Harvey's predecessors, is from the heart's right side along the pulmonary arteries to the lungs, where the dark, "stale" blood picks up fresh supplies of oxygen – and then returns, refreshed and bright red, along the pulmonary veins to the heart's left side. This is termed the pulmonary or lesser circulation. From the heart's larger, more muscular left side, blood surges with each pulsing contraction of a heartbeat, out along the major arteries. Like the bronchi in the lungs, these arteries divide and narrow repeatedly to supply all of the body's organs and tissues with blood. Gradually, the blood's pressure, speed of flow, and oxygen content fall – and then the blood returns along tiny veins that merge into wider ones, all the way to the great veins, and finally flows again into the right side of the heart. This is the greater or systemic circulation. Along the main veins and in the heart itself, one-way valves ensure a one-way current – there is therefore no "ebb and flow".

In all of this, the heart is a muscular pump – an amazingly tireless, highly adjustable, self-maintaining one, but chiefly a pump, requiring no such thing as a "pneuma", "animal spirit", or "vital force" to keep it going. Like Vesalius (see pp.116–25), Harvey knew that he would come under fire for contradicting Galenism – especially the idea that blood is manufactured in the liver, and that it ebbs and flows, to and fro, in two separate sets of vessels. But he was ready with mountains of evidence from his work with animals. In fact, he had already tested the main conclusions of De Motu Cordis 12 years earlier, in 1616, during a London lecture designed to "test the water" – and he had indeed received criticism then, which only strengthened his resolve.

One of Harvey's key pieces of evidence was a series of simple calculations involving the quantity of blood. He estimated how much blood was ejected by a heartbeat, and multiplied this by the beat rate. Since the blood could not return to the heart because of the valve system, it must be freshly and continuously made. Harvey's measurements were not particularly accurate, but they suggested that more than 240kg (540lb) of blood were pumped by the heart each hour – which is about three times the entire body's weight. He concluded that far more blood comes out of the heart than could be supplied by digested food. Simple observation supported this reasoning. For instance, if a single artery is cut, blood soon drains from the whole body, and is not replenished. Harvey summarized: "...The blood is driven into a round by a circular motion... it moves perpetually". Vein valves were another key to Harvey's arguments. In a famous illustrated sequence in De Motu Cordis, a ligature (tight band) is tied around the upper arm. The arteries and veins are compressed, and, without a supply of fresh, warm, oxygenated blood, the lower arm becomes cooler and pallid. Next, the ligature is slackened slightly. This allows blood to flow to the lower arm through the arteries, which are cushioned in muscles deep below the skin, but prevents it from returning along the veins near the surface. The lower arm now becomes engorged and florid. Blood can be seen queuing in the veins below the ligature, and the valves appear as little lumps here and there. Massaging the blood in these veins towards the hand has little effect, since the one-way valves prevent its motion. But stroking it the other way helps the blood to head back up the arm to the heart.

Why did blood circulate? Harvey suggested that it might be to distribute heat and nourishment, which is correct, but he went little further. Another vital feature of the circulation eluded him: how did blood travel from the tiniest arteries into the minute veins, as part of its complete circulation? If Harvey had used a microscope, rather than the simple magnifier lens he relied on, he might have discovered the capillary network. Early microscopes (see pp.150–51) were available at the time, but they were rarely used by physicians. The discovery of capillaries was left to Marcello Malpighi (see pp.145–46) in about 1661, 33 years after *De Motu Cordis*, and four years after Harvey's death.

Acceptance of Harvey's ideas was far from immediate. Galen's supporters were numerous and vociferous, especially in continental Europe. Harvey's findings also went against the theory, practice, and popularity of blood-letting (see pp.132–33). As a sign of those times, Harvey's medical practice in London suffered considerably after publication of *De Motu Cordis*. But gradually, sense prevailed. Physicians and surgeons accepted Harvey's findings well within his lifetime. Medicine would never be the same again, and patients would be eternally grateful.

CURE FOR SCURVY
Harvey prepared Aqua Cochlear, or "scurvy grass water", for his patients at St Bartholemew's Hospital. It was based on the vitamin C-rich herb, cochlear, also known as scurvy grass.

Pag: 81.

Figura: 3.

Fig: 4.

DE MOTU CORDIS
These illustrations from Harvey's *De Motu Cordis* show how the blood in the veins flows towards the heart (left), rather than away from it, and that the direction of flow is maintained by valves, which appear as bumps under the skin (right).

The Microscope Revolution

GERMS (SUCH AS BACTERIA AND VIRUSES), germ cells (including eggs and sperm), tiny parasites (such as malaria's plasmodium), and the smallest blood vessels known as capillaries – all these are invisible to the naked eye, and were unknown before the invention of the light microscope in the late 16th century. This simple device revealed the world of the very small, enabling medical researchers and doctors to explore afresh the human body's anatomy, both in health and disease. It was developed around 1590–1610, probably first in the Netherlands, and thought to be by either father-and-son lens experts Hans and Zacharias Janssen, or by Hans Lippershey. Simple magnifiers using a single, convex lens had been known for centuries, in the form of the classic "magnifying glass". The new microscope, however, was compound, using two or more lenses carefully shaped and distanced to make small things look much bigger. An early and enthusiastic user was astronomer Galileo Galilei, who built his own improved versions and demonstrated them to eminent academics and royalty.

One of the earliest works celebrating the microscope and illustrating its potential was the impressive *Micrographia* (1665), by English scientist, inventor, naturalist, philosopher, and architect Robert Hooke. His work portrayed all manner of fascinating tiny objects, from insect bodies, eyes, and legs to bits of blossom, seeds, and other plant specimens. *Micrographia* was one of the first bestselling books on science, and in it Hooke first used the word "cells" to describe tiny, box-like

ROBERT HOOKE'S MICROSCOPE
This illustration of the compound microscope used by Robert Hooke shows the oil lamp he employed to shed light on the specimens he examined.

ANTONI VAN LEEUWENHOEK
Dutch merchant and naturalist Antoni
van Leeuwenhoek was the first scientist
to observe single-celled organisms.

compartments in plant specimens of
cork. He likened them to the rows of
similar-shaped spartan chambers
or rooms occupied by monks.
His term soon passed into
general usage for the smallest
living components of plant
and animal bodies.

Perhaps the greatest pioneer microscopist, however, was Dutch
draper and businessman Antoni van Leeuwenhoek of Delft. Familiar
with the magnifiers used to count the threads in woven textiles, he
became fascinated with the design and construction of lenses, and
devised a secret way of producing tiny glass globules that could
magnify dozens of times, and eventually over 200 times. These were
in effect very powerful single-lens magnifiers, rather than compound
microscopes. Van Leeuwenhoek continually experimented, improved
his specimen preparation and lighting, and produced more than 500
lenses for use in a variety of holders. From the 1670s, his observations
and illustrations were published by The Royal Society of London, and
he kept contributing to its journals right up until his death.

Van Leeuwenhoek gathered specimens widely and observed
astutely. In water from ponds he saw what he termed "animalcules" –
in modern terminology, single-celled microorganisms. Looking at the
human body, he found what we now call bacteria in the fluid taken
from his mouth: "In the said matter there were many very little living
animalcules, very prettily moving. The biggest... had a very strong
and swift motion, and shot through the water (or spittle) like a pike
through water. The second sort... spun round like a
top". He also described blood cells, sperm cells in seminal fluid
from dogs and men, and the banded effect in striated (striped)
skeletal muscle cells.

A contemporary of van Leeuwenhoek was Italian scientist,
physician, and anatomist Marcello Malpighi. Working mainly at Pisa
and Bologna, he too employed the microscope to study the natural

MAGNIFICATION OF ANTONI VAN LEEUWENHOEK'S MICROSCOPES	MAGNIFICATION OF MODERN MICROSCOPES
275x	2000x

world and the human body. In the 1660s, he distinguished capillaries from surrounding tissues and saw tiny blobs moving through them, which he suggested were globules of fat. Capillaries were the "missing link" between small arteries and veins, whose existence had so perplexed William Harvey in his account of blood circulation (see pp.134–43). In the 1680s, with improved microscopes and better conditions for observation, Malpighi refined these ideas and described the beads as "red blood cells". His name lives on in several areas of microanatomy, such as the Malpighian layer at the base of the skin's outer layer (the epidermis), the Malpighian bodies (filtering units) in the kidney, and the Malpighian corpuscles (nodules of white blood cells) in the spleen.

Another pioneer microscopist, also Dutch like van Leeuwenhoek, was Jan Swammerdam. Reluctant to bend to his father's wishes and pursue a career in medicine, he became a leading entomologist (an expert on insects). His well-organized, systematic studies greatly advanced the understanding of the anatomy and life cycles of insects, especially how they change, or metamorphose (e.g. from caterpillar to chrysalis to butterfly). Swammerdam conceived many improved ways to preserve, prepare, and observe specimens under the microscope, which scientists would benefit from for two centuries.

In 1653, Italian philosopher-scientist Petrus Borellus published what may have been the first work on using microscopes for medical matters. Among some 100 procedures and observations, he described how to find and treat the tiniest of ingrowing eyelashes that produced otherwise puzzling inflammation and pain. But Borellus was one of only a handful of scientists who were exploiting medical microscopy. This was largely because physicians were conservative, and were worried about what the microscope might reveal. For instance, in

1761, Giovanni Morgagni, the foremost Italian anatomist of the day, published *De Sedibus et Causis Morborum per Anatomen Indagatis* (*The Seats and Causes of Diseases as Investigated by Anatomy*), in which he established the disciplines of pathology and morbid anatomy – the study of the body's structure and fabric as affected by disease. This was a century after Hooke and van Leeuwenhoek, yet this landmark work took little notice of microscopic anatomy.

Some 80 years later, Morgagni's opus was read in detail by German trainee physician and natural historian Rudolf Virchow, who was learning microscopy, among other things, at the Charité Teaching Hospital, Berlin. Virchow formed the opinion that the effects of disease should be visible not only to the naked eye, but also under the microscope. This was part of his great fascination with the cell as the basic building block of living tissues. He began to note the differences between cells in healthy and diseased specimens, such as the appearance of abnormal-looking white blood cells in various forms of leukaemia. For example, there could be an odd-shaped nucleus (control centre) in the cell, or suspicious granules, vacuoles, and other strange contents in the cytoplasm (the general bulk "jelly" of the cell), or a spiky, hairy, or crinkly cell membrane (outer skin). Such deformed cells might also react differently, compared with normal ones, to the stains or colouring substances used to highlight their different parts.

Virchow also read the works of French anatomist and surgeon Marie-François-Xavier Bichat, who first championed the concept of "living tissues" – layers, sheets, or membranes from which major body organs and parts were built. Today, a living tissue is regarded as a group of similar cells, such as bone cells, nerve cells, and so on. Bichat had little time for the latest compound microscopes and was wary of the concept of the cell. He trusted only his own eyes – aided by a simple magnifying lens, yet he managed to differentiate 21 different kinds of tissue, including muscle, skin, nerve and connective tissues, and grouped them into three main classes: fibrous, mucous, and serous (fluids). Bichat also turned to detailed autopsy as the route to discover the causes and consequences of disease. He carried out hundreds of autopsies, noting and describing the physical alterations in different tissues affected by morbid conditions. He used similar techniques to examine the effects of treatments such as drugs and surgery. Bichat came to the conclusion that abnormal changes in tissues, rather than changes in larger parts or whole organs, were the basis of disease.

Virchow appreciated Morgagni's contributions and the thrust of Bichat's approach. He then took Bichat's tissue-based ideas and applied them to the cellular level. Today, Virchow is famed as the author of *Die Cellularpathologie in Ihrer Begründung auf Physiologische und Pathologische Gewebelehre*, usually known in English as *Cellular Pathology*, and is viewed as the founder of this most essential and fundamental branch of medicine. Microscopic examination of tissues and cells, known as histology and cytology respectively, can reveal whether they are healthy or abnormal, and are invaluable tools that are widely used in modern medicine in the diagnosis of many diseases – for example, in the diagnosis of cancer, by identifying pre-cancerous changes in cells.

Virchow regarded cellular changes as the basis of many, if not most, diseases. Indeed, he went much further, decreeing in 1858 that cells, besides being the fundamental units of life, were the only way that life maintained itself. His celebrated pronouncement "*Omnis cellula e cellula*" is roughly translated from Latin as "All cells come from other cells". This statement was the third basic tenet of the cell theory that underpins all of the modern life sciences, including medicine. Previously, German biological researcher and embryologist Theodor Schwann, in correspondence with plant expert Matthias Schleiden, had formulated the first and second parts of classical cell theory: all living things are composed of one or more cells, and the cell is the basic unit of life in all living things. Even lifeless body parts such as hair and fingernails derive from once-living cells in the form of the tough protein they produce, called keratin.

However, Schwann and Schleiden's theories perpetuated the ancient idea of "spontaneous generation", whereby living cells or organisms can arise anew from non-living ingredients. In about 1855, spontaneous generation was denied by Polish-German physiologist Robert Remak, who declared that cells can only arise from the division of other cells – around the same time that Virchow first published a similar idea. Three years later, Virchow restated this view, and he is sometimes accused of taking credit for it without sufficiently acknowledging Remak's contribution. Later investigations by Louis Pasteur (see pp.196–203) and others consigned the idea of spontaneous generation as a medical phenomenon to history (conversely, modern evolutionary theory suggests that at some stage, probably more than three billion years ago here on Earth, life did indeed begin from a complex mix of non-living ingredients).

Through the groundbreaking work of early microbiologists, and the endeavours of Virchow and others, the light microscope is now an essential tool in medicine. However, light rays are too big or "wavy" to enlarge the view more than about 2,000 times clearly – to achieve greater magnification than this with clarity, an electron microscope is needed. Developed in the 1930s, the electron microscope has extended magnifying power to up to two million times, and enables the user to peer inside cells, to see the structure of their nuclei, membranes, "power-house" mitochondria, and other tiny parts known as organelles. Research into this realm of "ultrastructure" has yielded many breakthroughs in biological and medical knowledge, from how nerve signals travel and how drugs get into cells, to visualizing the changes in genetic material that signal inherited conditions, and how the most dangerous viruses multiply and wreak their destruction.

RUDOLF VIRCHOW OBSERVES
Pathologist and anthropologist Rudolf Virchow (centre, in black, seated) observes a cerebral operation in the Sorbonne, Paris, in 1900. Virchow himself never performed an operation.

Early Microscopes

The first microscopes were made in the early 17th century, in the Netherlands. Some were simple microscopes with a single lens, while more complex models with several lenses were known as compound microscopes. As lens-making techniques, precise focusing mechanisms, and clear illumination developed, scientists were able to use microscopes to see single-celled organisms for the first time, and to understand complex organic structures such as plant cells.

CAMPANI MICROSCOPE (c.1670–90)
Italian optical craftsman Giuseppe Campani was probably the first person to make a compound microscope with a screw-thread for more precise focusing.

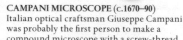

LEEUWENHOEK MICROSCOPE (1670)
Dutch scientist Antoni van Leeuwenhoek (see p.145) made simple microscopes with a tiny lens between brass plates, and a pin to hold the specimen. Some of his lenses achieved a huge magnification of x275.

HOOKE MICROSCOPE (1665)
British scientist Robert Hooke (see p.144) used this compound microscope to examine fleas and cork cells, publishing illustrations in his book, *Micrographia* (1665), a scientific bestseller.

CUNO HAND MICROSCOPE (c.1700)
This microscope, by Cuno of Augsburg, has two metal plates – one holding the lens, the other the specimen. A screw controls focus by adjusting the distance between the plates.

CULPEPER COMPOUND MODEL (1738)
British instrument-maker Edward Culpeper's
microscope used a concave mirror to
illuminate samples. With interchangeable
lenses, it could magnify up to x200.

NACHET COMPOUND MODEL (c.1860)
French scientist Louis Pasteur (see pp.196–
203) used this microscope to investigate the
diseases of silkworms. It has precision metal
construction, for perfect focusing.

Conquering the Dreaded Pox

THE BODY'S IMMUNE SYSTEM provides self-defence against diseases of many kinds. Chief among these are infestations and infections of tiny invaders such as minuscule worms and flukes, fungi and yeasts, single-celled protozoal parasites, even smaller bacteria, and tiniest of all, viruses. The details of how immunity works are fiendishly complex and still being unravelled. Yet well before this complexity was even guessed at, medical workers found ways of encouraging the body to build immunity against infections without actually suffering from them. Along with antibiotics and antiseptic surgery, the practise of vaccination is high on the list of medicine's all-time life-savers and is often quoted as the most effective.

In 1798, English country doctor Edward Jenner privately published *An Enquiry Into the Causes and Effects of the Variolae Vaccinae, a Disease Discovered in some of the Western Counties of England, Particularly Gloucestershire, and Known by the Name of the Cow Pox*. It described his treatment of 23 patients with the aim of protecting them against one of the greatest global infectious diseases, smallpox – then known by several names, including "variola" (from the Latin word for "pimples"), which is now the scientific name for the virus germ that causes the disease.

Jenner's slim volume established scientific evidence for what we now call vaccination: introducing a substance into the body that causes or increases immunity against a disease. Our term "vaccine" was first used somewhat later, by Louis Pasteur (see pp.196–203). It comes from the Latin word *vacca*, meaning "cow", and honours Jenner's use of the

EARLY VACCINATOR
The first vaccinators were simple devices, such as this wood-and-ivory model. The spike was dipped into the vaccine and then pressed into the arm of the patient.

infection known as cowpox to
protect humans against smallpox —
cowpox being similar to smallpox,
though rarely disfiguring, let alone
fatal, in humans.

Today, the term "vaccine" applies to
almost any substance that initiates or
bolsters immunity. The often-misused
term "inoculation" refers to administering,
implanting, introducing, or grafting a substance that will spread,
grow, multiply, or be similarly active in the body. Inoculating a
vaccine is called vaccination. Depending on the particular vaccine, it
may be inoculated by injection, by mouth (orally), jabbed through
the skin, or introduced by some other route. The whole process of
introducing a substance into the body to stimulate or boost the body's
immune system is known as immunization.

In his youth, Jenner had himself been inoculated against
smallpox. This process, then called "variolation", was well known,
having been brought to Britain from Constantinople (now Istanbul)
in the 1720s by Lady Mary Wortley Montagu, the wife of the British
Ambassador to the Ottoman Empire. She had suffered and been
scarred by smallpox a few years earlier, and her brother had previously
died from the infection. In Constantinople, she saw fluid being taken
from the blisters (or pus from the sores) of a person with a mild
case of smallpox, and then slipped into an incision or punctured
into the skin of the recipient. Another method was to jab or blow
dried, powdered smallpox blister scabs into the nose. Thereafter, the
recipient had a hugely improved chance of resisting the full force of
the smallpox infection. Overall, depending on the methods and
circumstances, variolation was estimated to reduce the death rate
from smallpox from as high as one-in-three, to one in 20 or below.

Variolation techniques had been known for many centuries, and
probably originated farther east, in India and China. Various claims
of an Indian origin go back more than 3,000 years to the Vedas

EARLY CHINESE INOCULATION
It is thought that by 1000, Chinese physicians were
inoculating against smallpox by scratching matter
from the sores of smallpox sufferers (above) and
inserting it into the arms of healthy people.

(ancient Indian texts), while Ayurvedic records describe the healer
Madhav and other wandering "variolators" during the 7th and 8th
centuries (see p.80). More concrete evidence comes from 16th-century
China, where the procedure became something of a traditional ritual,
with ornate pipes for puffing the material up into the nose. Further
versions of variolation were practised in the Middle East and Africa
during the 17th century. Some involved inoculating dried scab
material from smallpox sufferers, others pus and fluid from their
blisters and sores. The inoculation route into the recipient was
generally through cuts or scrapes in the skin of the arm. These
methods spread as far west and north as Turkey.

In 1701, Venetian doctor Giacomo (Jacob) Pylarini described
variolation in Constantinople in an article for the Royal Society. In
the 1710s, also in Constantinople, Greek physician Emmanuel Timoni
was seconded to the British Embassy. A member of the Royal Society,
he too became interested in the process of variolation and wrote a
treatise on the topic, which was published by the Royal Society in
1714. It set in train a series of reports by other widely travelled doctors.

It was a few years later, in around 1716–18, that Lady Montagu
observed variolation, again in Constantinople, during her husband's
time as ambassador there. She appreciated its effects and had it
applied to her own son before returning to London. In 1721,
another smallpox epidemic threatened England, and Lady Mary
persuaded her husband (Lord Montagu), the Princess of Wales, and

royal doctor Hans Sloane to support the idea of variolation. She also agreed to her daughter being treated. At the same time, variolation was tested on six London prisoners who had received the death penalty, and according to some accounts, on some orphan children too. When these people were later exposed to smallpox, none of them caught the disease. The prisoners were granted their freedom, and variolation caught on. Royalty took it up, and it spread through the fashionable English populace and gradually to continental Europe.

Variolation was also tried in Boston, America, which had a smallpox epidemic in 1721–22. Puritan minister and activist Cotton Mather had heard about the procedure from an African slave named Onesimus. He may also have read Timoni's article on variolation. To try and save residents from death and suffering – and to avoid the ensuing disruption to business and trade – he petitioned local physicians to carry out variolation. Doctor Zabdiel Boylston responded by testing the technique on his own son and two slaves, who survived. He then inoculated nearly 250 more people. Records show about six or seven of these succumbed to smallpox – a death rate of 2–3 per cent. In the general Boston population, nearly 6,000 people contracted the infection, of which some 850 died – a death rate of almost 15 per cent.

Such statistics reflected the positive results of variolation, but it was still a risky procedure. The recipient could die from the procedure itself, or not receive protection and die after encountering smallpox. Also, the variolated patient carried "live" smallpox germs and so was a source of infection, and was best kept away from others for two weeks. In 1783, faith in variolation was shaken when King George III's four-year-old son Octavius died after undergoing the process.

Despite such concerns, however, variolation was considered a great success. Jenner himself had survived the process when he was young, although it had made him very ill. Intrigued by the procedure, he also mused on the traditional country conviction that milkmaids who contracted a much milder form of the disease, called cowpox, rarely caught smallpox. Cowpox produced sores on a cow's udders and also on the milkmaid's skin, but it had no lasting effects. Jenner resolved to investigate further by embarking on a series of carefully calculated medical experiments that combined variolation and smallpox with cowpox.

Jenner was not the first to have such thoughts. More than 20 years previously, in 1774, Benjamin Jesty, a farmer from Dorset, had carried out what Jenner was now planning to do. Jesty saw how his milkmaids who had contracted cowpox were able to care for smallpox victims without themselves being affected. When a cowpox outbreak came to his area, Jesty attended infected cows in secret with his wife and sons, whom he inoculated with material from the cowpox sores, using a darning needle. The sons showed little reaction, but when his wife fell ill, the story became public knowledge. Even though Mrs Jesty recovered, Mr Jesty was ridiculed. Not only had the farmer deliberately tried to make his family ill, it was said, the cowpox material could have wreaked havoc on their bodies – and even given them horns.

The Jesty family eventually moved away and settled in Worth Matravers, Dorset. But after Jenner's success, Jesty's story prompted support and a campaign for his official recognition from the authority of the time, The Original Vaccine Pock Institute. In 1805, the Institute partially agreed. However, Jesty's lack of medical or other standing could not threaten Jenner, who was by now a lauded celebrity. Jesty's gravestone at Worth Matravers states: "… Particularly noted for having been the first Person (known) that Introduced the Cow Pox by Inoculation…"

In the two decades before Jenner's work, others besides Jesty had reported on the ability of cowpox infection to protect against smallpox. These included Doctor John Fewster and Doctor Rolph, both from Gloucestershire. Fewster's 1765 article "Cow Pox and its Ability to Prevent Smallpox" was presented to the Medical Society of London, but was thereafter sidelined. Also espousing the procedure around Europe were government official Jobst Bose of Göttingen, Germany, in 1769; a Frau Sevel in Germany, in 1772; Peter Plett, a teacher in Denmark, in 1791; and Herr Jensen, a farmer from Holstein, Germany, also in 1791. But none of these individuals had Jenner's authority, his number of case histories, or his profile in the scientific community.

The most celebrated of the 23 case histories described by Jenner in his 1798 *Enquiry* had occurred two years earlier. Of Case Number 17, he wrote: "The more accurately to observe the progress of the infection, I selected a healthy boy, about eight years old, for the purpose of inoculation for the Cow Pox. The matter was taken from a sore on the hand of a dairymaid, who was infected by her master's cows, and it was inserted, on the 14th of May, 1796, into the arm of the boy by means of two superficial incisions, barely penetrating the cutis [outer skin layer], each about half an inch long". The boy's name was James Phipps, and he was the son of Jenner's gardener; the milkmaid was Sarah Nelmes, herself the subject of Jenner's Case Number 16. Like the previous cases, Sarah had caught cowpox naturally, and not suffered from smallpox. James, however, had not caught the disease naturally. Jenner had given it to him on purpose — and the inoculation

SAVING LIVES
Edward Jenner vaccinates a child — one of the millions who would be saved by his work. Thanks to his pioneering vaccine, the science of immunology was born.

material was not from a cow, but from a human who had recovered from cowpox. About a week later, James suffered some minor swelling, fever, and chills, but then recovered. Six weeks after that, Jenner gave James a deliberate dose of smallpox, inserting the material fresh from a sufferer's pustule into several incisions on the boy's arms. With relief, Jenner recorded: "No disease followed".

As usual, there was initial opposition to Jenner's conclusions, especially from quarters of the generally conservative medical profession. Echoing Benjamin Jesty 25 years earlier, but on a national scale, popular mockery led to newspaper cartoons of vaccinated people mooing in Jenner's defence and morphing into cows (or, perhaps worse, humble milkmaids). But after the hit-and-miss history of variolation, the efficacy of the new procedure was soon recognized. Within three years, Jenner's work progressed into mainstream medicine and soon became government public health policy. With official organizations set up, researchers applied the idea of vaccination to other infections.

By 1840, the original variolation method using live smallpox material from human sufferers had been prohibited in England. Yet no one, including Jenner, his supporters, and his immediate successors, had any real idea how the whole thing worked. The variola virus was only discovered and characterized in the late 19th and early 20th centuries. More recently, some researchers have suggested that the vaccine material developed from Jenner's pioneering techniques may not have involved cowpox at all, but a related virus more similar to the smallpox one. It could be that vaccinators infected cows not with cowpox, but with human smallpox, leading to a variant virus that was similar to both but actually neither. Even horses and another variant, horsepox, have been implicated. Sadly no 19th-century vaccine samples survive for analysis.

Was Jenner justified in his work? Carrying out hopeful experiments on human subjects, without what we today would regard as official permission, risk analysis, and proper safeguards would now be regarded as unethical and unprofessional. Especially controversial was the use of James Phipps, a child. However, given the standards of the age, Jenner had already done a great deal of background work and completed similar trials on adults. He was confident of success, and saw the immense benefits to mankind. Giving James cowpox was not a great risk since it was a mild disease, although admittedly, Phipps may never have caught it naturally. Inoculating him with live smallpox material involved more serious hazards. Yet this was basically the procedure of variolation, which many people accepted because it provided an increased chance of

YEAR OF THE LAST KNOWN CASE OF SMALLPOX

1978

surviving smallpox when, rather than if, they were exposed to the disease. Also, from Jenner's accumulating evidence of previous case histories, the odds were that Phipps would have only a small reaction to the deliberately introduced smallpox, and then be resistant – immune – for many years after. In the event, Phipps had a possible minor reaction one week later, described by Jenner: "He complained of uneasiness in the axilla [armpit]... He became a little chilly, lost his appetite, and had a slight headache... He spent the night with some degree of restlessness, but on the day following he was perfectly well". Years later, as a thank-you for his involvement, Jenner provided the adult, newlywed Phipps with a house in their local village of Berkeley.

The move from variolation to vaccination was not only a great leap forward in the long, complex battle against smallpox, it was the start of research into vaccines against many other infections, which have since saved millions of lives (see pp.286–95). Jenner's legacy continued to grow after his death, and it came to fruition in 1980, when the World Health Organization announced the global eradication of "the smallpox".

Eradicating Smallpox

Smallpox was a deadly virus that ravaged populations throughout the world – it is also the only human disease to have been eradicated. Caused by the *Variola* virus, it attacked the small blood vessels of the skin, mouth, and throat, giving victims widespread blisters filled with fluid. Around a third of sufferers died; survivors were left with scars and sometimes went blind. Inoculation (see pp.292–93) could create immunity, but also risked causing full infection. Vaccination using the related disease cowpox was safer, and eventually led to the eradication of smallpox.

THE CHINESE GOD OF SMALLPOX

1796 British doctor Edward Jenner uses pus from the **cowpox blisters** of a dairymaid for his first successful smallpox vaccination on a boy called James Phipps.

1718 Lady Mary Wortley Montagu, living in Turkey, has her son **inoculated** against smallpox.

1520 Spanish **conquistadors** bring smallpox to the Americas.

1721 Physician Zabdiel Boylston brings inoculation to North America during a smallpox **epidemic** in Boston.

1803 The **Spanish colonies** in the New World receive vaccine from Spain.

1800 Harvard professor Benjamin Waterhouse carries out the **first vaccinations** in the US.

1661 Chinese physicians practise **variolation** by blowing powdered smallpox scabs up patients' noses.

1721 Lady Montagu brings inoculation to the UK and campaigns for it to be **widely adopted**.

1768 Physician Thomas Dimsdale successfully inoculates **Catherine the Great** of Russia.

1802 Massachusetts becomes the **first US state** to endorse smallpox vaccination.

TOTAL ESTIMATED NUMBER OF DEATHS WORLDWIDE FROM SMALLPOX BY THE LATE 20TH CENTURY

300 MILLION

c.1900 Material from vaccinated calves is used for human vaccination, reducing the chance of **accidentally transmitting** other diseases.

1967 The entire population of Costa Rica is inoculated against **smallpox, measles, and polio** in a campaign carried out by the government and US medical volunteers.

1820 Deaths from smallpox in London plummet to **fewer than half** the rate in the years before vaccination.

1918 The development of **freeze-dried vaccine** helps to control smallpox in tropical countries.

1949 The **last cases** of smallpox in the US are recorded, including one fatality.

1980 The World Health Assembly declares the world **free of smallpox** and in 1986 ceases vaccination.

1853 In the UK, vaccination becomes **mandatory** in the first three months of a child's life.

1864 French doctors experiment with material from vaccinated **livestock**.

1967 The **World Health Organization** launches its Intensified Smallpox Eradication Programme.

Medicine in the Industrial Age

1820–1920

Medicine gained momentum during the 19th century. The Industrial Revolution gathered pace in grimy cities, where overcrowding, malnutrition, and poor sanitation encouraged contagious diseases. English doctor John Snow's work on cholera in the 1850s was a landmark for epidemiology, although it was recognized at the time only with reluctance.

Other scientific disciplines fed into medicine. Taking cues from chemistry, US physicians in the 1840s investigated substances to make patients insensible to pain during operations. Two decades later in Scotland, surgeon Joseph Lister conducted research into chemicals for their infection-preventing powers. Within 40 years, these two operative advances, anaesthesia and antisepsis, had made surgery immeasurably safer. Meanwhile, in France, Louis Pasteur harnessed microbiology to medicine in a string of successes, including pasteurization of milk and wine, and vaccines for several animal diseases as well as for rabies in humans. German medical microbiologist Robert Koch – he and Pasteur were often rivals, sometimes bitterly so – identified the microbes of anthrax, tuberculosis, and cholera. At last, the coffins of the obsolete ideas miasmas and spontaneous generation were nailed firmly shut and replaced by the germ theory of disease.

The 19th century saw other welcome areas of progress. Elizabeth Blackwell in the US and Elizabeth Garrett Anderson in the UK campaigned successfully for women to receive equality in medical training and qualifications. They both set up medical schools for women. Although English nurse Florence Nightingale's feats in the Crimea in the 1850s have recently been debated, her subsequent founding of the modern nursing profession has not. And as the 19th century ended, Austrian neurologist Sigmund Freud's psychiatric approaches stimulated debates that continue today.

Women in Medicine

WOMEN HAVE ALWAYS PLAYED A VITAL ROLE in providing medical care – particularly as nurses (see pp.188–93), midwives (see pp.214–21), and herbalists – but throughout history, men have dominated the medical profession. In Renaissance Europe, women were effectively prevented from becoming doctors when a university qualification became a requirement – something women couldn't receive since they were already barred from universities. It was only in the 1900s that women won the right to study and practise medicine, and only later in the 20th century that they began to be treated on equal terms with men.

One of the first female physicians mentioned by name was Merit-Ptah, some 4,700 years ago, around the time of Ancient Egypt's physician-deity Imhotep (see pp.22–27). There are few clues to her abilities, save that her High Priest son placed the inscription "Chief Physician" on her tomb near Saqqara. During Ancient Egypt's lengthy history – it lasted longer than the millennia from its demise to today – the authority of women in medicine waxed and waned. Women mostly undertook caring roles, although 3,500 years ago, female students could attend medical school at Heliopolis. In Ancient Greece, more than 2,600 years ago, Homer's *Iliad* mentions Agamede, daughter of Augeas, King of the Epeians: "Fair-haired Agamede who knew of all the medicines that are grown in the broad earth". As in Egypt, a woman's place in medicine varied with time and place, since cities independently made their own rules through the centuries. Metrodora's *On the Diseases and Cures of Women*, written around 2,300 years ago, is one of the first medical books written by a woman. Metrodora covered gynaecology with a combination of personal experience and Hippocratic knowledge (see pp.30–39). Greek female physicians were generally limited to treating female conditions – a practice that Agnodice tried to avoid by assuming a male disguise (see p.214). This ruse has cropped up now and again throughout history. As late as 1865, the autopsy of British Army surgeon Dr James Barry showed that "he" – a medical graduate from Edinburgh, who had served in India, South Africa, the Mediterranean, and the Caribbean, become Inspector General of military hospitals, and enjoyed more than 40 years promoting diet, hygiene, and public health – was in fact a woman.

In the Islamic world, female healers are cited treating female conditions as early as the 8th century, and by the 15th century, female surgeons are depicted in the surgical manual *Cerrahiyyetu'l-Haniyye* (*Imperial Surgery*), produced by Sabuncuoglu Serefeddin. In the Germanic regions, the 12th-century abbess, poet, composer, and naturalist Hildegard of Bingen was one of the great physicians of her day. Her work *Liber Simplicis Medicinae* (*Book of Simple Medicine*), later called *Physica*, extols the medicinal values of hundreds of herbs, trees, animal parts, and minerals. Her *Liber Compositae Medicinae* (*Book of Composite Medicines*), which became *Causae et Curae* (*Causes and Cures*), also compiled in the 1150s, discusses the symptoms and treatments of physical and mental diseases holistically – as an interplay of body and soul. During a fever of humoral imbalance (see pp.106–107), for instance: "... the soul lies depressed in the body and waits... So it continues until the seventh day because it cannot yet free itself from its foul humours... However, if it notices that the intensity of these humours, through the grace of God, is beginning to recede somewhat... It gathers its forces again and by sweating it drives these foul humours out of its body".

Another great name of the time is Trotula di Ruggicro of Salerno, who lived during the latter half of the 11th century, although her personal life is shadowy and opinions vary on whether she was real or mythical. Salerno in southwest Italy boasted Europe's first generally recognized school of medicine (see pp.108–15), and one of its many innovations was allowing women to qualify as physicians – at the time, women were generally prohibited not just from formal medical training, but from most higher education. Trotula's name became attached to many publications that were a mainstay of medicine for several centuries; collectively known

HILDEGARDE OF BINGEN
Twelfth-century composer, philosopher, and Benedictine abbess Hildegarde of Bingen was one of the great physicians of her day.

as "The Trotula", these included *Diseases of Women, Treatments for Women,* and *Women's Cosmetics.* The style of the texts is direct and practical, and few references are made to the occult. The texts recommend diagnosing ailments by asking the patient questions and noting pulse rate, breathing, skin appearance, and urine analysis — all of which was unusual for the time. Remedies of herbs and animal parts are offered, and advice is given on rest, stress, cleanliness, exercise, diet — and how to disguise freckles. If Trotula was real, then she was a pioneer in gynaecology, obstetrics, and women's health. The texts cover feminine hygiene, menstruation, fertility, conception, pregnancy, and childbirth. Among her more radical ideas was that failure to conceive could be the fault of the man. She also advocated pain relief for childbirth — against the prevailing Christian view that women should endure the pain because of Eve's sinful behaviour in the Garden of Eden.

SALERNO MEDICAL SCHOOL
Duke Robert II of Normandy is received by a female doctor at the Salerno Medical School in the 11th century.

Sadly, Salerno's inclusive tradition did not persist, and a trend for barring women swept across Europe. In 1220, the bar was enforced at Paris University, and in 1390, women were effectively excluded from medical schools in London. There were a few exceptions – in 1390, Dorotea Bocchi succeeded her father to begin a 40-year stint as Professor of

RUSSIA HAD MORE WOMEN DOCTORS IN 1914 THAN ALL OF WESTERN EUROPE COMBINED:

1,600

Medicine and Philosophy at the University of Bologna – but by the 16th century, the bar was in place at most European universities. In 1732, Laura Bassi, the daughter of a well-connected lawyer, became Professor of Anatomy aged just 21 years, again at Bologna – and in 1755, Anna Manzolini succeeded her husband in the same position.

Bassi's achievement made a great impression on one Dorothea Erxleben of Quedlinburg, Prussia. When she was young, Erxleben decided to follow her father's profession and study medicine. Her father, who had a reputation for rebelliousness, even petitioned Frederick the Great to allow her to pursue her studies, and the Prussian king conceded. Erxleben wrote *Inquiry into the Causes Preventing the Female Sex from Studying*, and in 1754, graduated in medicine from the University of Halle as Prussia's first qualified female physician. Again, this was an isolated case; it was not until 1901 that another woman qualifed as a doctor at Halle.

In 1847, Elizabeth Blackwell was accepted as a student at Geneva Medical College, New York State, USA, having applied to many other medical schools to no avail. The college authorities were said to have shied away from making a decision about her request and offered it to a vote by the students – who thought it was a hoax, and gave a unanimous "yes".

Born in Bristol, England, Blackwell emigrated with her family to New York in 1830 and moved to Cincinnati eight years later. The family's sugar business involved a great deal of slave labour, but young Blackwell's instincts were for social reform, the abolition of slavery, and education for the poor and disadvantaged – especially women. A medical career would suit such ambitions, so Blackwell worked as a teacher to raise funds while studying medicine in her spare time.

At Geneva, Blackwell graduated in 1849 with a medical degree – the first awarded to a woman in the USA. However, hospital employment was hard to find, so she went to London, and then to Paris, where she found work in a maternity hospital. Her obstetric skills received great praise, and she moved to St Bartholomew's Hospital, London. However, the British attitude towards women doctors was even more intransigent, and by 1851, Blackwell was back in New York, where she set up a medical practice, and then a dispensary that provided free medications and treatments for poor women and children. In 1857, with her supportive sister Emily and like-minded reformer and Cleveland Medical College graduate Maria Zakrzewska, she opened the New York Infirmary for Indigent Women and Children. This was so successful that in a year it needed bigger premises, eventually becoming what is now the New York University Downtown Hospital.

The movement started by Blackwell gathered pace, and soon medical schools for women were opening in Boston, Philadelphia, and New York. Then, in 1869, Blackwell left the US to return to England, where she was instrumental in founding the London School of Medicine for Women in 1874, along with Sophia Jex-Blake and Elizabeth Garrett Anderson. Jex-Blake was one the first women doctors in Britain, and she went on to establish the Edinburgh School of Medicine for Women in 1886. Elizabeth Garrett Anderson had met Blackwell in 1859, and been immediately inspired to pursue a career in medicine. She started as a nurse at London's Middlesex Hospital in 1860, and with her family's financial and moral backing, she had private lessons in related fields such as anatomy, physiology, and materia medica (medicines), and attended chemistry lectures. The following year, she graduated in materia medica and chemistry, and in 1862, she enrolled with the Society of Apothecaries, again engaging private tuition. Three years later, the Society approved her licence for medical practice – the first for a British woman – although it too then changed its rules and banned the admission of women.

ELIZABETH BLACKWELL
The first woman to receive a medical degree in the USA, Elizabeth Blackwell founded the New York Infirmary for Indigent Women and Children.

ELIZABETH GARRETT ANDERSON
English feminist Elizabeth Garrett Anderson passes
her examination to obtain an MD from the University
of Paris in 1870.

Women were still being treated unequally in hospitals, so like Blackwell, Garrett Anderson opened a private practice, and in 1866 founded the St Mary's Dispensary for Women and Children. In 1872, the dispensary gained in-patient beds and became the New Hospital for Women – renamed the Elizabeth Garrett Anderson Hospital in 1918. Garrett then co-founded the London School of Medicine for Women, and became the first female member of the British Medical Association in 1873. From 1883 to her retirement in 1902, she was the first female dean of the London School of Medicine for Women, and for many years she strenuously campaigned for the suffragette movement.

In 1876, British Parliament at last approved a bill allowing women to enter the medical profession fully. Other nations did the same. In 1875, Madeleine Brès became the first woman to receive a French medical licence, and in 1900, Japanese physician and women's rights campaigner Yoshioka Yayoi founded Tokyo Women's Medical University. Two years later, the Hackett Medical College for Women opened in Guangzhou, China. Finally, women had opportunities – but it was well into the 20th century before anything like equality between the sexes was established.

NURSES AND MIDWIVES
A group of trainee nurses and midwives pose for the camera at a training college in London in 1908. In Britain, women were finally allowed into the medical profession in 1876, following the tireless campaigns of Elizabeth Blackwell and others.

Anaesthesia

TODAY, NO PERSON OF SOUND MIND would choose to be operated on in filthy, germ-ridden conditions, and without pain relief. But before the mid-19th century, which heralded the monumental advances of anaesthesia and germ-killing antiseptics (see pp.206–13), this was the reality faced by patients. General anaesthesia renders the body temporarily unconscious and unresponsive to stimuli, even great pain; it allows the surgeon to work on the quietened body without the patient screaming and writhing in agony. The first successful public medical demonstration of anaesthesia, in which dentist William Morton used the gas ether, occurred on 16 October 1846. This date marks the era of modern anaesthesia, and is celebrated each year as World Anaesthesia Day. But, like most other medical practices, anaesthesia has a long and colourful history.

The first anaesthetic of sorts was stumbled upon 6,000 years ago by winemakers of Eastern Europe and West Asia. Doubtless enjoying the fruits of their labours, they found that overindulgence resulted in blunted sensibilities, and that alcohol masked stimuli such as pain. Another ancient option was opium, prepared from the sap of the opium poppy. Its mind-altering, sleep-inducing properties were mentioned on tablets from Ancient Sumer, and opium became a part of life in many Asian cultures. From the 16th century, opium became popular in Europe, too. Luminaries such as Paracelsus (see pp.110–15) and, in the 17th century, Thomas Sydenham, combined opium, alcohol, and other ingredients to produce laudanum. Patent medicines based on laudanum achieved a degree of analgesia (pain relief) and anaesthesia, along with other consequences – notably, addiction.

Other plants long used for their narcotic qualities – having a stupefying effect, reducing pain, and causing loss of consciousness – include cannabis, henbane and other nightshades, mandrake, bryony, hemlock, metel, thorn-apple, saw-wort, and wild or opium lettuce. In the Americas, coca plants were exploited for analgesia and other properties (see pp.82–87). Ancient Egyptian pain-relief practices were described in *Incantations of Analgesia* from the Ebers Papyrus (see pp.26–27), and Greek physician Dioscorides listed the properties of mandrake extracts. In 2nd-century China, physician-surgeon Hua Tuo performed operations using a mysterious substance

FIRST USE OF ETHER
Dentist William Morton's demonstrations of anaesthesia took
place here in the surgical amphitheatre at the Massachusetts
General Hospital. The amphitheatre is now known as the
Ether Dome and is a designated US historical landmark.

known as mafeisan. Much later, in the early 1800s, Japanese
physician-surgeon Hanaoka Seishu revisited the idea of mafeisan to
create tsusensan, using nightshade extracts. Hanaoka's patients
reportedly drank the tsusensan, sinking from consciousness before
the surgeon got to work.

In the Middle Ages, sense-nullifying potions multiplied unchecked.
Methods of administering included the "soporific sponge", where
preparations were soaked into rags or sponges and held over the
patient's nose and mouth. This way, if things went wrong, the sponge
could be rapidly removed. Arab physician Ibn Sina mentioned the
sponge in his epic *Al-Qanun fi al-Tibb* (see pp.100–105). The major flaw

in using such potions was the unpredictable quantity and quality of active compounds. With no way of securing a standard dose, the effects veered from virtually nothing to helpful anaesthesia or even sudden death. As a result, non-chemical methods of anaesthesia were attempted. These ranged from packing the body in ice or giving a knockout blow to the head to strangling the patient to the point of collapse. Taking a rather less violent approach, hypnotic anaesthesia and analgesia rose to prominence in Europe during the 19th century, thanks to Franz Anton Mesmer. Physicians reported some success with "mesmerism", but the procedures were far from reliable.

All these methods were overshadowed by the events of the 1840s, which changed the course of anaesthesia for good. A number of discoveries, beginning in 16th-century Europe, led up to this moment. In about 1540, German scientist Valerius Cordus discovered how to make ether from ethanol and sulphuric acid, and consequently, this volatile liquid became more available. Wandering physician Paracelsus, who had earlier created laudanum, noted that adding sweet oil of vitriol (ether) to food "... quiets all suffering without any harm and relieves all pain, and quenches all fevers, and prevents complications in all disease". But he made these observations in chickens. By the late 18th century, ether vapour was being inhaled for pain relief – and, later, at "ether frolics". At these gatherings, participants inhaled the gas and entertained the audience with their giddy, confused antics. Nitrous oxide was another fashionable inhaled drug of the time. This gaseous compound was first produced by English chemist-theologian Joseph Priestley in 1772, who was also an early pioneer of isolating oxygen. In 1800, another eminent English scientist, Humphry Davy, reported that inhaling nitrous oxide not only caused uncontrollable laughter – he dubbed it "laughing gas" – but also helped to deaden pain such as toothache. One day, he mused, might this gas be used to alleviate pain during surgical procedures?

In the US, ether frolics and laughing-gas parties became popular in the early 19th century, especially with students of chemistry and medicine. Some students noticed that painful injuries sustained during frolics seemed not to trouble the participants. Going on to qualify in medicine and dentistry, and remembering the apparently analgesic effects of the two gases, they reasoned that a larger dose could work as an anaesthetic during surgery. In January 1842, in

LAUGHING PARTY
Nitrous oxide was used as a recreational drug in the
19th century. Guests inhaled "laughing gas" at parties
and revelled in its euphoric, pain-numbing effects.

Burlington, Vermont, William Clarke allowed a dental patient to
inhale ether from a towel during a tooth extraction. Two months later,
in Jefferson, Georgia, another physician, Crawford Long, administered
ether by inhalation while removing a tumour from patient's neck. But
neither Clarke nor Long reported their actions at the time.

In December 1844, dentist Horace Wells watched a nitrous oxide
stage demonstration in Hartford, Connecticut. He was intrigued to
see that one of the participants was injured, yet seemed not to notice.
The next day, Wells asked another dentist, John Riggs, to remove
Wells's painful wisdom tooth, while the show's organizer, Gardner
Quincy Colton, put Wells "out" with nitrous oxide. The experiment
worked, and Wells started to use nitrous oxide on his patients. Keen
to prove his success, he arranged a public demonstration of his new
technique at Boston's Massachusetts General Hospital in January
1845. Sadly, the plan backfired, and the patient moved and groaned
during the operation. Wells was distraught: "The gas bag was by
mistake withdrawn much too soon… Several expressed their opinion
that it was a humbug affair". His reputation plummeted. Despite his
continued efforts to champion the method, he failed to regain his
credibility, and committed suicide three years later.

The following year, in September 1846, Wells's former partner and
fellow dentist William Morton — who had helped to arrange Wells's
failed demonstration — began using ether to anaesthetize his patients.

Encouraged by early successes, he too set up a staged demonstration at Massachusetts General Hospital. On 16 October, Morton administered ether to patient Edward Abbott while leading surgeon John Collins Warren partly removed a lower-jaw tumour. The ether worked – Abbott did not cry out or react to the surgery. Warren noted that the patient "... sank into a state of insensibility... did not experience any pain at the time, although aware that the operation was proceeding..." Medical observers were impressed, and news spread rapidly: the era of controlled general anaesthesia had begun.

Meanwhile, across the Atlantic, Europeans reacted to the news by creating their own anaesthetic. Their gas of choice was chloroform. In March 1847, French physiologist Marie-Jean-Pierre Flourens showed that animals that inhaled chloroform experienced a temporary state of insensibility. Eight months later, Scottish physician James Young Simpson introduced chloroform anaesthesia for humans, using it on women in childbirth. Simpson had first tried it himself with friends – a risky business that he was lucky to survive. Pioneer epidemiologist and anaesthetist John Snow (see pp.180–87) helped to determine safe amounts of chloroform, and later, ether, for varying levels of pain relief and unconsciousness. In 1853, under Snow's supervision, Queen Victoria of England took chloroform for the birth of her son Leopold, and, four years later, for her daughter Beatrice. She wrote: "Dr Snow gave that blessed chloroform and the effect was soothing, quieting, and delightful beyond measure". Encouraged by this royal endorsement, the general public rapidly took to the idea of anaesthesia.

Back in the US, ether anaesthesia faded as chloroform became the favoured drug. But chloroform had dangerous – sometimes fatal – side effects, so by the early 20th century, it was replaced. Intense research has since brought safer, more effective general anaesthetics, including ethyl chloride (1903), ethylene (in the 1920s), halothane

CLOVER AND CHLOROFORM
Joseph Thomas Clover invented an apparatus for administering quantities of chloroform through a face mask.

(1950s), methoxyflurane and enflurane (1960s), isoflurane (1970s), desflurane (1987), and sevoflurane (1990s). As the gases used for anaesthesia improved, so too did ways of administering them. In the wake of hit-and-miss sponges and towels came inhaler designs with flasks, tubes, and pumps. In the late 18th century, English doctor Thomas Beddoes devised several innovative designs, aided by steam-engine expert James Watt and Humphry Davy, of laughing gas fame. In the 1860s, wire face masks were developed, onto which an anaesthetic liquid was dripped, which then vapourized. Joseph Thomas Clover, an English physician, added regulators and bags to face masks. In 1917, Henry Boyle, at St Bartholomew's Hospital, London, introduced an "anaesthesia machine" – a wheeled trolley with gas supplies, pumps, reservoirs, valves, flow and pressure meters, masks, and other equipment needed to administer a continuous flow of anaesthetic gases and monitor the patient's condition. By this time, gas tubes were being placed into the trachea (windpipe), enabling more accurate control, and in the 1930s, the barbiturate sodium thiopental became the first general anaesthesic to be given intravenously (directly into the blood circulation).

As well as "knock-out" general anaesthesia, other types were developed. In the 1870s, the first local anaesthetic – one that removes sensation from a small area – was cocaine. This had been purified from coca plants in 1860 by Albert Niemann at the University of Göttingen, Germany. The subsequent discovery of cocaine's toxicity led to the introduction of safer "locals", such as procaine in 1905 and lidocaine in the 1940s. Regional anaesthesia numbs a larger or deeper part of the body, such as the abdomen. In the 1890s, German surgeon August Bier introduced spinal anaesthesia to remove sensation from the body below the injection site; and in the 1940s, an improved method, the epidural, entered mainstream practice (see pp.214–21).

Our expectations of medicine have been shaped by the advances of anaesthesia. Imagine a major operation – or even a visit to the dentist – without it. The quest for safer, more effective anaesthesia continues. Estimates vary widely, but with the latest care, the risk of death directly linked to general anaesthesia ranges from one in 7,000 to one in 200,000.

APPROXIMATE DEATH RATE AFTER OPERATIONS BEFORE THE 19TH CENTURY

80%

Early Anaesthetics

In the 1840s, the use of anaesthetics – substances that cause temporary loss of sensation or consciousness – developed rapidly. Patients inhaled substances such as chloroform, ether, or nitrous oxide in the form of a vapour, to render them insensible to pain. As the use of anaesthetics during surgery became more commonplace, both physicians and manufacturers devised improved equipment so that chemicals could be administered more safely.

SKINNER'S IMPROVED MASK FOR ANAESTHESIA (1862–1901)
Gynaecologist Thomas Skinner designed this mask to be portable and easy to use. Liquid chloroform or ether was dropped onto a flannel covering, which the patient held or clipped onto the nose before inhaling the anaesthetic.

MURPHY-TYPE CHLOROFORM INHALER (1850–1900)
This inhaler, which contained a sponge soaked in chloroform, was widely used as an anaesthesic for women in childbirth during the second half of the 19th century.

SNOW'S CHLOROFORM INHALER (c.1848)
James Simpson discovered chloroform was an anaesthetic in 1847 (see p.176). John Snow, Britain's first specialist anaesthetist, then devised this inhaler. The top of the tube was attached to a lead mask worn by the patient.

NITROUS OXIDE CYLINDER (1840–68)
In 1868, a way was found to turn nitrous oxide (also known as "laughing gas") into liquid form, so that it could be stored in cylinders. When it was sold in this form, the gas became popular as an anaesthetic, especially in dentistry.

MORGAN-TYPE ETHER INHALER (1881–90)
British surgeon John H. Morgan developed this inhaler. A sponge soaked with ether was placed in the narrow end of the cone and the patient inhaled through the wide end.

HYPODERMIC SYRINGE (1885–1900)
Hypodermic syringes such as this American model became increasingly popular in the 19th century, especially for dental anaesthesia.

HYPODERMIC SYRINGE SET (1885–1910)
Packed in a compact aluminium case, this syringe has two needles and a supply of anaesthetic tablets. The surgeon crushed these and diluted them before injection.

ETHER (1891–1930)
Using ether as an anaesthetic caught on quickly after it was demonstrated in public in the US in the 1840s. It was used in a wide range of procedures, from tooth extraction to removing tumours.

TRICHLOROETHYLENE (1940–60)
Marketed as Trilene, this volatile liquid chemical was inhaled through a mouthpiece to provide pain relief during labour. Although popular for decades, it was later replaced by nitrous oxide.

"ESO" CHLOROFORM APPARATUS (1945)
Designed to deliver chloroform vapour through a mouthpiece, this device was developed during World War II and made robust enough to withstand parachute drops and use on the battlefield.

John Snow and
Epidemiology

EPIDEMIOLOGY IS THE STUDY of the patterns, causes, and effects of disease (and health) in populations. It investigates and analyses the patterns of diseases, and looks for ways of controlling them and preventing their return. However, identifying diseases with any accuracy has only been possible since the discovery of bacteria in the late 19th century (see pp.222–27). Before that, it was widely thought that epidemics were caused by "noxious air", or "miasma" (see p.196–97), which was believed to emanate, among other things, from rotting organic matter. One of the first people to challenge this idea was English physician John Snow, who, during an outbreak of cholera in London, England, in 1854, suggested that there was a link between the disease and the water supply. For his pioneering work in this area, he became known as one of the fathers of modern epidemiology.

Cholera's long history is often confused by the fact that there are many conditions that have similar symptoms. Such symptoms are described in the *Susruta Samhita* of Ancient India (see pp.77–79), the Hippocratic Corpus (see pp.30–39) – in which *chole*, bile, is one of the four humours (see pp.106–107) – and the works of the 11th-century Arab physician Ibn Sina (see pp.100–105). Today, we know that cholera is caused by a bacterium called *Vibrio cholerae*, which affects the intestines, causing copious, watery vomiting and diarrhoea. This can so disturb the body's balance of fluids and salts that dehydration and even death may follow.

One group of cholera deaths in London in 1854 occurred in the west-central area of Soho. John Snow lived just a few streets away and knew the area well. He had also come across cholera during an epidemic in 1831–32, and recalled vividly the suffering it had caused in crowded, working-class mining areas. After his early upbringing in York, Snow had been apprenticed to Newcastle surgeon William Hardcastle. By 1930, Snow was in London, and in 1836 he set up a practice in Soho. The following year he went to Westminster Hospital, where he became a member of both the Royal College of Surgeons (in 1838) and the Royal College of Physicians (in 1850). In late 1846, Snow became interested in developments in anaesthesia taking place in the USA (see pp.172–79). He took up this new speciality, designed new equipment, and published *On the Inhalation of the Vapour of Ether* in 1847. By 1853, his reputation as an anaesthetist was so good that he was asked to administer chloroform to Queen Victoria during the birth of her son Leopold.

Snow maintained his interest in epidemic diseases, especially cholera, and deliberated on the patterns of outbreaks he had experienced in northeast England, London, and other regions, and on factors such as overcrowding, hygiene awareness, the quality of food and drink, and general living conditions. From Snow's point of view, the evidence pointed not to "miasmatic air", but to something in the water, partly because cholera's initial symptoms were in the gut, rather than in the lungs or the blood. In 1849, the same year of another cholera outbreak, Snow published *On the Mode of Communication of Cholera*, in which he argued that cholera "is contained in the evacuations, and communicates the disease by being swallowed", principally through drinking water – but his work was largely ignored by the medical establishment.

During the summer of 1854, cholera flared up around London. The Soho outbreak was sudden and vicious, starting on August 31. Three days later, more than 100 people were dead, and after two weeks, the toll had exceeded 500. Hoping to prove that contaminated water was the cause, Snow identified the dwellings where people had died, and investigated the local street pumps that raised water from the wells. Much of the mortality was clustered around Broad Street and on questioning local residents, with the help of the Reverend Henry Whitehead, Snow learned that the water from the Broad Street water pump had been cloudy and smelling odd for several days. To stop the spread of the disease, Snow proposed removing the pump handle to prevent people from using the water. This was done, and the cholera cases subsided immediately. Snow conceded that the number may already have been falling, if only because so many

JOHN SNOW
British physician John Snow correctly deduced that cholera was transmitted through fluids, including drinking water.

MICROCOSM dedicated to the London Water Companies

MONSTER SOUP commonly called **THAMES WATER**

"MONSTER SOUP"
This satirical engraving of 1828 shows a lady viewing
disease-riddled river water, but it was years before
people were convinced of the direct link between
polluted water and diseases such as cholera.

people had fled the area or died, but he plotted the locations of those
who had died on a map, visually demonstrating the link between the
deaths and the water pump.

Investigations eventually showed that the Broad Street well, which
was 9m (30ft) deep, was very close to an old cesspit, and that leakage
of contaminated excrement from this had polluted the water from
the well. It was also discovered that those who had survived the
disease had used water from their own wells – and that a family that
died some distance away had relied on water from the Broad Street
well. Nevertheless, once the outbreak had faded, very little changed
in Soho. The pump handle was replaced, and a Board of Health report
recorded: "In the general use of one particular well... at Broad
Street... having (it was imagined) its waters contaminated... After
careful inquiry we see no reason to adopt this belief". There were no
public health changes of note.

In 1855, Snow published a hugely expanded, revised edition of
On the Mode of Communication of Cholera, in which he noted: "Within 250
yards of the spot... there were upwards of 500 fatal attacks of cholera

in 10 days... I suspected some contamination of the water of the much-frequented street-pump in Broad Street". However, his ideas continued to be ignored, and cholera continued its deadly attacks. The miasma theory prevailed, and was only questioned after it was challenged by the experiments of Louis Pasteur in the 1860s (see pp.196–203). Unfortunately, Snow had already died by then, from a stroke at the age of 45, shortly before the publication of his book *On Chloroform and Other Anaesthetics and Their Action and Administration*.

Snow's work, then, did not overturn the standard view of his day – despite its proof of the contrary – nor did Snow "invent" epidemiology as such. Other pioneers included Dane Peter Anton Scleisner, who reduced the incidence of newborn babies in Iceland dying of tetanus by introducing hygiene measures, and Hungarian Ignaz Semmelweis, who also brought down infant mortality rates, this time in Vienna, by bringing in disinfection methods. Back in England, Snow was a founding member of the Epidemiological Society of London, the establishment of which was first mooted after an earlier epidemic. The society's aims included "rigid examination into the causes and conditions which influence the origin, propagation, mitigation, and prevention of epidemic diseases". It was founded in 1850 and was subsumed into the Royal Society of Medicine in 1907. One of its primary tools was the study of death certificates and similar civic records, the use of which, for medical purposes, was pioneered by amateur scientist John Graunt in the 17th century. Historically, each parish was responsible for its own birth, death, and marriage records, but England and Wales introduced a nationwide information bank in 1837, thus enabling scientists to track mortality rates and disease trends more effectively. In the 19th century, many other countries established similar systems

"As great a benefactor in my opinion to the human race as has appeared in the present century"

REVEREND HENRY WHITEHEAD, ON JOHN SNOW

to help with social surveys, public health needs, and economic planning. These changes were of enormous help when epidemiologists began studying international trends in the spread of diseases. When the International Epidemiological Association held its inaugural meeting in Noordwijk, the Netherlands, in 1957, 20 nations were represented; today, it has members in more than 100 countries. In 1983, the Association stated: "The ultimate aim and purpose of epidemiology [is] to promote, protect, and restore good health".

The chief job of the epidemiologist is to compare health-related data between given groups of people, using numerical expressions such as "XXXX per YYYY people" to express the rates of occurrence of certain health conditions. These "raw" figures might be refined by making adjustments for factors such as gender, age, season, occupation, lifestyle factors such as smoking, and so on. Two major phenomena measured by such comparisons are incidence – the number of new cases of a condition or symptom per group during a specified time period – and prevalence – the total number of cases at a specific time. So if two people in 100,000 develop a condition each year, its incidence is two per 100,000. If this condition lasts for one year, its prevalence is also two per 100,000, but if it lasts for ten years (and does not cause death in this period), its prevalence is eventually 20 per 100,000. Such data analysis led to one of the 20th century's greatest medical advances – revealing the links between smoking tobacco, lung cancer, and other serious diseases. In the 1920s, German clinicians noted the increase in the incidence of lung cancer and investigated factors such as industrial air pollution, road asphalting, exposure to fuel with the spread of motor vehicles,

MARLBORO MAN
The "Marlboro Man" image was used to advertise Marlboro cigarettes from 1954 to 1999. Three of the men who modelled the figure over the years later died of lung cancer.

the influenza pandemic of 1918, and even exposure to gas warfare in World War I. In 1929, German physician Fritz Lickint, who invented the term "passive smoking", published epidemiological evidence that lung cancer patients were especially likely to be smokers, and advocated anti-tobacco measures. In 1939, a German survey by Franz Müller reported: "the extraordinary rise in tobacco use was the single most important cause of the rising incidence of lung cancer". By 1950, despite the best diversionary attempts of the tobacco industry, more statistical evidence had accumulated, and a British team led by Richard Doll and Austin Bradford Hill published results showing that the common factor among lung cancer patients was the inhalation of tobacco smoke. Doll worked tirelessly to raise the status of epidemiology, turning it from one of medicine's backwaters to one of its most vital branches.

By 1955, a huge US epidemiological study of almost 200,000 men, led by E. Cuyler Hammond and Daniel Horn, concluded that cigarette smoking increased the death rate overall, the lung cancer rate by ten times, and the death rate from coronary artery disease by a similar factor. The risks of smoking were exposed, an achievement that has saved millions from suffering and premature death.

John Snow was passionate about hygiene, sanitation, and public health measures, which figure greatly in epidemiology. He paved the way for the work of bacteriologists such as Russian-born Waldemar Haffkine, who introduced cholera vaccinations to India. Today, Snow would be astounded by the ease with which data can be collected, the immense analytical powers of computing, instant global communications, and fields such as evidence-based medicine (see p.383–84). Soho's Broad Street, with which he will always be associated, was renamed Broadwick Street in 1936, and in 1992, a memorial pump was installed near the site of the original – the place where, it could be said, epidemiology was born.

ANTI-CHOLERA INOCULATION
Waldemar Mordecai Wolff Haffkine inoculates
a community against cholera in Calcutta, India,
in 1894. One of epidemiology's first case-study
infections was cholera, and Haffkine pioneered
vaccines against both cholera and bubonic plague.

Florence Nightingale

NURSING TODAY IS THE ULTIMATE caring profession, but until the 19th century, nurses required neither skill nor training. Instead, their motivation ranged from fashionable fancy or family obligation to feelings of guilt or a religious vocation. Nursing tasks – such as cleaning or feeding a patient – were seen as a servant's role and traditionally took place in the home. As hospital treatment became more common, the need for better sanitary conditions and higher levels of care and training became apparent. Florence Nightingale was instrumental in bringing about these reforms.

Ancient references to nursing abound. Egyptian papyri mention temple attendants who cleansed patients and implemented regimes of diet and exercise. Greeks and Romans used terms such as "assistants", "caretakers", and "helpers". The Greek god of healing was Asclepius, whose daughters Hygieia (meaning "health") and Panacea (meaning "all-healing") were worshipped for their caring attitudes to the sick (see p.32). Nursing and religion were closely intertwined, and the earliest hospitals were established by religious institutions. Towards the end of the 4th century, the noble Roman matron Fabiola converted to Christianity and used her family riches to establish a hospital for all-comers in Rome. There, she cared for patients, working alongside male physicians. Similarly, at the Hôtel Dieu (hospital) in Lyons, France, which was set up in around 542, both men and women tended to patients' daily needs. The Hôtel Dieu in Paris was founded about a century later, staffed by one of the first Christian orders created specifically to provide nursing care – the Augustinian Sisters. But it

NURSE FLORENCE
Florence Nightingale eschewed marriage and children to dedicate her life to nursing. She founded the first formal nursing training school.

was men, especially the Benedictine monks, who dominated nursing in the European Middle Ages. The Crusades saw the arrival of first aid and post-emergency nursing care for the battle-wounded (see pp.356–57).

Elsewhere in the world, nursing skills flourished. Dating from about 2,500 years ago, the Sanskrit text *Susruta Samhita* (see pp.77–78) recounts: "... The physician, the patient, the drugs and the nurse are four feet of... the medicine, upon which cure depends". In 7th-century Islamic hospitals, known as bimaristans, teams of staff included physicians, nurses, porters, and cleaners. Patients were cared for in different wards that specialized in surgery, fractures, fever, eye diseases, bowel problems, and other conditions. One of the first female nurses of this era was Rofaidah, the daughter of a physician, who was praised for her empathy, clinical skills, kindness, and her ability to organize and inspire others. Back in Europe, the Protestant Reformation of the 16th century saw many European nations break with the Roman Catholic Church. Through the ensuing conflicts, the Catholic caring orders went into decline. In England especially, conditions in hospitals – many attached to now-closed monasteries and convents – worsened. Standards of hygiene and sanitation declined, and nursing skills faded. Matters had degenerated further by the mid- to late 18th century, as the Industrial Revolution created overcrowding in already unsanitary cities.

Against this backdrop of industrial grime and disease, Florence Nightingale was born into a wealthy English family in 1820, and named after the Italian city of her birth. The Nightingales returned to England the following year. Blessed with money and connections, Florence grew into an independent, strongly religious young woman. She relished learning and was especially adept at mathematics; she was also a talented writer. In 1837, Nightingale had the first of several religious experiences that would guide her life and work. She began to show an interest in nursing, citing the example of the Catholic nuns who helped others in hospitals. Several years later, despite eligible suitors, she announced her decision not to marry and have children. Instead, she pursued her new interest, reading widely about hospitals, nursing, medicine, hygiene, and sanitation. She gained some practical experience in hospitals and convalescent homes, and even travelled to Egypt to spend time with the Sisters of Charity of St Vincent de Paul in Alexandria – an offshoot of the original Sisters of Charity community, which had been established in Paris in 1633. Rather than remain in convents, the sisters visited the sick in their homes. Nightingale was impressed by

LADY WITH THE LAMP
Florence Nightingale in the military hospital at Scutari, where she gained an almost saintly reputation for her efforts to improve care.

"… the very first requirement in a hospital [is] that it should do the sick no harm"

FLORENCE NIGHTINGALE

their nursing work and high standards of care, compared with their lax, ill-educated English counterparts. In 1851, she enrolled on a three-month nursing training course at a Protestant deaconry in Kaiserwerth, near Düsseldorf, Germany. Founded by Pastor Theodor Fliedner, the course was run by deaconesses, and followed the Catholic tradition of helping the sick, poor, and children, as well as prisoners and ex-prisoners. Deaconesses had been around for centuries; the Bible describes Phoebe, who offered care, food, and medicine as an early visiting nurse. As well as providing care, the deaconesses of Kaiserworth encouraged self-reliance and female emancipation through teaching and mentoring. Greatly struck by her experience in Germany, Nightingale returned to England, and in 1953, took her first post as the superintendent of the Establishment for Gentlewomen During Illness on Harley Street, London. By now, she was already becoming an acknowledged authority on hospitals and nursing.

As Nightingale settled into her new role, the Crimean War began. Russia threatened Turkey, and France and Britain sent armies to assist the Turks. The main battles took place on the Crimean Peninsula (now part of Ukraine). Reports of the war's progress arrived in record time via the relatively new telegraph; war photography was another recent feature that enabled the public to connect closely with the unfolding drama. Nightingale read about the horrific conditions in the hospitals for the war-wounded, and was eager to do something to help. Secretary of State at War and close friend Sidney Herbert asked her to prepare a group of nurses. In November 1854, Nightingale and her 38 female charges arrived at Scutari's Selimiye Barracks Hospital (today part of Istanbul) in Turkey. Conditions there were even more terrible than anticipated. Aside from patients, almost everything was in short supply: "There were no vessels for water or utensils of any kind; no soap, towels, or clothes, no hospital clothes; the men lying in their uniforms, stiff with gore and covered with filth to a degree and of a kind no one could write about; their persons covered with vermin…" Nightingale set about restructuring the facilities and improving food and water supplies. She reorganized the orderlies (assistants) and demanded more, and better, equipment. Using her contacts in England, she summoned the Sanitary Commission, who arrived the following spring to clear sewers and upgrade general hygiene. She also campaigned for better nutrition, recognizing the importance of a healthy diet. Death rates at Scutari dropped. By how much, how quickly, and why, has been much disputed since; Nightingale herself never claimed any special responsibility. Nevertheless, back in England, the public followed *The Times* reports of her tireless dedication: "When all the medical officers have retired for the night and silence and darkness have settled… she may be observed alone, with a little lamp in her hand, making her solitary rounds". She thus acquired her title of the "Lady with the Lamp".

When the Crimean War ended in 1856, Nightingale arrived home, and soon after petitioned Queen Victoria to prioritize military hospital reforms. Determined to prevent the return of such appalling conditions, she used her skills with statistics to convince the authorities of the importance of cleanliness in avoiding infection. She invented a mathematical chart, similar to a modern pie chart, to compare how soldiers had died – whether from wounds, preventable diseases, or other causes. Nightingale lived quietly and wrote prodigiously, and her accounts of the Crimea in *Notes on Matters affecting the Health, Efficiency and Hospital Administration of the British Army* (1858) were instrumental in bringing about better sanitation, updated nutrition, and overall improved care in military hospitals. Her talents were applied elsewhere, too: news of the Indian Mutiny drew her attention to conditions for the British troops there, and to the poverty and malnutrition suffered by local people. Nightingale was able to use her influence to convince the government of India to establish a sanitary department. In 1859, she published her famous work *Notes on Nursing*: "It is recognized as the knowledge which every one ought to have – distinct from medical knowledge, which only a profession can have". The following year, she founded the Nightingale Training School and Home For Nurses at St Thomas's Hospital, London. The school established nursing as a formal occupation, with proper training, accreditation, career progression, and payment. Teaching methods were theoretical and practical, records were kept of student progress, and the carefully selected students would reside in nurses' houses designed to "encourage discipline" and "form character".

Nightingale campaigned tirelessly, writing thousands of letters over the years despite being hampered by her own health. In 1855, on a visit to the Crimea, she had contracted a 12-day illness, known as Crimea fever, that was to cause periods of disability and bed rest throughout the rest of her life. But Nightingale was not alone in her efforts to improve levels of care and sanitation. Mary Seacole was a Crimean War contemporary, who went to the Crimea in 1855. There, she set up the British Hotel near Balaklava, offering care, food, and rooms to wounded European Allies soldiers, albeit on a commercial basis. Although she did not have the impact of Nightingale with regard to the formal nursing system, she gained a reputation for her nursing prowess and bravery in visiting battlefields, along with the nickname "Mother" Seacole.

In line with the medical establishment at the time, Nightingale's attitudes to medical progress were conservative. She was wary of the germ theory of disease (see pp.222–27), but even so, in Quain's Medical Dictionary of 1882, she advised: "Always have chlorinated soda for nurses to wash their hands, especially after dressing or handling a suspicious case. It may destroy germs at the expense of the cuticle, but if it takes off the cuticle, it must be bad for the germs".

Florence Nightingale's ceaseless work launched the nursing principles and practices of today. Her long career inspired many others to establish professional nursing schools, and she was the first woman to be awarded an Order of Merit, in 1907. Her name lives on in the form of many Nightingale nursing colleges and organizations, and in various awards. Each year, International Nurses' Day is celebrated on her birthday – 12 May. Yet in life, Nightingale was ever reluctant to seek recognition or appear in public, and her burial was a quiet family affair in Hampshire.

MARY SEACOLE
Half-Jamaican nurse Mary Seacole was also influential in improving conditions for wounded soldiers.

Measuring Blood Pressure

Blood pressure is the pressure that is exerted on the artery walls by circulating blood, and it is measured using instruments and the pulse to help diagnose a patient's health. High blood pressure (hypertension) results from a high volume of blood or narrowing of the arteries, and can be caused by lack of exercise, alcoholism, high salt intake, and other factors. It puts stress on the heart and arteries, and can increase the risk of strokes, heart attacks, kidney disorders, and other diseases. Low blood pressure (hypotension) can be caused by age, illness, or blood loss, and may result in dizzyness, fainting, and, in extreme cases, shock. Both conditions can also be hereditary. Blood pressure varies during each heartbeat, and so is measured as a range (see opposite).

Pulse and pressure in history

For thousands of years, physicians have used the pulse as a diagnostic tool. The Ancient Egyptians took simple pulse readings, and ancient cultures from China to Greece theorized about its strength, rhythm, and quality. Blood pressure was discovered in 1733 by clergyman Stephen Hales, who inserted tubes into animals' arteries and measured how far the blood rose. From the 19th century, measuring devices arrived that used a cuff and did not break the skin, such as the tonoscillograph and the sphygmomanometer (see opposite).

CHINESE PULSE
DIAGNOSIS CHART,
LATE 17TH CENTURY

The cuff fits around the patient's arm. It incorporates a valve, so that the physician can let out the air during use

TONOSCILLOGRAPH
BRITAIN, 1931–40
Hungarian scientist and
doctor Janos Plesch, a friend
and physician of Albert
Einstein, developed the
tonoscillograph, which
was widely used during the
1930s. Featuring an inflatable
cuff, it was a precursor
of the instruments in
use today. It was easy
to use and produced a
record in graph form.

How it works

Blood pressure is measured at its highest (systolic) and
lowest (diastolic) points, today with a sphygmomanometer
(blood pressure gauge). An inflatable cuff is fitted around
the upper arm, and a listening device called a stethoscope
(invented by René Laennec in 1816) is placed below the
cuff. The inflated cuff closes the artery and stops blood
flow. Listening through the stethoscope, the physician
slowly deflates the cuff, noting the first sounds as the
artery opens under systolic pressure, and when blood
flows freely under diastolic pressure.

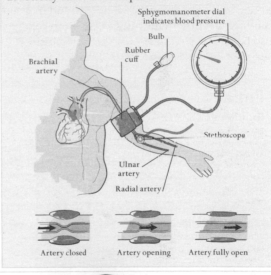

Sphygmomanometer dial
indicates blood pressure

Bulb

Rubber
cuff

Brachial
artery

Stethoscope

Ulnar
artery

Radial artery

Artery closed   Artery opening   Artery fully open

The patient's blood pressure
is recorded on a removable
graph, known as
a tonoscillogram

The device contains a
mechanism to measure
pressure that works like
a barometer: changes in
pressure make a metal cell
expand or contract, and
levers transmit these
movements to the dial

The bulb is used to
inflate the cuff with
air, to stop the blood
flow temporarily in
the patient's artery

Pasteur and Microbiology

GERMS ARE INVISIBLE ENEMIES. These miniature life forms can harm the human body and other living things, but they are so small that they can only be seen under a microscope. Not just any old micro-organisms or microbes, germs are pathogenic — they multiply in the body and cause infectious diseases or infections. In the 17th century, early light microscopes (see pp.150–51) revealed multiple microbes of countless kinds. But it wasn't until the 19th century that these miniscule invaders were shown to cause illness, leading to the germ theory of disease. French scientist Louis Pasteur's extraordinary achievements were pivotal to this development, as were those of German scientist Robert Koch (see pp.222–27).

For centuries, infectious diseases and other ill health were blamed on a variety of causes, which included revenge from angry gods or a sinful existence. Two major theories prevailed. The first, miasma, was a general notion that foul, poisoned air somehow spread diseases. The idea was not wholly ridiculous — nasty smells from soil or water polluted with decaying matter and excrement invariably accompanied cholera, dysentery, and similar diseases. In Ancient Greece, Hippocrates considered noxious air akin to pestilence. Similarly, Vitruvius, a Roman architect and engineer from the 1st century BCE, mused on the harmful effects of nostril-wrinkling air from sources such as swamps, stagnant water, and sewers. Two centuries later, Galen linked bad air and disease with his concept of humours (see p.43). Galen's popular theories persisted through the Middle Ages, and were adapted to explain pandemics such as those of smallpox and bubonic plague. The toxic gases that were thought to spread disease became known as miasms. Air was supposedly

LOUIS PASTEUR
Together with his long-term rival, German physician and scientist Robert Koch, Pasteur is considered a founding father of microbiology.

charged with an "epidemic influence", and when this encountered emissions of decay, it was believed to turn into malignant miasms that led to disease. Restless minds in Renaissance Europe began to probe the mystery. In the 1540s, Italian physician and scientist Girolamo Fracastoro suggested that minute particles – spores – might be responsible. A century later, the microscopes of Antoni van Leeuwenhoek and others revealed "animalcules" (see p.145). In 1700, French practitioner Nicolas Andry recorded his observations of tiny, wriggling "worms", which he thought might cause disease. Some of these worms were known parasites, such as tapeworms. Others, which Andry suspected might cause venereal disease, were actually sperm cells, or spermatozoa. A keen proponent of the miasma theory, he suggested that bad air might contain "seeds of worms".

The second theory was first recorded by Aristotle in Ancient Greece. He believed in spontaneous generation or abiogenesis, in which living matter could arise from non-living ingredients due to some manner of "life-force". It seemed a sensible explanation for mould that suddenly sprouted on old bread, maggots that seemingly appeared from nowhere on rotting meat, and infestations of lice and fleas where there had been none. As new microscope technology revealed more about microbes, existing theories were questioned by sceptical scientists seeking evidence. In 1668, Italian naturalist-physician Francesco Redi described his experiments with jars containing old meat. He left some jars open, covered some with close-mesh cloth, and stoppered others with cork. Redi noted that maggots appeared in the meat only if flies could actually land on it; therefore, maggots were not arising spontaneously from the dead meat. At the time, however, belief in spontaneous generation was so widespread that Redi's work made little headway. In the mid-18th century, English priest and biologist John Needham tried a different approach, first boiling chicken broth to destroy any life, then sealing it from air. The broth became cloudy, which Needham attributed to spontaneous generation of microbes. He claimed that "vital atoms" harboured the quality of life, permeated the natural world, and animated their surroundings to create life. In retrospect, it is likely that Needham's boiling time did not destroy all of the microbes in the broth, and that flies may have landed on the broth and contaminated it as it cooled in the open air. Another priest, Italian Lazzaro Spallanzani, took Needham's experiments further in the 1760s. He boiled the broth for longer, and ensured that it was then sealed quickly and securely in glass phials. The sealed broth samples remained intact and uncontaminated, whereas those open to air soon swarmed with small life. Clinging to the belief in spontaneous generation, opponents countered that such severe treatment destroyed Needham's "vital atoms", which needed contact with air for their gift of life.

A disease affecting silkworms (silk moth caterpillars) that spread through Europe in the early 19th century piqued the interest of Italian insect expert Agostino Bassi. He embarked on a laborious series of experiments, eventually concluding in 1835 that the disease was caused by some kind of contagion or transmissible particle – a microbial life form, spread as powdery spores by contact or close proximity. Ten years later, he postulated that microbes could act as disease agents in humans, too. Bassi's work provided early sound evidence of contagion as a cause of disease, and the fungus that attacked the silkworms was later named *Beauveria bassiana* in his honour. By now, he was far from alone. In Germany, rising star in anatomy and histology Friedrich Gustav Jacob Henle penned an article supporting the contagium vivum ("living germ") proposal: "The material of contagions is not only an organic but a living one... [it] is, in relation to the diseased body, a parasitic organism". Two other significant advances helped the contagion cause. In Vienna, obstetrician Ignaz Semmelweis reasoned in 1847 that "cadaverous particles" carried by doctors and medical students were the cause of an unusually high incidence of puerperal fever (see p.220). Seven years later, in London, John Snow carried out his celebrated removal of a water pump handle during a cholera outbreak, suspecting that contagions were at work (see pp.180–87). The contagion or germ theory of disease gained ground, but even so, the concept of miasma still held sway in 1860s Europe. Miasma appeared to explain, for example, why cholera was so prevalent in cities with crowded, deprived neighbourhoods, and poor hygiene and public health. According to this theory, the foul air, reeking of decay and human waste, was highly charged with miasms, so more people succumbed to the disease.

France was one of many countries across Europe and Asia that suffered regular cholera outbreaks; the disease raced through Paris in 1832 and again in 1849. Enter Louis Pasteur, future giant among microbiologists. Born in Dole, eastern France, in 1822, Pasteur gained his bachelor's

CLOUD OF CHOLERA
The belief in miasma – that diseases were spread by
"bad" air – was so strong in the 19th century that
germ theorists struggled to make themselves heard.

degree at the regional Royal College of Besançon. It was not until 1843,
however, when he was admitted to the prestigious École Normale
Supérieure in Paris, that Pasteur's aptitude for chemistry was
acknowledged as more than mediocre. He graduated and became a
chemistry assistant, then briefly taught physics in Dijon before
becoming professor of chemistry at the University of Strasbourg.
Having married Marie Laurent in 1849, Pasteur moved with his family
in 1854 to Lille, where he was appointed professor of chemistry and
dean of the science faculty. Two years later, he returned to his old
school in Paris, taking on the role of director of scientific studies. From
his base in the capital, Pasteur's reputation soared. He had high
standards and a hawk-like eye for detail, which he applied with great
success to diverse problems within the fields of livestock farming,
veterinary science, and human health and medicine, among others.

Pasteur's work evolved through several main phases, beginning
with research on how light passes through different shapes and
arrangements of crystals. By the mid-1850s, his interests had turned
to fermentation and why liquids go sour. During his time at Lille, he
was asked to investigate beer spoilage, with a view to saving the

"Never will the doctrine of spontaneous generation recover from the mortal blow struck by this simple experiment"

LOUIS PASTEUR

brewing industry huge losses. Working with wine and beer, Pasteur demonstrated that, contrary to popular belief, fermentation was not a purely chemical process, but involved microbial forms of life. He also noted that a particular sort of microbe – rounded yeasts – had to be present in normal fermented beer. Samples of sour beer contained the wrong sort of microbe. In 1859, recalling the work of Needham and Spallanzani, Pasteur carried out a decisive set of experiments, using boiled meaty broth and glass flasks that were variously sealed or open to air, like his predecessors. Some of Pasteur's flasks had extended, downward-curving necks, which allowed air to flow in and out, but kept out airborne dust and passing contagion particles. The broth in these flasks stayed uncontaminated for longest. In flasks with the neck bent up to allow potentially contaminating particles to enter, the broth developed moulds much sooner. These results, from such a respected scientist, dealt a huge blow to supporters of spontaneous generation, bolstered the case for germ theory, and furthered the argument that contaminating particles might cause human diseases. Pasteur went on to work with acclaimed French physiologist Claude Bernard in the early 1860s, and between them they devised an answer to the drink spoilage problem: heat to kill the contaminators without altering the product's flavour. This form of heat treatment is now known universally as pasteurization.

From about 1865 to 1871, Pasteur also researched silkworm diseases. In an echo of Bassi's earlier work, described above, Pasteur showed that the diseases were caused by microbes (one later established as fungal, the other viral), and thereby helped to revive the French silk industry. Emperor Napoleon III offered his grateful thanks to Pasteur for his contributions to the drink and silkworm industries, which enhanced Pasteur's escalating reputation still further.

By the 1870s, Pasteur had developed an interest in vaccination. This was already widely practised for smallpox (see pp.152–61), but Pasteur's ambition was to find vaccinations for other human and livestock diseases, especially cholera and anthrax. He assembled a team that included promising young physicians Emile Roux and Charles Chamberland, and carried out tests on fowl cholera – the form that affected chickens, turkeys, and similar birds. Roux went on to work on diphtheria, while Chamberland invented a filter to trap bacteria from a solution. Both later worked at the Institut Pasteur, which was founded by Pasteur in 1887. Pasteur and his team cultured – purified and grew in the laboratory – the germ that causes fowl cholera, a bacterium since named *Pasteurella multocida*. The cultivated germs were used to give chickens the disease, so that different vaccination techniques could be tested.

In 1879, partly as a result of Chamberland's forgetfulness, one batch of these microbes failed to thrive as normal. They produced only mild symptoms in the birds, which then, unusually, recovered. Puzzled by this, Pasteur inoculated these same chickens with a full-strength bacterial preparation. The birds did not develop fowl cholera. He suspected that the strange culture consisted of germs that had somehow become weakened or attenuated. Normally, the batches were not exposed to air, but the forgotten culture had been. Did this weaken them? To test his theory, Pasteur grew some new cholera microbe cultures. Some were exposed to air, while others were sealed in tubes, where the oxygen was rapidly used up. Pasteur then tested their virulence by inoculating chickens to see how many of them became ill and died. The results were conclusive: "Remarkably, the experiment shows that the virulence under these conditions [with no oxygen] is always the same as that which was used to inoculate the original closed tubes [the full-

BLOOD BANK
These test tubes from the museum at the Institut Pasteur in Paris, France, contain samples of blood from hens that died as a result of being inoculated with fowl cholera.

FOAMING AT THE MOUTH
Knowing that rabies is transmitted by saliva, Pasteur
investigated the disease further by taking samples of
foam from the mouth of a rabid dog.

strength microbes from the first set of experiments]. Meanwhile, the
cultures which have been exposed to air are either dead or possess a
very weak virulence… Our problem is therefore solved: it is the oxygen
which brings about the attenuation in virulence". Pasteur had
succeeded in producing an artificially weakened strain of an infectious
microbe that could be used for vaccination. This differed from the
smallpox vaccine, which was a naturally occurring version. Poultry
farmers were grateful, the discovery stimulated much research into
other diseases, and vaccines for human cholera arrived by 1900.

Around the same time, Pasteur was also investigating anthrax, a
serious disease of cattle, sheep, other livestock, and wild animals that
can also be deadly in humans. The causative *Bacillus anthracis* had already
been isolated and identified in the mid-1870s by Pasteur's rival Robert
Koch (see pp.222–27). Working from several farms, Pasteur adopted the
approach he had taken for chicken cholera, developing a weakened
strain to use in a vaccine against the full-strength version. In 1881, he
carried out a trial at a farm at Pouilly-le-Fort near Melun, southeast of
Paris. He used two groups of livestock, each containing 25 sheep, along
with a few cows and goats. Each animal in the first group was given

two inoculations of the new anthrax vaccine, 15 days apart. The animals in the other group received none. Fifteen days after the second inoculation, the animals from both groups received a dose of live anthrax bacteria. The results were startlingly clear. All of the vaccinated stock survived – they "frolicked and gave signs of perfect health". The rest of the animals died within two days. Doubters of vaccination were deflated, as were supporters of spontaneous generation and miasma. Farming quickly benefitted, although a human vaccine for anthrax did not become available until 1954.

The final main phase of Pasteur's vaccination work focused on the dreaded disease of rabies (see pp.204–05). Rabies is best known for afflicting dogs, but any warm-blooded animal can be infected and it can be passed on to humans if they are bitten. Pasteur studied writings on rabies by Girolamo Fracastoro, mentioned earlier, and by German scientist Georg Gottfried Zinke, who, in 1804, proved that rabies is transmitted by saliva. The rabies microbe – a type of virus – affects the nervous system, especially the central nervous system (the brain and spinal cord). Pasteur's colleague Roux developed a method of producing vaccine by infecting rabbits, and then dissecting out and drying the spinal cord to weaken and kill the microbes. By 1885, the vaccine was being tested on dogs. That same year, nine-year-old Joseph Meister was mauled by a rabid dog. Desperate for help, his mother took him to Pasteur. Rabies was so feared at the time that some people committed suicide after rabid dog bites rather than endure the agony. Pasteur considered the situation and consulted others: "The opinion of our wise colleague and of Dr Grancher was that by the intensity and the number of bites, Joseph Meister was almost inevitably to come down with rabies". Despite not being qualified to treat humans and risking the wrath of the authorities, Pasteur administered the vaccine. Joseph did not develop rabies, so the vaccine was assumed to be successful. Trials proceeded rapidly, and Pasteur's reputation ascended to new heights.

Joseph Meister later became caretaker at the Institut Pasteur in Paris. This world-renowned institution has led the way in medical research against infectious diseases and is a lasting tribute to the great man's achievements.

The Horror of Rabies

Rabies is a dangerous viral disease that inflames the brain, producing a hideous range of advanced symptoms, from thrashing out and biting to phobias and hallucinations. It is fatal if the patient is not swiftly vaccinated. Rabies can be passed between species, and humans often catch it from the bite of an infected dog; the disease was untreatable until the first human vaccine in the late 19th century. Vaccines are now also available to prevent the disease in animals, but 55,000 people die from rabies globally every year.

VIAL OF RABIES VACCINE

1548 Italian physician Girolamo Fracastoro attributes rabies **transmission** to a substance in the sufferer's saliva. Fracastoro also named the virus after the Latin word for "rage"; both human and animal victims slather at the mouth and act aggressively.

1885 Pasteur and Roux produce a rabies vaccine; several hundred patients are successfully **vaccinated** within the year.

1271 Thirty people are killed by an outbreak of rabies in Germany, after **infected wolves** invade a village.

1804 German scientist Georg Gottfried Zinke **injects animals** with rabies, proving that the disease is infectious.

1884 Pasteur and Roux describe how rabies is found in the **spinal cord** and brain.

1881 French scientists **Louis Pasteur** and Emile Roux begin research on rabies.

1793 Physician Samuel Argent Bardsley proposes a **quarantine** system in the UK for isolating animals and eradicating infection, but this idea is not implemented.

1881 French professor Pierre-Victor Galtier injects sheep with rabies-carrying saliva; this seems to make them **immune** from further infection.

1883 Emile Roux publishes a paper on his and Pasteur's **research**.

MORTALITY RATE FOR UNVACCINATED PATIENTS DIAGNOSED WITH RABIES

100%

1936 Leslie Webster and Anna Clow grow the rabies virus in the lab; it has a distinctive **bullet-like** shape.

Impfgebiet

TOLLWUT

In diesem Gebiet sind z. Z.
Impfköder mit Tollwut-Impfstoff so ausgelegt,
daß Füchse sie aufnehmen und damit gegen Tollwut
geschützt werden.

Bitte beachten:

- Impfköder nicht berühren
- Hunde nicht frei laufen lassen
- Haustiere von Impfködern fernhalten
- Bei Kontakt Arzt oder Tierarzt befragen
- Informieren Sie bitte Ihre Kinder

1970S–80S European authorities use **oral vaccination** via food left for foxes to control high numbers of rabid animals.

1902 The UK is declared **free of rabies**, although there have since been isolated cases.

1932 Dr Russ Pfister discovers rabies in **vampire bats**.

1976 The HDCV vaccine is licensed in Europe; it requires a shorter course of **injections** than previous vaccines.

1979 Scientists in the Philippines produce a **vaccine for dogs** that gets rid of rabies in parts of the country.

2015 Western Europe declared **free of rabies** from non-flying animals by World Organization for Animal Health.

1955 Vaccinating dogs against rabies becomes a **legal requirement** in nearly all parts of the USA.

1967 The highly effective **human diploid cell** vaccine for rabies is developed.

2017 A total of **106 countries** report no cases of rabies within the previous 12 months.

1984 The **VR-G vaccine**, which can be given to animals orally, is developed at the Wistar Institute in the US.

Lister and Antiseptics

"**O**PERATION SUCCESSFUL, PATIENT DIED" was a common entry in 19th-century hospital records. The revolution in medical anaesthesia in the 1840s meant that surgeons no longer had to struggle with victims writhing in agony, or work in double-quick time to minimize the torment (see pp.172–77), and with their patients at rest and insensible, surgeons could explore new procedures using greater care and caution. Yet even in the best hospitals, many patients still died soon afterwards, usually from infection.

By the mid-1860s, the germ theory of disease had started to infiltrate medicine, thanks to the work of Louis Pasteur (see pp.196–203). John Snow's insight into the London cholera epidemic a decade earlier (see pp.180–87) contributed, as did the experience of Ignaz Semmelweis with puerperal fever in 1840s Vienna (see p.220). Even so, it took a long time for the idea to be widely accepted. Traditional theories had held sway for centuries: these included miasma, in which some kind of malignant chemical quality in foul air set off disease; and spontaneous generation, in which parasites and pestilence arose from inanimate matter (see pp.196–98). The medical establishment, notoriously suspicious of even slight change, took a cautious stance. Some surgeons still did not accept the advantages of anaesthesia, insisting that pain was integral to treatment and recovery. They argued that circumventing pain with anaesthesia, or even the anaesthetic agents themselves, could lead to problems such as post-surgical festering wounds, oozing pus, or the rotting flesh of hospital gangrene. Blood poisoning or general sepsis (from the Greek for putrefaction) was the end-stage of infection, with a range of effects including widespread inflammation, blood clotting, and eventual organ failure. With such a high mortality rate from post-surgical infection, something had to change.

JOSEPH LISTER
Lister worked hard to banish filth from operating theatres and destroy the germs responsible for high post-operative death rates.

British surgeon Joseph Lister revolutionized surgery and immeasurably improved patients' fortunes by demonstrating that infecting microbes could be tackled by germ-destroying substances called antiseptics.

Joseph Lister gained his early medical qualifications in 1852 at University Hospital, London, becoming a Fellow of the Royal College of Surgeons. In 1853, he moved to Edinburgh, and the following year began working with celebrated surgeon and medical reformer James Syme, whose daughter Lister later married. Guided by Syme's pioneering spirit, Lister was a keen researcher, studying and writing reports on muscle action, blood coagulation (clotting), and inflammation. He was appointed Regius Professor of Surgery at the University of Glasgow in 1860, and started to practise at the attached Glasgow Royal Infirmary. Today's onlookers would be horrified by a typical operating theatre of the time. Surgeons, nurses, and other staff took little or no notice of hygiene. Their hands, clothes – ordinary working ones – and instruments were rarely cleaned before, after, or between patients. In the recovery wards, seeping pus, the stench of gangrene, and the dreaded sepsis were commonplace. At the time, it was widely thought that oxygen in the air had a direct chemical effect on exposed flesh, triggering gangrene. The solution was to dress and bind the area tightly to keep air out. This reduced blood flow to and oxygen levels in the tissues – ironically, conditions that gangrene-causing microbes loved. Keen to make an impact on such a depressing situation, Lister tried a different approach. He began to keep himself clean in theatre, along with his attire and his instruments; he also used tourniquets to reduce blood loss and provide a clearer view of the operative area. Other surgeons smirked at Lister's efforts, and a few even openly ridiculed him, since blood and gore on their apparel was symbolic of their great status. Lister persevered; his measures began to yield results and his operating success rate crept up.

In the mid-1860s, a professor of chemistry at Glasgow University, Thomas Anderson, showed Pasteur's work to Lister, suggesting how microbes might be responsible for hospital gangrene and other infections. Lister also learned of Semmelweis's campaign for cleanliness to foil puerperal fever. He conjectured: "... Decomposition of the injured part might be avoided... by applying in a dressing some material capable of destroying the life of the floating particles". Pasteur had identified three measures against spoilage organisms: filters, heat, and chemicals. Lister, ever keen to help his patients and boost his own success rate, began looking round for an appropriate chemical substance to experiment with. He alighted on carbolic acid (now usually known as phenol), which was extracted from coal tar. First produced in the 1830s, carbolic acid had already found various uses as a preservative, and in neutralizing effluent in sewers. Its powerful and distinctive smell, sweet and tarry, was intended to destroy the foul disease-causing vapours known as miasms. Lister recalled: "In the course of the year 1864 I was much struck with an account of the remarkable effects produced by carbolic acid upon the sewage of the town of Carlisle [North-West England]... Not only preventing all odour from the lands irrigated with refuse material, but as is stated destroying the entozoa [worms and similar parasites] which usually infest cattle fed upon such pastures... I saw that such a powerful antiseptic was peculiarly adapted for experiments... The applicability of carbolic acid for the treatment of compound fracture [see below] naturally occurred to me". Lister researched carbolic acid's effects on human skin and flesh, obtained supplies from Anderson, and carried out preliminary trials. Encouraged by the results, he began to use carbolic acid liquid before, during, and after surgery, for cleaning his hands and instruments, and for soaking bandages.

An accident on 12 August 1865 brought 11-year-old James Greenlees into Glasgow Royal Infirmary. Injured by a cart, he had sustained a compound fracture of the left tibia (shin bone). In a compound or open fracture, not only is bone broken, but also skin, allowing in dirt, germs, and other contaminants. In Lister's time, such injuries usually progressed via sepsis to death, unless the limb was amputated – another risk-ridden procedure. Lister himself cleaned the break and wound, dressed it with lint soaked in carbolic acid solution, and splinted the leg. Every few days, he repeated the cleaning and dressing process. In six weeks, against all odds, James was infection-free, and able to walk on two good legs. Following this triumph, Lister decreed that all surgery under his supervision should follow the new procedures involving carbolic acid. Meanwhile, he

CHANCES OF SURVIVING
SURGERY BEFORE
ANTISEPTICS ARRIVED

50%

SPRAY CLEAN
Lister invented a machine for killing airborne germs
with a fine mist of carbolic acid. He would direct the
distribution of the spray before an operation.

continued to search for improvements. Neat, crude carbolic acid caused
problems such as skin irritation and sloughing, so he requested purer
forms, tested dilutions, and mixed them with other substances such as
linseed oil and carbonate of lime. Increasingly confident, he also began
to lecture and publish his results, summarizing his early methods in
Antiseptic Principle of the Practice of Surgery, which was published in
an edition of the *British Medical Journal* in 1867: "In conducting the
treatment, the first object must be the destruction of any septic germs
which may have been introduced into the wound... by introducing the
acid of full strength into all accessible recesses of the wound by means
of a piece of rag held in dressing-forceps and dipped in the liquid...
Limbs which otherwise would be unhesitatingly condemned to
amputation may be retained with confidence of the best results".
Mortalities from major surgery under Lister's supervision fell from
nearly 50 per cent to 15 per cent. Antiseptic methods were applied more
widely to contusions (bruising), lacerations, and abscesses.

In 1869, Lister returned to Edinburgh as Professor of Clinical
Surgery. Around this time, he devised a spray to kill floating
contaminants in the operating theatre – and cover everyone and
everything there with a fine mist of diluted carbolic acid.

FRENCH SPRAY MACHINE
Lister's techniques were promoted in France by Just Marie Marcellin Lucas-Championnière, who reinvented Lister's spray machine.

Lister's spray machines went through several incarnations: the first were laboriously hand- and foot-pumped – these were known as "donkey engines" – but, by 1871, they were steam-powered. These were later phased out when airborne contamination was found to be less of a risk than breathing in the carbolic spray. Some British surgeons remained unconvinced, even dismissive, and proposed other reasons for Lister's results – from better diet and nursing care to the local climate. They were reluctant to admit that their time-honoured practices could actually cause infection by transferring germs, or to alter their habits for little creatures they could not even see.

Antisepsis – the process of killing or inhibiting the growth of any germs present – was adopted faster and more enthusiastically in continental Europe, especially Germany, than England. As the germ theory of disease gradually became accepted, other antiseptics were tried in place of carbolic acid. Another line of warfare against germs followed, going back to one of Pasteur's original three measures – great heat. In 1879, Pasteur's assistant Charles Chamberland (see p.201) invented an oven-like device called the autoclave, which killed germs with high-pressure saturated steam. Seven years later, in Berlin, Latvian-born surgeon Ernst von Bergmann introduced steam sterilization for surgical instruments and dressings. He had previously adopted Lister's methods while a military surgeon, with great success. Von Bergmann's sterilization initiative marked a shift away from antisepsis to asepsis – in which there is a complete absence of germs. Along came the operating theatre's familiar white masks, gowns, and trays of sparkling, clean instruments.

Lister was not the first to use antiseptics – microbe-killers or inhibitors that can be applied to living tissues with relative safety. But he did formalize their use and demonstrate their efficacy in medicine. Disinfectants do much the same, but for inanimate objects such as instruments, beds, or floors. Since ancient times, some substances have filled both needs. Alcohol (ethanol) and vinegar were recorded in Ancient Greece, India, and China, while in Rome, Aulus Cornelius Celsus (see pp.111) used vinegar and thyme oil. For millennia, pitch or oils were poured on to open injuries or hurried amputations (see pp.126–31). Compounds of copper, silver, and mercury were also tried, although some of these proved rather toxic. Today, hand-sanitizers in many hospitals are based on alcohol or iodine. The latter, isolated in 1811, was incorporated into an iodine solution in 1829 by French physician Jean Guillaume Auguste Lugol. Lugol's iodine went on to become a widespread antiseptic, disinfectant, and cure-all for a great variety of health and hygiene problems.

The *British Medical Journal* finally acknowledged Lister's achievements in 1879: "… The man who has done the most to take the 'disgrace' out of surgery is Mr Lister". By this time, he was already Chair of Clinical Surgery at King's College, London, and Personal Surgeon in Ordinary to Queen Victoria. Royal approval was sealed when he had the privilege of lancing a large abscess in the queen's left armpit. She recorded: "… I bear pain so badly. I shall be given chloroform… The abscess, which was six inches in diameter, was very quickly cut… Mr Lister, whose great invention, a carbolic spray to destroy all organic germs, was used…" In 1883, Lister was made a baronet; in 1891, he co-founded and became chairman of the British Institute of Preventive Medicine (now called the Lister Institute of Preventive Medicine); and in 1897, he was the first surgeon to be made a baron for his medical achievements.

Lister may not have had exceptional surgical skills, nor did he have much of a sense of humour: medical students met with a muted response when they joked about his carbolic spray machine, saying before an operation, "Let us-s-pray". But however private and emotionally detached he may have been as a man, Lister's quest to rid the operating theatre of its septic legacy saved the lives of many patients, and secured his place in history.

IODINE TINCTURE
Iodine, first incorporated into iodine solution in 1829, was one of the most widely used early antiseptics. It is still used in hospitals today.

SPOTLESS SURGERY
Despite initial scepticism, Lister's methods of
using cleanliness to combat germs spread rapidly
across Europe. This Austrian painting from about
1900 depicts the disinfection process in a hospital
operating theatre of the time.

SPIRITUS   KARBOL   SUBLIMAT

Mother and Baby Medicine

IN TODAY'S CONVENTIONAL MEDICINE, the central figures in the care of mothers and babies during the postnatal period are the obstetrician and the midwife. Obstetricians are qualified doctors who specialize in the medical care of pregnant women and new babies. Midwives are qualified professionals who provide care and advice that usually extends from mother and baby to partners and family, taking in emotional and social care in a more holistic and rounded way. In general, the midwife's role is to support and monitor women during a "normal" healthy pregnancy and birth; the obstetrician is there for women experiencing more difficult or complex problems, which may need more specialist intervention.

From the earliest times in Babylonia and Egypt, female birth attendants were depicted helping the new mother. Egyptian images from more than 2,500 years ago show mothers squatting or sitting to give birth, and midwives are described in the Ebers Papyrus (see pp.26–27). A prominent name in Ancient Greece, more than 2,300 years ago, was Agnodice (see p.164), although it is unclear whether she was mythical. At the time, women were allowed to treat other women during pregnancy and birth, but could do little else in medicine. It is said that Agnodice cut her hair and dressed as a man to qualify as a general physician. As recounted by Gaius Julius Hyginus three centuries later: "She heard a woman crying out in the throes of labour so she went to her assistance. The woman, thinking she

AGNODICE REVEALED
Agnodice shows herself to be a woman after years pretending to be a man in order to practice medicine.

was a man, refused her help; but Agnodice lifted up her clothes and revealed herself to be a woman and was thus able to treat her patient". Female patients learned to ask for "him" by name, which made doctors suspicious. Angered by accusations, Agnodice finally came clean by raising her robes in public. She was accused of deception and condemned to death, but patients' lobbying brought her pardon, and women were then allowed to practise medicine more widely.

In the 1st century CE, Greek physician Soranus of Ephesus wrote *Gynaikeia* (*Gynaecology*), which contained a great deal of detail on obstetrics and midwifery. He described the difficulties of breech presentation, in which the baby is positioned to exit the womb bottom- or feet- first, and showed how a baby can be "turned" by manipulating it inside the womb. He recommended that the midwife sat in front of the mother on her birthing chair, ready to receive the baby, with bandages, oils, and herbs at the ready. She would encourage the baby to breathe, cut the cord, and sprinkle the stump with healing substances, and then check and clean the infant so that it was ready to present to the mother – some of which are classic midwifery procedures still practised today. Parts of Soranus' *Gynaikeia* were adapted in the 6th century by an author named Muscio (Mustio), and were again recycled in the 16th century by Eucharius Rösslin (also known as Rhodion; see below).

One of the oldest known surgical procedures is Caesarean section – the delivery of a baby through an incision in the mother's abdominal wall and womb. In Greek mythology, the sun god Apollo removed Asclepius, the god of healing and medicine, in this way. The name is popularly believed to originate from the birth of Roman Emperor Julius Caesar by this method – however, in Roman times, the operation was usually performed to save the baby when the mother was dead or dying, yet Julius's mother, Aurelia, lived. It is more likely that the name comes from the Latin word *caedare*, meaning "to cut". In 1598, influential French royal surgeon Jacques Guillemeau published a work on midwifery in which he used the term Caesarean "section" rather than "operation", which then passed into common usage.

In East Asia, around 850, Chinese physician Zan Yin compiled the 52-chapter *Jing Xiao Chan Bao* (*Treasured Knowledge of Obstetrics*, or *Tested Prescriptions in Obstetrics*). The first major Chinese work on gynaecology and obstetrics, it incorporated many aspects of Chinese traditional medicine, such as the conditioning of qi energy (see pp.64–73), as well as more than 300 herbal formulas and prescriptions. Zan Yin covered

ANATOMICAL MODEL
This ivory model of a pregnant woman
with removable parts, of a type common in
17th-century Europe, was used by midwives
to educate women about giving birth.

miscarriage, excessive bleeding, hyperemesis
gravidarum (a severe form of morning sickness),
premature birth, and difficult presentations,
such as breech presentation. Texts from ancient
India indicate that Indian midwives were from well-
to-do families and had great expertise. The *Susruta
Samhita* (see pp.77–79) recounts how the expectant
mother should lie on her back with pillows for
support, thighs flexed, and be aided by four older,
experienced midwives with well-trimmed nails.

Midwifery as the formally organized speciality
we know today began to take shape in Europe
during the 16th century. Famed French battlefield surgeon Ambroise
Paré (see pp.126–31) was one of many eminent medical men who began
to take an interest in obstetrics. He used a method of "podalic version",
whereby a baby lying sideways in the womb could be repositioned for
an easier, feet-first birth. The recently invented movable-type printing
press, and the tendency of eminent medical men like Paré to write in
the language of the day rather than in scholarly Latin, opened the
study of medicine and health care to the public, giving budding male
physicians opportunities in pregnancy and childbirth. In Germany,
apothecary and physician Eucharius Rösslin was dismayed at the low
standards of midwifery, and published *Der Schwangeren Frauen und
Hebammen Rosengarten* (*The Rose Garden for Pregnant Women and Midwives*) in
an attempt to raise standards. In 17th-century France, Louyse
Bourgeois became the first woman to write a scholarly book on
obstetrics, *Observations diverses sur la stérilité, perte de fruits, fécondité,
accouchements et maladies des femmes et enfants nouveaux-nés* (*Various
Observations on the Sterility, Fruit loss, Fertility, Childbirth and Diseases of Women
and Newborn Infants*), published in 1609 – but the encroachment of men
into the traditionally female world of the midwife continued, giving
rise to the term "man-midwife", or *accoucheur*, in French. Historical
accounts from the Netherlands tell of how the local surgeons' guild
organized midwife training under its appointed *accoucheur*, whom the

midwife had to call for professional advice if birth complications arose. Midwives' status was eroded and numbers fell. The Dutch city of Leiden was typical in having only ten active midwives on its registers during the 17th century, a number that halved during the 18th century.

In the first half of the 1700s, obstetric forceps, which fitted around the baby's head to make delivery easier, became widely available, largely thanks to Scottish obstetrician William Smellie. Smellie trained in Glasgow, Paris, and London. He greatly improved knowledge of labour and showed how forceps could be used to deliver a baby safely, even if the mother's life was not threatened. This shifted the emphasis towards saving the lives of both mother and infant, rather than just the infant.

MAN-MIDWIFE
In the 18th century, cartoonists caricatured the male midwife, or man-midwife, as a half-male, half-female figure.

CAESAREAN CHILDBIRTH
Before the introduction of anaesthetics and
antiseptic surgical techniques in the 19th
century, Caesarean childbirth was extremely
risky for the mother. This woodcut shows the
operation being performed in the 16th century.

Jonas Arnold
Delineavit

He published widely, including *A Treatise on the Theory and Practice of Midwifery,* which appeared in the 1750s. The vaginal speculum, which had existed since at least Roman times (see pp.46–47), also came into greater use in the 18th century. It permits an interior view of the vagina, particularly during childbirth. Again, it was an instrument for the obstetrician rather than the midwife – one benefit being that the doctor had less need to touch a woman's genital area.

By now, queens and other aristocratic women were requesting the obstetric services of male doctors, exacerbating the trend away from midwives. The shift in birth patterns from home to hospital also played into the hands of obstetricians. Some members of the medical establishment even suggested that midwifery should be abolished. In 1842, the renowned British medical weekly *The Lancet* carried a letter stating: "It is notorious that the attendance of midwives… is in many respects positively injurious, and in numberless cases women would be much safer if intrusted entirely to nature". The same attitudes were spreading across several other European countries and North America.

Around this time, Hungarian doctor Ignaz Semmelweis was working in obstetrics at Vienna General Hospital. He puzzled over the pattern of cases for the common and dreaded "childbed fever" – puerperal fever, now known to be a bacterial infection. One clinic in particular had an unusually high incidence. In 1847, Semmelweis reasoned that "cadaverous matter" could be the cause, since those staffing the high-incidence clinic were medical students, who often came from autopsies, cadaver dissections, and other similar duties. Semmelweis recommended that students clean their hands with a chlorine-based handwash – and the effects were immediate. Within a year, cases of puerperal fever in the clinic plummeted, a fact that helped establish the germ theory of disease (see pp.222–27), and the use of antiseptics in hospitals (see pp.206–13). In 1860, Florence Nightingale founded the first modern-style school of nursing (see pp.188–93). Midwives received similar recognition in

"… midwives ought to be… sober, patient, and discreet, free from external deformity…"

WILLIAM SMELLIE

**A MIDWIFE
ON CALL**
A female midwife
transports an
analgesic gas-air
machine on the
back of her bicycle
in 1938. At the time,
men still dominated
both obstetrics
and midwifery.

1881, when wealthy Russian-born philanthropist Louisa Hubbard set
up the Midwives' Institute, which aimed to "raise the efficiency and
improve the status of midwives and to petition parliament for their
recognition". In 1902, the Midwives Act in England and Wales made
midwifery an established profession, complete with systems of
supervised training, certification, and registration. The profession
was still dominated by men, but it was now illegal for anyone to
practise as a midwife without qualification.

Internationally, midwifery progressed in different ways. In the
Netherlands, it benefited from having training schools much earlier
than elsewhere in Europe, so it avoided being marginalized; the first
Dutch training school was established in 1861. French midwives
gained considerable status, being allowed to diagnose and treat a wide
range of conditions. The American College of Nurse-Midwifery was
chartered in 1955. By the mid-20th century, the profession had a
sound footing in most developed nations, ensuring the future well-
being of mothers and babies alike.

The Germ Theory of Disease

DISCOVERIES ABOUT BACTERIA and other disease-causing micro-organisms multiplied almost as fast as bacteria themselves in the late 19th century. Scientific researchers peering into microsocopes recorded all sorts of new bacteria, yeasts, protozoa (single-celled, animal-like organisms), micro-worms, and others. Microbes were grown or cultured, fixed, and preserved in new ways, and they could now be coloured or stained for easier study. These tiny life forms gained a new significance as their roles in fermentation, decomposition, disease, and the whole of the natural world became apparent. Along with Louis Pasteur (see pp.196–203), a key founder of bacteriology was hard-working German physician and microscopist Robert Koch. Although the two scientists had much in common, they soon took strenuously against each other. Mirroring the political rivalry of France and Germany at the time, their battles were conducted chiefly through the medical press. While Koch insulted Pasteur's "poor methods", Pasteur retaliated by accusing Koch of being "a debtor of French Science". But whatever Pasteur's opinion, there is no doubt that Koch made colossal leaps in the field of medical microbiology.

Born and raised in Clausthal, northwest Germany, Robert Koch studied medicine at the University of Göttingen and qualified with distinction in 1866. Koch's career would soon lead him away from treating people to his main passion – microbes. He was doubtless inspired by the professor of anatomy at Göttingen, Jacob Henle, who had conjectured in 1840 that certain diseases were caused by parasitic organisms (see p.198). After several hospital and general practice jobs, Koch volunteered for medical duties in the Franco-Prussian War. He moved to Wollstein

ROBERT KOCH
Koch was famous for his pioneering work on anthrax and cholera, and for identifying the germ that causes human tuberculosis.

(now Wolsztyn, Poland) in 1872, as District Medical Officer. Between his official duties, Koch worked on his research at home. His wife, Emmy, had given him a microscope as a present; the rest of his equipment he begged or improvised. It was here, in his cramped, home-made laboratory, that Koch made his first set of radical findings – on anthrax.

In 1850, French physicians Pierre Rayer and Casimir Davaine had observed microbes in the blood of diseased sheep; German doctor Aloys Pollender had seen "staff-shaped little bodies" a year earlier. No one really knew if these microbes were the cause of the disease, a side effect, or a result of it. More than a decade later, Davaine showed that transferring infected blood between animals also transferred the disease, anthrax. Anthrax was a real problem at the time, with regular outbreaks among livestock, and the occasional but serious human case. Even isolating animal herds did not work because the disease seemed to pop up at any time. Koch decided to investigate. Using improvised splinters of wood, he inoculated mice with samples from the spleens of healthy and diseased farm animals. Those inoculated with diseased samples developed anthrax, but those inoculated with healthy samples did not, confirming that the disease can be transmitted by blood. Koch then set about purifying the microbes and growing them away from host animals, in a laboratory culture created using the fluid from the inside of ox eyeballs. Over the course of his career, he would try a host of different nutrient substances for breeding bacteria, from potato slices to meat broth, eggs, bread, and seaweed extracts. Koch also pioneered photography through the microscope, testing the technique with the anthrax germs, and he invented ways to add pigmented substances – stains to colour microbes, making them easier to identify.

Koch grew multiple generations of anthrax microbes, noting that when they were put into animals, they still caused anthrax. He also observed that in less favourable conditions, each microbe seemed to form inside itself a rounded object. This resisted adverse conditions such as heat, cold, dryness, and lack of oxygen; as conditions improved, the object – an endospore – gave rise to the bacterium again. This explained how anthrax could suddenly reappear in livestock that had had no contact with infected animals: the endospores survived in the soil. In 1876, Koch demonstrated his work to a number of eminent scientists, including botanist and microbiologist Ferdinand Cohn, who had already studied the anthrax

BOTTLED GERMS
These samples of
different bacteria were
recorded by Ferdinand
Hueppe, one of Koch's
co-workers. Figures 7
and 8 show the
tuberculosis culture.

FIG. 5   FIG. 6   FIG. 7   FIG. 8

microbe *Bacillus anthracis*. The word *Bacillus* stems from the Latin for a small staff, stick, or wand, indicating the bacterium's rod-like shape; *anthracis* comes from the Latin for coal or anthracite, and refers to the areas of dead, dark skin in some forms of the disease. Koch explained his findings about the microbe's life cycle and transmission, and control measures. Cohn was impressed and arranged publication, to great acclaim. It was another great step for the germ theorists, while the supporters of spontaneous generation and miasma (see p.196) had been dealt a further crushing blow.

Koch moved to the Imperial Health Bureau in Berlin in 1880. Later in the decade, he devised a set of conditions known as Koch's postulates – a set of criteria used to establish that a microbe causes disease. Over time, he would apply these to each new germ he discovered. Koch's postulates can be summarized in four points: an infected organism (plant, animal) or tissue contains the microbes in question in abundance, while healthy ones do not; the microbes must be isolated from infected organisms or tissues and grown as pure cultures; when the cultured microbes are introduced into a healthy organism, that organism develops the disease; and lastly, these "second generation" microbes are extracted and isolated again, and shown to be identical to the original microbes. With his postulates, Koch was trying to ascertain whether the microbe and the disease were inseparable. But medicine is never so clear-cut. For instance, some humans or animals are "carriers" of a disease – outwardly healthy with few or no symptoms, while their bodies are reservoirs of the germs to pass to others. So, rather than absolute rules, Koch's postulates became an ideal set of criteria, and remain as such today.

In Berlin, Koch finally had a proper laboratory, with assistants, and it marked the start of his second great phase of work, on tuberculosis. He and his team continued to develop new methods and techniques: a significant innovation in about 1881 was the growth of microbes on a jelly-like nutrient substance, gel agar, using agar-agar extracted from seaweed. The microbes grew visibly in small patches that could be conveniently accessed – far better than swishing around in nutrient broth or buried deep in test-tubes. This method was developed by one of Koch's assistants, Walther Hesse, whose wife Angelina had suggested including agar as a gelling agent after making jellies and jams. Another of Koch's assistants, Julius Richard Petri, gave his name to his invention – Petri dishes. The agar was spread on these shallow, circular glass plates with close-fitting lids, so the microbes within could be easily observed. Both agar and Petri dishes are still used in experiments worldwide.

By now, Koch was on the trail of the germ that caused one of the world's most common, long-term, and often deadly diseases – tuberculosis. This germ is smaller than its anthrax counterpart, and also reacts differently to coloured stains. The work was detailed and painstaking. On 24 March 1882, a triumphant Koch announced that he and his team had found and identified the germ, tubercle bacillus: "If the importance of a disease for mankind is measured by the number of fatalities it causes, then tuberculosis must be considered much more important than those most feared infectious diseases, plague, cholera, and the like". Koch went on to describe his new staining methods and other techniques, and explain how he used guinea pigs as experimental laboratory animals, as well as studying tissues from humans, apes, and

PROPORTION OF ALL DEATHS IN EUROPE IN THE 19TH CENTURY DUE TO TUBERCULOSIS

25%

farm animals. The germs were taken from one animal source, grown in culture, and put into other animals, each time causing tuberculosis. For added proof, Koch produced microscopes, glass slides with stained microbe cultures, jars with tissue samples, and other equipment, so that members of the audience could see for themselves. Within a month, the news had spread across Europe, followed by North America, Africa, and Asia. Initially known as Koch's bacillus, the microbe is now called *Mycobacterium tuberculosis*.

Next, Koch turned his attention to the cholera germ. In 1883, he was sent by the government as Leader of the German Cholera Commission to study an outbreak in Alexandria, Egypt. There, he identified a suspicious, comma-shaped bacterium. Another trip took him to India, where he continued his investigations. Eventually, he was able to pinpoint the causative germ. He described its spread – through contaminated drinking water and contaminated food (see pp.180–87) – and recommended prevention and control measures. These achievements earned Koch a huge reward of 100,000 Deutschmarks and further boosted his global reputation. The cholera microbe – since named *Vibrio cholerae* – had, in fact, been discovered almost 30 years earlier, in 1854, by Italian anatomist Filippo Pacini. But the germ theory of disease was so unfashionable then that Pacini's achievements went unrecognized.

After his epochal work with anthrax, tuberculosis, and cholera, Koch finally stumbled. In 1890, amid great fanfare, he introduced tuberculin – a remedy for tuberculosis. He refused to disclose its origins and said it had been tested on animals. Initial reports from human trials were positive, but tuberculin induced severe reactions in some – and death in others. This so-called cure was anything but; Koch admitted that tuberculin was a particular extract of the bacteria, but he was unable to describe its exact contents. Public opinion swung against him. Matters worsened when it became known that he was financially involved with the tuberculin producers, even though his research was government-paid. Having drifted apart from his wife, his new relationship with teenager Hedwig Freiberg did not help. Koch left the country and embarked on his travels once again. He visited Italy, Africa, India, and New Guinea, studying bubonic plague, leprosy, malaria, rabies, and exotic fevers in humans and livestock. In 1897, he presented a new version of tuberculin; this too failed, but it would in time make a useful diagnostic test for tuberculosis. An

MOTHER CARE, 1918
This poster was produced by the American Red
Cross to raise awareness of child mortality rates
from diseases such as tuberculosis.

effective vaccine against tuberculosis in humans was finally
developed in the 1920s – ironically at the Institut Pasteur, founded
by Koch's great rival Louis Pasteur.

Despite his later failures, Koch had inspired a new wave of medical
research into germs and infection. His students included Friedrich
Loeffler, who identified and cultivated the diphtheria germ in 1884;
Kitasato Shibasaburo, who was also involved with diphtheria, and
who, in 1894, was co-discoverer of the bubonic plague microbe; Emile
von Behring, who was awarded the first Nobel Prize in Physiology or
Medicine in 1901 for his work on diphtheria; August von Wassermann,
who formulated a diagnostic test for early syphilis infection in 1906;
and Paul Ehrlich, who discovered the anti-syphilitic drug
arsphenamine (Salvarsan) in 1909. In 1905, Robert Koch received the
Nobel Prize in Physiology or Medicine for "his investigations and
discoveries in relation to tuberculosis". It was a testament to his
groundbreaking discoveries, which were fuelled by his ceaseless work
ethic. A motto he had attached to a prize-winning essay at medical
school read *Nunquam Otiosus* – Never Idle.

Viruses in Action

Viruses are tiny infectious particles – about a thousand times smaller than bacteria – which can only be seen with an electron microscope. Each particle contains a set of instructions on how to make thousands of identical copies of itself. There are millions of different viruses and they cause illnesses ranging in strength from the common cold and flu to deadly diseases such as AIDs, polio, and hepatitis.

Viruses lie in the environment, waiting to invade bacteria, plants, and animals. They can be spread in the air, in fluids, or via insects. Antibiotics have no effect on viruses, but vaccination (see pp.286–93) can help to provide immunity against some of them.

Dmitri Ivanovsky

In 1890, Russian biologist Dmitri Ivanovsky went to the Crimea to study a disease in tobacco plants. He crushed infected tobacco leaves and passed an extract through a filter with microscopic holes that would exclude bacteria. Yet he found that the source of the infection was still present: he had discovered something infectious that was even smaller than bacteria – a virus.

IVANOVSKY IS CONSIDERED ONE OF THE FATHERS OF VIROLOGY

HOW A VIRUS WORKS

A virus has no cells of its own, so in order to live and make more viruses, it has to invade a cell of a bacterium, plant, or animal and take over its replication mechanism. The virus usually kills the host cell in the process.

1 Attachment – the virus binds to the cell membrane of the host cell

Host cell

3 Replication – the virus's genetic material enters the nucleus of the host cell

2 Penetration – the virus enters the cell, and its casing breaks down to release the genetic material inside

Host nucleus

Virus shapes

In 1931, the electron microscope was invented in Germany, and by the end of the decade German physician Helmut Ruska was using it to examine viruses. Scientists soon established the basic structure of a virus. They found that viruses vary enormously in form and structure, to enable them to target and penetrate the right host cells, and resist attack from the host organism's immune system. Four main virus shapes have been identified.

ICOSAHEDRAL
Many animal viruses take the form of a polyhedron.

SPIRAL-HELICAL
Some viruses have a casing in the shape of a helix.

COMPLEX
Complex viruses show variations to the casing, such as a "tail".

ENVELOPED
Some viruses coat themselves in the host-cell membrane.

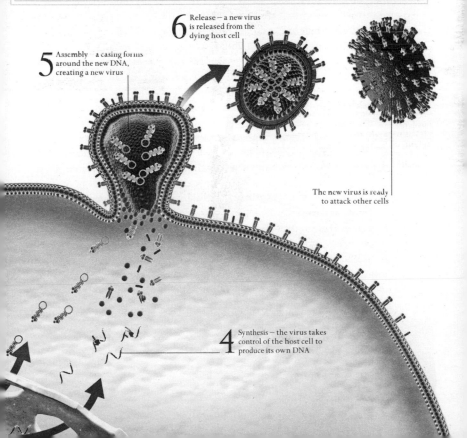

5 Assembly – a casing forms around the new DNA, creating a new virus

6 Release – a new virus is released from the dying host cell

The new virus is ready to attack other cells

4 Synthesis – the virus takes control of the host cell to produce its own DNA

Medicine and the Mind

THE NAMES OF CONDITIONS HAVE CHANGED, but mental illness has been with us throughout history, and may have been one of the reasons for the earliest form of Stone Age surgery – trepanning (see pp.20–21). In early civilizations, mental disorders were generally seen as punishments from the gods, and were sometimes linked to the phases of the Moon – hence the term "lunatic". The sufferer tended to be the family's responsibility, which often brought shame and stigmatization, and there was little in the way of treatment, other than a calming environment and some soothing herbs and minerals. At best, if the disorder was brief and episodic, the sufferer could be considered to be a conduit through which the gods could communicate their prophecies and decisions – at worst, he or she might be physically restrained or isolated. In Mesopotamia and Egypt, priest-physicians performed ritual incantations and sacrifices to rid the sufferer of demons, and in Babylon, patients were encouraged to sing, dance, and paint to purge themselves of evil. This supernatural view of mental illness held sway in many societies for millennia, and in some parts of the world it even persists today.

In Greece, 2,300 years ago, the physician Hippocrates (see pp.30–39) had other ideas. He suggested that mental problems were rooted entirely in the body, particularly in the balance of the four humours (see pp.106–107). Slight humoral disparities between people generated the normal range of human personalities, it was thought, but a marked imbalance in a single individual could result in mental disturbance. Hippocrates described several conditions that we recognize today, including paranoia, mania, and depression – the latter known as melancholia, since it was believed to be caused by an excess of the black bile humour, called melanchole. As ever, Hippocrates recommended gentle remedies for melancholia, such as calm, quiet surroundings and relaxing herbal potions. Galen of Ancient Rome (see pp.40–45), whose medicine endured throughout the Middle Ages, followed the Hippocratic trend, although he tended to focus on major symptoms rather than overall conditions. The traditional Ayurvedic medicine of India (see pp.74–81) has a version of humoral theory in which an imbalance in the fluid-like doshas can lead to mental problems. In Ancient China, texts such as the *Huang-di Nei'Jing* (see pp.64–68) advocated treatment by negating a

REMOVING THE STONE OF MADNESS
Trepanning – boring holes into the skull
– has been practised throughout history
as a way of surgically alleviating madness.

mental condition with opposing moods or emotions – so a person with depression might receive gifts and treats, while anxiety could respond to intense support and reassurance.

Societies that emphasized respect for the family and the honour of ancestry were extra-sensitive to the indignity and dishonour of mental disorders. Suspicions that such illnesses might be contagious or run in the family could lead to the isolation of a family within the community. In China, for instance, sufferers were quietly removed from public life, and often hidden, or even abandoned. These attitudes hardened in Europe during the Middle Ages as the stigmatization of the mentally ill increased. Despite Christianity urging goodwill to all people, sufferers who were too difficult to care for in the family risked being abused, beaten, and locked up. The lucky ones were taken in by monasteries and convents – others found their way into workhouses or general hospitals, survived on charity, or undertook the most lowly, menial tasks to earn a crust. All kinds of quacks and charlatans offered treatments, including protective charms and amulets that were worn to relieve, or prevent the onset of, various mental illnesses. Worn around the neck or forehead, these amulets bore biblical images or quotations, and were adorned with therapeutic herbs such as Saint John's wort. Their power relied on the wearer reciting prayers and chants, frequenting church, and making pilgrimages to saints' shrines.

Thoughtful, humane treatment of the mentally ill emerged during the Golden Age of Islam (see pp.100–105). As the Qur'an states: "Do not give to [those weak of understanding] their property that God has assigned you to manage: provide them and clothe them out of it, and speak to them honourable words". In the 8th century, soon after Baghdad was founded, a hospital ward was put aside for such patients, and similar facilities were set up in Fez, Cairo, Damascus, and Aleppo over the next few centuries. However, this more enlightened attitude spread only sporadically across Asia – it was unusual in cities, and even rarer in rural areas. In Europe, from the 15th century, events took a different

PROTECTION AGAINST EVIL
Amulets bearing biblical images were worn throughout Christendom to protect against all kinds of mental and physical illness.

LUNATICS' TOWER
Vienna's fortress-like Narrenturm (Lunatics'
Tower), built in 1874, had 139 cells in which
the mentally ill were incarcerated.

turn. Sufferers who were not cared for by a family, religious order, or
charity were gathered together into asylums. One of the first of these
was established in Valencia, Spain in around 1410. More asylums
followed in Spain and throughout Europe, notably La Maison de
Charenton in Paris, in the early 1640s, and the Narrenturm (Lunatics'
Tower) in Vienna, 1784. So began a notorious period in which the
mentally ill suffered all kinds of horror and degradation. Visitors told of
barbaric conditions, neglect, and cruelty. In crowded, cold, dark,
stinking rooms, which were often worse than prison cells, the sick were
manacled, or shackled, or put in stocks and left for days at a time.
Clothes, food, cleanliness, and sanitation were desperately inadequate.
Asylums also became dumping grounds for criminals (both sane and
insane), syphilis sufferers, and the rest of society's unwanted.

   Treatments, if any, were harsher than ever before. Under the humoral
view of mental illness, ways to restore a sound body and mind included
purging with emetics and laxatives, cupping, blistering, and bloodletting
(see pp.132–33), the favoured treat-all. Bloodletting from the jugular
vein in the neck removed blood that came directly from the brain, which
was thought to contain the worst humoral imbalance. Drenching in

HUMANE TREATMENT OF THE SICK
Pioneering doctor Philippe Pinel releases the
mentally ill from their chains at the Hospice
de la Salpêtrière for women, Paris, in the 1790s.

scalding or icy water, subjection to deafening noises, whipping, hanging
by the arms or the feet, starving, burning with acids and other chemicals,
semi-suffocation, and semi-drowning – almost every form of torture
was tried in the name of therapy. Many of these "madhouses", as they
were known, were paid for and run by the state, but some, most
notoriously in Britain, were privately owned. Families paid to have their
mentally ill relatives incarcerated, and the owners grew rich as greed
produced ever-worsening conditions. One profitable sideline was
charging the public to view these "inmates" and their antics. Infamous
for this was London's "Bedlam", as the St Mary Bethlehem hospital, or
Bethlem, came to be known. French traveller and letter-writer César de
Saussure wrote of Bethlem in 1725: "On the second floor is a corridor…
reserved for dangerous maniacs, most of them being chained and
terrible to behold. On holidays numerous persons of both sexes, but
belonging generally to the lower classes, visit this hospital and amuse
themselves watching these unfortunate wretches, who often give them
cause for laughter". The hospital itself, now regarded as a pioneering
institution, moved premises several times, and continues today as the
Bethlem Royal Hospital near London.

Despite – or perhaps because of – such horrors, attitudes gradually changed. Public visiting at Bethlem ceased around 1770, and in 1793, French doctor Philippe Pinel took over L'Hôpital Bicêtre, an asylum for men in Paris, inaugurating an era in which the mentally ill began to be treated more humanely. According to Pinel, residents of asylums should be called patients, rather than inmates, and should be given normal food and clothing, as well as sunlight and fresh air, rather than dank darkness. In 1794, he read out his paper titled *Memoir on Madness* to the Paris Natural History Society, in which he explained his "psychologic treatment" and belief that mental illnesses could be cured. He urged physicians to spend time with their patients, to interview them, and to take notes and write case histories, which should include a record of any events that precipitated their patients' conditions. Of the severely mentally ill he noted: "I cannot here avoid giving my most decided suffrage in favour of the moral qualities of maniacs. I have no where met... fonder husbands, more affectionate parents... than in the lunatic asylum, during their intervals of calmness and reason". *Memoir on Madness* was one of the earliest works of what we now call psychiatry – the diagnosis, treatment, and prevention of mental illness.

SPECTATORS VISITING BETHLEM EACH WEEK BEFORE 1770

2,000

In 1795, Pinel assumed the role of chief physician at the huge Hospice de la Salpêtrière for women, and continued to apply his philosophy. At Bicêtre, he had been greatly helped by the hospital's like-minded superintendent, Jean-Baptiste Pussin. In 1797, Pussin decreed that patients, except in extreme cases, should no longer be chained, and soon after that he joined Pinel at Salpêtrière. In 1804, Pinel was elected to the French Academy of Sciences and became a founding member of the Academy of Medicine in 1820. His work *Nosographie* concerned the medical field of nosology (the classification of diseases), while his *Traité Médico-Philosophique sur l'Aliénation Mentale* (*Medical-Philosophical Treatise on Mental Alienation*) furthered his "psychologic approach".

Advances were also made in other areas. In the mid-19th century, outstanding French physician Jean-Martin Charcot laid the foundations of neurology, the study of the nervous system, which had particular relevance to psychiatric disorders. In Italy, in the late 1780s, physician Vincenzo Chiarugi had instituted improved

"You never saw a very busy person who was unhappy"

DOROTHY DIX

conditions at Santa Dorotea Hospital and then at San Bonifacio Hospital, both in Florence. In 1796, in England, William Tuke, a Quaker and well-to-do merchant dealing in teas and coffees, had set up the York Retreat, a charitable organization that provided a humane environment for the mentally ill. Others joined the movement for reform, which became known as *traitement moral*, or moral management, since it emphasized moral virtue and religious duty in its treatments. After visiting England and experiencing these Quaker-inspired reforms, teacher and American campaigner Dorothea Dix returned to the US in 1840 and pushed long and hard for change, establishing a movement that became known as the "mental hygiene movement".

Back in the 1770s, hopes for a radical new way of treating mental disorders had risen with the "animal magnetism" movement of Franz Anton Mesmer, who believed that there was a "life energy" in each individual that could be passed to the sick through a Christian-style "laying on of hands". This idea gained popularity and spawned offshoots such as hypnosis, but it faded from the science-based medical community by the early 20th century. Phrenology came to the fore in the early 19th century with the work of German physician Franz Joseph Gall. This involved feeling and measuring the contours of the skull to determine the sizes and relative development of the brain regions or "organs" underneath. Each brain "organ" controlled a particular mental, intellectual, or moral faculty. Neurology has since shown that regions of the brain are indeed specialized, but not in the way phrenology proposed. Despite its phenomenal popularity, it had no scientific basis, and by about 1900 it too had drifted out of conventional medicine.

Another chapter opened in 1895, when Austrian physicians Josef Breuer and Sigmund Freud published *Studies in Hysteria*. They described a new form of therapy, called psychoanalysis, which Freud developed in detail over the coming decades. *Studies in Hysteria* investigated several women with a condition then called hysteria. Patient "Anna O" had symptoms including a nervous cough, disordered vision and hearing, partial right-side paralysis, and fainting. In conversation, Breuer and

Anna talked about all the possible causes of her condition, and she recalled events from her youth, some traumatic. One technique that Breuer used was "free association", in which the patient said anything that came to mind, and then – guided by the doctor – spoke about what it might mean or symbolize. It was treatment simply by talking.

Freud developed these and other techniques into his own brand of psychoanalysis, according to which the most important events of a patient's life happened in childhood and have since been repressed. Freud also proposed three basic components to the mind: the "id" was in effect the unconscious – the realm of the primal sexual and aggressive drives; the "superego", both conscious and unconscious, resisted the id and tried to exert a civilizing effect; the "ego" mediated between the two, balancing basic desires with social acceptance. Conflict between these elements of the mind, or psyche, could trigger mental problems, and delving into the unconscious to expose its deep-seated content was part of treatment. Techniques for access to the unconscious included analysing dreams, or working through fantasies, as described in *The Interpretation of Dreams* (1900), and *The Psychopathology of Everyday Life* (1901).

During this time, asylum conditions were improving and the number of asylums grew rapidly, especially in the West. In the USA, the number of people in asylums increased from some 40,000 in 1880 to more than 250,000 in 1900. This led to the increasing problem of institutionalization. New treatments for mental illness continued to surface, including insulin shock therapy, lobotomy, electroconvulsive ("electroshock") therapy, and the administration of chlorpromazine and other antipsychotic drugs. As for "talking cures", psychoanalysis had its supporters and detractors. Inspired or alarmed by Freud, others developed alternative systems, such as the individual psychology of Alfred Adler and the analytical psychiatry of Carl Jung. Their ideas still provoke debate, even as millions of people daily consult their "analysts" for help with mental health problems today.

SIGMUND FREUD
The founding father of psychoanalysis, Freud believed that many mental disorders were caused by the suppression of childhood traumas.

"SCENE IN BEDLAM"
Satirist William Hogarth depicted Bedlam in his
1730s series *A Rake's Progress*, as the resting place of
the disgraced hero. In the background, well-
dressed visitors amuse themselves at the antics
of the insane, as was customary at the time.

Modern
Medicine
1920–2000

Medicine took giant strides through the 20th century. An early breakthrough was Karl Landsteiner's work on blood groups, which helped emergency treatment and surgery of all kinds. In 1921 and 1922, Frederick Banting and his team in Toronto started insulin treatment for diabetes and, a few years later, Alexander Fleming noticed mouldy growths contaminating his bacterial samples. The "culprit" was penicillin, but it took the pressures of World War II to ensure that this first antibiotic was mass-produced.

Just after this came the first major inroads of chemotherapy into cancers. The vaccine for polio put it on the growing list of preventable diseases that already included smallpox, diphtheria, tuberculosis, and influenza. Urgent vaccine research continues for diseases that threaten globally, from the old enemy malaria to serious infections that have recently emerged, especially HIV/AIDS. Elsewhere, immunosuppressant drugs led to greater success for transplanted organs – in 1967, South African surgeon Christiaan Barnard shook the world with the first heart transplant. Medical technology and biomechanics also made the headlines. John Charnley's work brought artificial hips to millions and, in 1969, the world reeled at more heart news, this time of a (temporary) artificial implant. From the 1970s, CT, MRI, and other computerized scanners created new generations of body images.

The work of pioneer geriatricians such as Marjory Warren, and Cicely Saunders' founding of the modern hospice movement, transformed the end of life for elderly and terminally ill patients. In 1978, there was a new approach to the start to life too, with Patrick Steptoe, Robert Edwards, and the first test-tube IVF babies.

Blood Groups and the Sugar Disease

MOST BLOOD LOOKS THE SAME – whether from humans or animals – so early physicians wondered whether it was possible to replace lost blood with blood from another living being, and in particular, whether blood from animals could be used as transfusions for humans. After William Harvey's discovery of blood circulation in 1628 (see pp.134–43), physicians started to experiment with blood transfusion. In 1665, English physician Richard Lower demonstrated that blood could be transferred between two dogs, and in 1667, French physician Jean-Baptiste Denys infused lamb's blood into a feverish teenage boy. Denys carried out several more animal-to-human transfusions, until he was charged with murder after the death of his fourth patient. Later that year, Lower and Edmund King attempted the first animal-to-human blood transfer in England, on "freakish" scholar Arthur Coga, observed by Samuel Pepys. Coga's brain "was sometimes a little too warm", according to King, and the aim of the experiment was to cool it with lamb's blood. Similar experiments were conducted in Italy. One problem was that as soon as blood was exposed to air, it clotted. With no way of preventing this, early transfers were made directly along a tube from one body to the other. That these

ANIMAL-TO-HUMAN BLOOD TRANSFUSION
In England and France, transfusion was attempted from both lambs and calves, as shown in this engraving based on a drawing of 1679.

early transfusions succeeded at all – without any knowledge of anticoagulants, blood groups, or modern procedures – was probably due to the small amounts of blood involved. But the frequency of deaths led to experimental transfusions being prohibited in France, England, and Italy, and they were abandoned for 150 years.

Experiments began again in around 1820, when London obstetrician James Blundell attempted transfusions to save new mothers from excessive bleeding during or after childbirth (puerperal or postpartum haemorrhage). Blundell rigged up human donors – often the husband standing by the bedside – whose blood was transfused along tubes to the patient. He also experimented with transferring blood using syringes or containers. The results were mixed: some patients died and others survived. This was sufficiently encouraging for physicians to try new methods of transferring blood, using hand-squeezed rubber bulbs, pumps, stopcocks, and adding ingenious valves to tubes. Others attempted to forestall clotting by diluting blood with saline solution (saltwater) or mixing it with other chemicals. However, results remained stubbornly inconsistent.

Then, in the mid-1870s, German physiologist Leonard Landois made a breakthrough regarding blood clotting. Using blood samples, laboratory reagents (substances that force a chemical reaction), and microscopes, he showed that mixing animal blood with human blood made the red blood cells clump together (agglutinate). In some cases, the red cells also ruptured, which may have led to a type of anaemia. A further advance was made by Austrian Karl Landsteiner, who first identified the existence of different blood groups. Landsteiner had qualified in medicine from Vienna University in 1891 and joined research staff at the Vienna Hygiene Institute, one of the university's pathology departments. He was particularly interested in immunity – the way in which a body defended itself against germs, cancerous cells, and "foreign" substances such as allergens – and how it made antibodies to counteract these (see pp.286–91). Immunity also involved the new field of serology – the study of blood serum, which is plasma (the liquid part of blood) with the clotting substances removed.

In around 1900, Landsteiner began experimenting with mixing human blood samples. He observed that red blood cells clumped together and ruptured only when samples from certain individuals were mixed together. He painstakingly tested each blood sample against a range of others in order to determine the effects of each combination. From the results, he deduced that each person had one of three different types or groups of blood – A, B, and C (which we now know as O). Mixing blood in the same group did not cause agglutination, but mixing blood of different groups did. This was because of the different antibodies that each blood group carried in the blood serum. In 1902, a fourth blood group, AB, was identified by Landsteiner's Viennese co-workers, researcher Adriano Sturli and kidney transplant pioneer Alfred von Decastello. Landsteiner refined this work through the 1900s, while another team of researchers, Ludwig Hirszfeld and Emil von Dungern at the Heidelberg Institute for Experimental Cancer Research, demonstrated that blood groups show a pattern of inheritance. Landsteiner had suspected this, and proposed that these patterns could be used to resolve cases of disputed paternity.

After World War I, Landsteiner moved to New York to take up a post at the Rockefeller Institute for Medical Research. His enthusiasm was undimmed as he continued to identify more blood groups – the MN group and P group, both discovered in 1927 in collaboration with Philip Levine. In 1940, along with Alexander Wiener, an innovator in forensic medicine, he helped to discover the rhesus (Rh) factor in blood. This has an indirect connection with the rhesus macaque monkey, a well-known laboratory animal. Rhesus monkey blood mixed with rabbit serum caused agglutination, as did human blood and rabbit serum. The Rh factor is involved in haemolytic disease in newborn babies, in which a baby suffers jaundice, anaemia, and other severe symptoms, due to incompatibility between the Rh factors in the baby's blood and that of its mother.

Landsteiner received the 1930 Nobel Prize in Physiology or Medicine for his 1901 "discovery of human blood groups". The lapse of 29 years reflected the time it had taken to turn his discoveries into practical, life-saving measures. Landsteiner's work paved the way for safer transfusions by matching the blood groups of the donor and the recipient, but two further grouping systems had confused the issue – Czech professor Jan Jansky's I, II, III, and IV groups (equivalent to O, A, B and AB) in 1907, and William Moss's in the US in 1910, which reversed Janksy's I and IV. This nomenclature problem was not resolved until the late 1930s, when the ABO system became standard.

As is often the case with medical advances, it took a massive conflict, in this case World War I, to boost the technology of transfusion. Surgeons discovered that blood could be chilled, and sodium citrate added as an anticoagulant to slow its natural tendency to clot. This overcame the need to have a live donor on the spot. From January 1916, recipients could receive stored blood, which gave medical staff sufficient time to make sure that the blood groups matched. By World War II, blood transfusion was routine, and civilians were called upon to donate blood to treat wounded soldiers.

As Landsteiner was discovering blood groups, another line of research was heading towards a breakthrough in our understanding of how energy is transferred from the blood (in the form of glucose) to the billions of cells around the body. It was discovered that the process was controlled by insulin, a hormone produced in the pancreas, and that disruption of this process led to diabetes – a fatal disease that had already been known to the Ancient Egyptians by 1500 BCE. The full name of the disease, "diabetes mellitus", meaning "to pass honey", was coined by the 2nd-century Greek physician Aretaeus because an early test of the illness was to taste a person's urine for sugar. This sugar, or blood glucose, is the body's main source of energy, and it is replenished by stores from the liver and elsewhere with the help of insulin. In type 1 diabetes, the pancreas is unable to make enough insulin because the body's immune system attacks the beta cells that produce it (as opposed to type 2 diabetes, in which the body becomes insulin-resistant). These beta cells are produced in

IF HE SHOULD FALL

IS YOUR BLOOD THERE TO SAVE HIM?

THE EMERGENCY BLOOD TRANSFUSION SERVICE NEEDS

BLOOD DONORS

GIVE BLOOD!
During World War II, posters were used to call upon civilians to donate blood for soldiers to the blood transfusion service.

a million or so tiny structures in the pancreas called the islets of Langerhans – named after Paul Langerhans, the German medical student who first described them in 1869. Lack of insulin results in cells being unable to take up glucose from the blood, and so ceasing to function properly. The unused glucose then builds up in the blood, a condition known as hyperglycaemia. To provide energy for the body, the liver breaks down fats instead, leading to a dangerous build-up of acidic substances called ketones in the blood (ketoacidosis). This in turn damages tissues and organs and can be severe enough to cause a "diabetic coma". The excess blood glucose is filtered out by the kidneys into the urine (glucose in the urine is called glycosuria) – hence the age-old urine taste test for diagnosing the "sugar disease".

In 1889–90, Lithuanian-born pathologist Oscar Minkowski and German physiologist Joseph von Mering at Strasbourg University first established the vital role that the pancreas plays in glucose regulation, by removing the pancreas from dogs. Over the next 35 years, dogs remained at the forefront of diabetes research. In 1891, American pathologist Eugene Lindsay Opie, who was based at Johns Hopkins University, Baltimore, US, observed that the islets of Langerhans seemed to degenerate in people who had diabetes. A series of experiments showed that if the tube carrying digestive enzymes from the pancreas into the intestine (the pancreatic duct) was ligated (tied), the parts of the pancreas (acini) that made these enzymes deteriorated. The islets of Langerhans, however, remained intact, and glucose did not pass into the urine. These findings focused researchers' attention on the islets themselves.

Today, the term "hormone" is familiar – it refers to chemical substances that circulate in the blood and control the various body processes. The name was originally used in 1905 by British physiologist Ernest Henry Starling, who, with William Maddock Bayliss, had discovered secretin, the first known hormone, in 1902. Another British physiologist, Edward Albert Sharpey-Schafer, had proposed in the 1890s that pancreatic islets might make a substance that affected blood glucose. The hormone concept fitted this idea well and, in 1913, Sharpey-Schafer proposed that the sugar-affecting substance could be called "insuline". In fact, the name "insuline" had been suggested in 1909 by Belgian physiologist Jean de Meyer.

Minkowski and other researchers were already trying to extract and purify the substance produced by the islets. When tested, some extracts did lower blood glucose, but they also had adverse side effects, causing

GLUCOMETER
Invented by Joseph Long,
an instrument-maker in
London, this early glucometer
was used to check a patient's
urine for signs of glucose.

abscesses and fever. In 1920, Canadian
researcher Frederick Banting read
about the link between islets and the
conjectured hormone "insuline". Since the
pancreas made digestive enzymes, he wondered
if the enzymes might be digesting the hormone.
Would the ligated ducts of dogs, in which the enzyme-manufacturing
parts of the pancreas degenerated but the islets did not, yield a purer
extract? He noted, with erratic spelling: "Diabetus. Ligate pancreatic
ducts of dog. Keep dogs alive till acini degenerate leaving islets. Try to
isolate the internal secretion of these to relieve glycosurea".

Banting took his idea to Toronto University's Head of Physiology,
John J. R. Macleod, who was working on glucose and diabetes.
Banting and Macleod did not get along well, but Macleod agreed to
furnish Banting with laboratory facilities, dogs, and an assistant,
Charles Best. In May 1921, Banting and Best set to work, overseen by
Macleod. The pace was rapid – others were chasing the same goal.
The duo tried chemical techniques to purify the hormone extracted
from ligated dog pancreases, and tested it by injecting dogs that had
been made diabetic by having their pancreases removed. Step by step,
their results improved. One dog – known as Marjorie, or lab dog 33
– was kept alive by injections for ten weeks, but the results were
inconsistent. Eventually, Banting and Best refined their methods to
obtain greater yields of the active ingredient, to which they gave the
working name "isletin". However, to their frustration, the research
was delayed by Macleod asking for trials to be repeated – leading to
tension and clashes with Banting. The team knew that dog pancreases
would never yield enough hormone for human use, and devised
techniques to extract it from the pancreases of cows instead.

At last, they felt ready for a human trial. On 11 January 1922, at Toronto General Hospital, the latest cow pancreas extract was injected into 14-year-old diabetic patient Leonard Thompson. The results were sadly disappointing: his blood glucose levels showed only slight improvement and he suffered some side effects. At this point, Canadian biochemist James Bertram Collip joined the team to lend expertise in the extraction process. A week after the first human trial, Collip found an improved way to purify the extract. He injected it into healthy rabbits, and it lowered their blood glucose levels.

A few days later, daily injections of the new extract were given to the same patient – this time with success. Leonard's blood glucose, ketoacidosis, and other features normalized; the side effects were greatly reduced; and his overall condition improved dramatically. Over the following weeks, more young patients at Toronto General Hospital were treated and recovered from diabetic coma, to the delight of staff, family, and friends. The early results were published in March 1922 in the *Canadian Medical Association Journal*: "These results taken together have been such as to leave no doubt that in these extracts we have a therapeutic measure of unquestionable value in the treatment of certain phases of the disease in man". As the project grew, the team produced a more detailed account, presented in May 1922 by Macleod to the Association of American Physicians. They named the active ingredient insulin, unaware that this name had already been suggested. However, there were still many obstacles to surmount: scaling up production, reducing contaminants, standardizing strengths, and working out suitable doses. Pharmaceutical companies came on board: Eli Lilly and Company solved many of the problems, especially how to prepare extracted insulin within a certain acidity range to boost yield and purity. By early 1923, Lilly's facilities were manufacturing enough insulin of sufficient quality to help hundreds, then thousands of people with diabetes. Within two years, type 1 diabetes had been transformed

NUMBER OF PEOPLE WITH DIABETES TODAY

422,000,000

MARJORIE, LAB DOG 33
Frederick Banting (right) and Charles Best
on the roof of the University of Toronto's
Medical Building, with Marjorie, the dog kept
alive for weeks with insulin injections.

from a potentially fatal condition into one in which insulin treatment allowed a normal life.

Sadly, running parallel to this life saving work was a tale of resentment and jealousy. Banting and Macleod never got on and Collip was an uneasy participant. In 1923, the Nobel Prize in Physiology or Medicine was jointly awarded to Macleod and Banting "for the discovery of insulin treatment". Banting was enraged that Best had been excluded and shared his own prize money with him; Macleod did the same with Collip. Other scientists working with insulin also claimed recognition. In later years, the Nobel committee revisited the insulin episode, gave Best fuller credit, and also recognized the prior achievements of Romanian professor of physiology Nicolae Paulescu. He had discovered insulin (or "pancreatine") in cows in 1916, but had not found a way to use it in humans.

Progress in insulin treatment continued. In 1982, human insulin was the first major therapeutic agent produced by recombinant DNA technology, or "genetic engineering" (see pp.338–49), and, by 2000, more than 300 insulin analogues were available – including 70 derived from animals, 80 derived from humans, and 150 synthesised by DNA technology. These various types of insulin, and the sophisticated blood glucose meters now available, have made it possible for doctors to customize treatment and for diabetics to monitor and control their own blood glucose levels more successfully. These advances in diabetes care have greatly improved diabetics' quality of life and significantly increased their life expectancy.

Receiving Blood

Physicians first tried blood transfusions as a treatment in the 17th century, with little success. By the 19th century, scientists suspected that blood differed from one person to another, so before transfusion, they mixed blood from the donor and recipient to see if there was any clotting. By 1902, physician Karl Landsteiner and his team (see pp.243–44) had defined four different human blood groups: A, B, AB, and C (now called O). He realized that transfusion went wrong when antibodies in the recipient's blood – which neutralize foreign bodies – attacked the donated blood, causing a fatal allergic reaction. Today, transfusion is a common and safe procedure, with around 92 million blood donations collected every year.

Tourniquets

Mounting plate

Interchangeable needles

The first transfusions

After William Harvey described blood circulation in 1628 (see pp.134–43), there were some early transfusions, often from animals. Many recipients died as a result. A few survived, either through luck or because only a tiny amount of blood was transfused, which limited the detrimental effects.

CONTEMPORARY ILLUSTRATION FROM AROUND THE 17TH CENTURY SHOWING A MAN RECEIVING A BLOOD TRANSFUSION DIRECTLY FROM AN ANIMAL

Blood groups

The variation in blood groups is due to antibodies and antigens present in the blood. Antibodies – in the plasma – detect unusual or dangerous substances in the body and attack red blood cells that do not match their own. Antigens – found on the surface of the red blood cells – bind with antibodies of the right type. In modern transfusions, patients are given only red blood cells, rather than whole blood, which limits the chance of harmful immune responses.

A antigen

GROUP A
Blood in group A has A antigens and anti-B antibodies. It cannot be given to people with groups B or O.

Anti-B antibody

GROUP B
Blood in group B has B antigens and anti-A antibodies. It cannot be given to those with groups A or O.

B antigen   Anti-A antibody

GROUP AB
Blood in group AB has both A and B antigens, but no antibodies. It can be donated only to people with blood of the same group.

B antigen   A antigen

Anti-B antibody

GROUP O
Group O has no antigens but both anti-A and anti-B antibodies. Group O blood can be donated to people of all groups.

Anti-A antibody

Plunger handle

Central chamber

The plunger is inserted into the top of the central chamber

TRANSFUSION SYRINGE
FRENCH, c.1940
This transfusion apparatus is double-ended, meaning that blood could be transferred directly between donor and recipient. Before the use of "blood banking" and refrigeration in the early 20th century, all transfusions were done person to person.

The First Antibiotic

MOST MEDICAL DISCOVERIES ARE THE FRUITS of diligent and exhaustive research by teams of scientists and physicians. One of the most significant breakthroughs in medical history, however, came about by chance. In 1928, Scottish medical researcher Alexander Fleming returned to his unseasonably cold, messy laboratory from holiday and noticed the strange effects of a patch of mould. He had inadvertently stumbled upon penicillin, the very first antibiotic. The drug would go on to save millions of lives, as it still does today, but it did not come into widespread use until the 1940s. Why was there such a long gap?

The germ-killing properties of moulds have a long history. For centuries, medical experts regarded oozing pus and foul discharge as a sign that the body was expelling noxious material. For centuries too, folk remedies recommended the use of mouldy bread, cakes, or fruit to treat suppurating wounds. Many of these anecdotes could have been referring to the antibiotic effects of the *Penicillium* mould – tiny, unprepossessing fungal cells found in the soil and many other places. In established medicine, sporadic notes by John Tyndall, Louis Pasteur, Joseph Lister, and others had recorded that moulds prevented bacterial infection of laboratory samples and damaged the bacterial cultures they were trying to grow (see pp.201–203). In 1896–97, a young French physician, Ernest Duchesne, went so far as to find that injections of a *Penicillium* mould seemed to counteract the bacterial infection typhoid in laboratory animals. He could not establish a definite correlation, however, so the French medical establishment took no notice and Duchesne was subsequently whisked away on army duty.

The term "antibiotic", meaning "against life", dates only from 1942, when it was first used by US-based microbiologist Selman Waksman (see p.258). It is usually used to refer to agents that act against bacteria, but while plenty of substances, such as hot tar and strong acids, kill bacteria, the term antibiotic is generally reserved for a substance produced by another living thing, often another microbe. The similar term "antibacterial" is usually applied to substances not produced by living processes. These include the sulfonamide (sulfa) drugs, which opened a new era in medicine in the 1930s. They were not antibiotics as they were synthesized in the laboratory, but they were antimicrobials

– a category of substances that kill or inhibit microorganisms. The first sulfonamide on the market was Prontosil, quickly followed by many similar antibacterials before World War II. German bacteriologist Gerhard Domagk was awarded the Nobel Prize in Physiology or Medicine "for the discovery of the antibacterial effects of Prontosil" in 1939 – six years before Fleming and his team were awarded the same prize for pioneering penicillin.

Alexander Fleming grew up in a farming family in Ayrshire, Scotland, where he attended Kilmarnock Academy. At the age of 13, he moved to London to live with his older brother Tom. Alec, as he was known, worked for a shipping company until he inherited a small sum of money from an uncle four years later and decided to follow Tom into medicine. In 1906, he qualified with distinction as a doctor at St Mary's Hospital Medical School, West London. St Mary's was his working home for the rest of his peacetime career. During World War I, Fleming joined the Royal Army Medical Corps. Based at the military hospital in Boulogne, France, he was struck by how many soldiers died from infected wounds. Antiseptics had a limited effect because they could not penetrate deeply enough, and Fleming became convinced that they were in fact harmful to the blood corpuscles that destroyed bacteria.

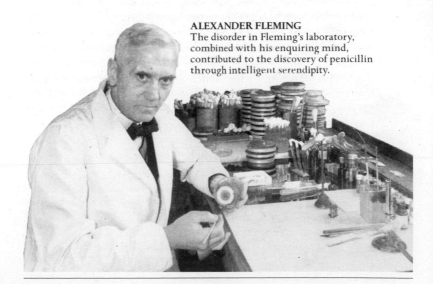

ALEXANDER FLEMING
The disorder in Fleming's laboratory, combined with his enquiring mind, contributed to the discovery of penicillin through intelligent serendipity.

At the end of the war, Fleming returned to to his research post at St Mary's. Encouraged by his mentor, eminent bacteriologist and immunologist Almroth Wright, he started to research bacteria-killers. In 1922–23, he identified a naturally occurring substance that he called lysozyme; this enzyme, found in saliva, tears, mucus, and egg white, had antibacterial effects. Its action, however, was limited and it proved difficult to purify and concentrate.

On Monday 3 September 1928, Fleming returned from a holiday with his family at their residence in Suffolk. Back at work, he set about tidying his laboratory – Fleming was not known for his neatness. He had been working with the bacterium *Staphylococcus*, whose harmful strains cause abscesses, boils, respiratory infections, and food poisoning. Test tubes, flasks, and Petri dishes were put aside in piles, ready for cleaning. Exact accounts of what happened next vary, but while he was chatting to colleague and former research assistant Mervyn Price, Fleming noticed something odd. On one of the dishes where colonies of bacteria were supposed to grow, there was also a colony of mould with a bacteria-free area around it. Something – apparently the mould – had stopped the bacteria from growing. How the mould had arrived on the dish was unclear. Microscopic fungal spores float almost everywhere, but the laboratory windows were fixed shut.

Intrigued, Fleming kept the dish, took samples, and grew them. This was the turning point. A colleague from the mycology unit, Charles La Touche, identified the fungus as a type of *Penicillium*, provisionally *P. rubrum*. In fact, La Touche was also growing moulds, including *Penicillium*, as part of an asthma research project, and the spores may have drifted up from his lab. Fleming embarked on a standard series of experiments to test his findings, refining extracts of the fungus into a broth, which

1950s PENICILLIN
By the 1950s, penicillin was being manufactured on a large scale. British drug companies such as Glaxo, producers of this penicillin, relied on US technology to improve their output.

"One sometimes finds what one is not looking for"

ALEXANDER FLEMING

he called first "mould juice", then penicillin. In 1929, he summarized some of his early results in the report "On the antibacterial action of cultures of a *Penicillium*, with special reference to their use in the isolation of B. *influenzae*", which was published in the *British Journal of Experimental Pathology*.

Penicillin killed or inhibited the growth of many bacteria, including *Staphylococcus* and *Streptococcus*, which were responsible for illnesses that ranged from sore throats to pneumonia. These bacteria were all Gram-positive – they reacted to a dye known as Gram's stain by turning dark blue or purple. Most bacteria harmful to humans are Gram-positive, but some are Gram-negative – they turn pink or red in reaction to Gram's stain. Penicillin seemed largely ineffective against Gram-negative bacteria. Later research demonstrated that penicillin works by damaging the way in which Gram-positive bacteria build their cell wall, so that as each bacterium grows and divides, its weakened cell wall disintegrates, spilling the contents. Gram-negative bacteria, on the other hand, have an additional layer around the cell wall that penicillin is unable to penetrate.

Fleming's early hopes that he had discovered a wonder cure faded. Further investigation showed that penicillin was toxic neither to animals nor humans, which was good. However, it did not remain in the body for long, as it was rapidly excreted in urine; it was hard to obtain and purify, and it tended to deteriorate in storage rather than remaining stable. Furthermore, the mould did not always yield the desired antibacterial substance. Unknown to Fleming, *Penicillium* only does this in adverse conditions, as a survival trick to neutralize bacteria that might compete for the same food source. It was only years later that Fleming's research assistant Ronald Hare demonstrated that a cold spell in August 1928 had stressed the *Penicillium* while Fleming was on holiday, producing the antibiotic effects that he observed. Although the results were not all that Fleming had hoped for, he still thought penicillin might be useful as an antiseptic and it was kept at St Mary's as a useful laboratory "tool" for several years. Because it inhibited some bacteria, but not others, it was helpful in purifying bacterial cultures for research and vaccines. Elsewhere, Cecil Paine, a former student of Fleming's, had some success in curing eye infections with penicillin at Sheffield Royal Infirmary in 1930, but never reported his results. Fleming, in the meantime, began to research other areas, including sulfonamides. As he later admitted in 1940, he "forgot about [penicillin] some years ago".

In 1939, the story shifted to Oxford University, where Howard Florey was Professor of Pathology at Lincoln College. Originally from Australia, Florey had moved to England in 1921, taking up his position at Oxford in 1935. Ernst Boris Chain was also working in pathology there. A chemistry graduate born of Jewish parents in Berlin, he had emigrated to England in 1933 after the Nazis' rise to power. In 1938, Chain took on a project to find out how antibacterial substances worked. With Florey, he read Fleming's work and selected penicillin as a subject. The third key member of the Oxford team was biochemist Norman Heatley, a research associate with an aptitude for laboratory equipment and techniques. Like Fleming, Chain and Florey found penicillin hard to extract and purify. Despite its promise, it yielded only tiny amounts. World War II had started and funding in Britain was scarce, so the research team appealed to the US Rockefeller Foundation for funds. With its support, they had produced enough penicillin by mid-1940 to test on mice; four injected with the antibiotic did not succumb to a lethal dose of *Streptococcus*, whereas four untreated mice died overnight. Work began to standardize dose strength, with all kinds of equipment – milk churns, bottles, rubber and glass tubing – commandeered to grow the moulds.

In February 1941, the first trial of penicillin on a human was carried out, on 43-year-old policeman Albert Alexander. An infected scratch had produced terrible abscesses affecting his face and lungs – the type of infection that is rarely seen today because of antibiotics. Injections of penicillin set him on the road to recovery, but the supply ran out before he was fully cured, and he died. However, out of the next five patients, four recovered. After these results were published in *The Lancet*, the Northern Regional Research Laboratory (NRRL) in Peoria, Illinois, part of the US Department of Agriculture, backed the research. Drug companies Merck, Squibb, Pfizer, Lilly, and Lederle also showed an interest. A search began for higher-yielding strains of *Penicillium*, with fruit and soil samples sent to Peoria from all over the world, especially by the US military. In 1943, a Peoria housewife contributed a mouldy cantaloupe with a huge *Penicillium* yield. Shining ultraviolet light on samples to cause genetic changes increased yields further. Improved ways of growing the mould were also found and companies in the US and the UK were soon producing penicillin on an industrial scale. More supplies and intense demand from the battlefield led to more clinical trials and, in 1944, supplies of penicillin to troops at the D-Day landings dramatically reduced the death toll from infected wounds. Wider use among the military and civilians followed. By the end of the war, enough penicillin was produced each month to treat hundreds of thousands of cases. Fleming, Florey, and Chain were jointly awarded the 1945 Nobel Prize in Physiology or Medicine for their research, and Fleming and Florey were both knighted. Ever modest, Fleming insisted: "I did not invent penicillin. Nature did that. I only discovered it by accident".

The story of antibiotics is not over, but nor is it an entirely happy ending. While penicillin and the drugs developed in its wake are still used all around the world, their effectiveness has been undermined by their inappropriate use for diseases that are viral rather than bacterial, and patients' failure to complete courses of treatment. There are now 150,000 deaths globally every year from multi-drug-resistant tuberculosis, and antibiotic-resistant bacterial illnesses such as the hospital-acquired infection MRSA pose major health issues.

WORLD WAR II POSTER
Treatment of infected war wounds stimulated research into penicillin in the 1940s. Use of the antibiotic reduced deaths from infection in the later stages of the war.

Antibiotics at Work

By the late 19th century, scientists understood that many diseases were caused by bacteria, and researchers tried to find ways of killing these microbes or impeding their growth. In 1928, Alexander Fleming (see pp.252–57) discovered that a *Penicillium* mould inhibited the growth of *Staphylococcus* bacteria. In the early 1940s, a team derived a stable form of the antibiotic penicillin suitable for mass production from the mould, and soon it was being used to treat many diseases, including pneumonia and syphilis. Further types of antibiotics were produced in the 1950s. Scientists classify antibiotics into groups, according to the ways in which they act on the cells of bacteria.

A flagellum acts like a tail to propel the bacterium

Bacterium DNA – the quinolone group of antibiotics stops DNA replicating, so bacteria cannot multiply

Ribosome – streptomycin restricts the bacterium's protein growth by binding to the ribosomes (where protein synthesis occurs). Without proteins, the bacterial cell rapidly dies

Selman Waksman

American microbiologist Selman Waksman came up with the term "antibiotic". In 1943, he and a colleague, Albert Schatz, were working on organisms that live in soil. This led to the production of streptomycin, an antibiotic that proved to be effective against tuberculosis. Waksman's laboratory at Rutgers University in New Jersey synthesized several other antibacterial drugs.

A US CITIZEN FROM 1910, WAKSMAN CAME FROM A PART OF THE RUSSIAN EMPIRE NOW IN UKRAINE

Plasma membrane – the drug polymixin binds to the membrane around bacterial cells, making it permeable: pressure drives water into the bacterium, which eventually kills it

Messenger RNA – rifamycin drugs block RNA, which conveys genetic information to synthesize proteins

Protein, essential for the bacterium to survive

Plasmid ring, a small DNA molecule

Peptoglycan sheet – a mesh-like layer that forms part of the bacterial cell walls; bacteria cannot grow without complete cell walls, so penicillin and several other widely used antibiotics work by preventing bacteria forming the peptoglycan sheet

Pilus (hairy projection) can connect to another bacterium

ANTIBIOTICS IN ACTION
This diagram shows the different actions of some types of antibiotics on a bacterium. These actions include inhibiting the cell's protein growth, interfering with the working of its DNA, preventing the cell wall from developing, and damaging its protective membrane.

How drugs work

Many drugs work by imitating a chemical that controls a particular biological process in the cell. Drugs that stimulate a process are called agonists, while those that supress a process are called antagonists. This was discovered in 1940 with experiments on sulphanilamide, a compound similar to a bacterial nutrient. When introduced to bacteria, it took the place of the nutrient; deprived of the actual nutrient, the bacteria died.

Cell
Body chemical
Cell receptors
Agonist drug in cell receptor stimulates activity

AGONIST DRUGS
Most cell activity is controlled by natural body chemicals that fit into receptors on a cell's surface. An agonist drug can mimic one of these chemicals, triggering the receptors, which in turn stimulate a process inside the cell.

Body chemicals acting on cell
Body chemicals cannot enter receptor
Antagonist drug blocks receptors

ANTAGONIST DRUGS
Antagonist drugs, including antibiotics, also mimic natural body chemicals and fit into receptor sites in the cell. Unlike agonists, they do not trigger the cell's receptors, instead blocking them. As a result, the natural process controlled by the receptors is reduced or stops completely, damaging or killing the cell.

The Fight Against Cancer

ATTITUDES TO ILLNESS CHANGE OVER TIME. In the mid-20th century, cancer was a word to avoid. Public perception and stigma meant knowing glances and hushed whispers, as if the diagnosis were an automatic death sentence. This was far from true then, and even less so today. In the mid-1970s in the US, the five-year relative survival rate (relative to the rest of the population, taking into account that they might have died even without cancer) for adults for all forms of cancer was around 50 per cent. Thirty years later it was approaching 70 per cent. For children, these numbers were 60 per cent and 80 per cent respectively. Other developed nations saw similar improvements. The trend today is for five-year survival rates to increase in some regions by more than one per cent per year – although ageing populations may affect future figures.

Advances in the past half-century include hugely increased understanding of cancers, groundbreaking discoveries about their causes, the boon of earlier diagnosis, and a wider range of improved treatments. In 2012, the American Cancer Society stated: "Scientists have learned more about cancer in the last two decades than had been learned in all the centuries preceding."

There are more than 200 different types of cancer. Underlying them all are microscopic cells multiplying out of control to form tumours (growths) that are malignant – that is, they have the potential to spread to other parts of the body. In a healthy body, each type of cell continually divides to make more of its kind in a controlled, organized manner. In the small intestine lining, cell turnover is measured in days; in skin, about one month; in the pancreas, a year or two. When cells become cancerous, they ignore the usual restraints and multiply faster, which can create pressure on neighbouring cells, disrupting how they function. Cancerous cells may fail to carry out their own specialized tasks and start to look more like unspecialized stem cells (see pp.364–69). Unlike the cells of a benign (non-cancerous) tumour, cancer cells can invade adjacent tissues. They can break away from the primary site and travel, usually in the blood or lymph system, to other places where they lodge, continue to multiply, and set up secondary growths. This process, which is so characteristic of cancer, is known as metastasis.

One way of classifying cancers is by their primary site – bone, skin, liver, and so on. Another system is by the types of cell affected, since most organs are made from several kinds of cell and tissue. Lymphomas involve the white blood cells known as lymphocytes (see pp.286–91); carcinomas affect epithelial cells, which form the coverings and linings of body parts and organs; sarcomas affect the connective tissues, such as bone, cartilage, and muscle; and melanomas derive from pigment-making skin cells known as melanocytes. Such details about cancer were unknown until the invention of the microscope made it possible to study cells and tissues and then, in the mid-19th century, cellular pathology

METASTASIS IN THE SPINE
This scan shows a malignant secondary tumour (grey mass, centre-right) on a disc between two thoracic (middle) vertebrae.

(see pp.144–49). Before that, there were only vague notions about what cancers were and how they arose. In ancient Greece and Rome, they were attributed, like most diseases, to an imbalance of the bodily "fluids" called the four humours (see pp.106–107). The term "cancer" (Latin for "crab") arose at this time, probably because Hippocrates and others likened the appearance of some tumours, which had a dense centre and radiating lines of blood vessels, to the shape of a crab's body and legs.

Most cancers occur more frequently with advancing age. In medieval and Renaissance times, people died younger, so cancers were less prominent than today. They were also less well documented. With no knowledge of cancers' common feature – uncontrolled cell proliferation – there were few reasons to link the different kinds of tumour. In the 18th century, indicators of the causes of cancer were first spotted. Italian physician Bernardino Ramazzini, who pioneered occupational medicine with his book *Diseases of Workers*, noted in around 1713 that breast cancer occurred more frequently in nuns than in other groups of women. He speculated that this was linked to lack of sexual activity. The causes of breast cancer are still unclear today, but factors that reduce its likelihood include having children, and having them sooner rather than later. In general, women who have children are about 30 per cent less likely to develop breast cancer than those who do not. In the 1770s, surgeon Percival Pott, at St Bartholomew's Hospital, London, described cancer of the scrotum (the skin bag containing the testes) in chimney sweeps – since classified as a form of skin cancer known as squamous cell carcinoma. It was the first conventional medical report of a carcinogen, a substance that causes or triggers cancer – in this case, soot.

Momentous 19th-century strides in surgery included anaesthesia and antisepsis/asepsis (see pp.206–213). Operations such as surgical removal of tumours grew longer and more complex. Surgeons found that cutting out only the growth could allow recurrence, but removing the surrounding tissues as well, especially lymph glands (channels and nodes), reduced the likelihood of this. Radical surgery developed – excision of the cancerous growth, plus the local blood and lymph supplies, and neighbouring tissues. Professor of Surgery William Stewart Halsted started performing radical mastectomy for breast cancer in the US in the 1880s at Johns Hopkins University, Baltimore (although a surgeon called Bernard Peyrilhe had undertaken the first such operation a century earlier in France). Around 1900, London surgeon Sampson Handley showed that lymph channels were the main route for breast cancer to spread.

The radical approach for breast and other types of cancer continued until the mid-20th century. More conservative operations, removing the tumour alone, guided by sophisticated imaging techniques (see pp.302–311), and supported by drugs and radiotherapy, became the treatment of choice from the 1950s in Europe, and the 1970s in the US.

FRESH HOPE ON CANCER
The cover of *Life* magazine in 1958 heralds radiation therapy as a ray of hope in the search for cancer treatments.

Radiotherapy, in which cancerous tissues are exposed to X-rays, gamma rays, or similar forms of energy, is one of the main forms of cancer treatment today. This treatment dates back to Wilhelm Röntgen's discovery of X-rays in late 1895 (see pp.302–303). Within weeks, doctors noticed that X-raying patients to view their bones also seemed to shrink or obliterate some skin tumours, so they quickly adapted the new X-ray machines for cancer treatment. At first the radiation was given in one massive blast, but it had dire side effects, including skin burns, bleeding from the orifices, pain, inflammation, confusion, hair loss, and fatigue, collectively known as radiation sickness. Worse, new cancers sometimes appeared. The double-edged nature of X-rays became clear – they could kill as well as cure. The X-ray energy damages molecules within cells, including gene-containing DNA, which duplicates itself as each cell divides. Cancer cells generally divide faster than healthy cells, so they are more affected, but exposed normal cells are also damaged.

During the 1910s and 1920s, French physician and radiotherapy pioneer Claudius Regaud experimented with animal, and then human trials to show that a series of shorter, lower-dose X-ray bursts could be effective while reducing side effects. Another French physician, Henri Coutard, continued his work and, by the 1930s, had established the principles of fractionated radiotherapy – controlled low doses given at regular intervals – that are still in use today. Regaud also helped to develop therapies using the radioactive metal radium, discovered in 1898 by French physicist Marie Curie. Radium became all the rage, and not only to treat cancer. It found its way into all manner of products from bath salts and toothpaste to bracelets and belts. But mounting evidence showed that this "treatment" was, in most cases, at best ineffective and at worst deadly.

The infamous 1920s case of the Radium Girls involved women who added glow-in-the-dark paint containing radium to watch and clock dials at a factory in New Jersey, US. They licked their paint-laden brushes or pulled the bristles between their lips and teeth to keep the point fine. Many of these women went on to develop diseases and cancers of the lips, teeth, and mouth, and suffered general radiation sickness. By the 1930s, the damaging effects of radium and similar substances had become well known. Using radium for radiotherapy became more limited, specialized, and controlled. The same principle of radiation from a substance (rather than X-rays) is used today, most often with caesium-137, iridium-192, and iodine-125. Small seeds (containers) are implanted around the growth to control and shrink it. This is known as internal radiation therapy, or brachytherapy. Other methods include radiation-dosed tubes or wires and swallowed or injected liquids that contain radioactive substances that accumulate naturally in the target tissues.

Radiotherapy using X-rays improved throughout the mid-20th century, with more controlled doses targeted at cancerous tissues. As with cancer surgery, a new era of radiotherapy became possible in the 1970s, in the form of image-guided radiation therapy (IGRT), which used techniques such as computerized tomography (CT) and magnetic resonance imaging (MRI) to show the position, shape, and size of growths. This made it possible to analyse the cancerous area in three dimensions for conformal radiation therapy (CRT), in which radiation machines with devices called multi-leaf collimators "mould" several beams into the same shape as the tumour, thus avoiding the healthy surrounding tissue. More recently, intensity-modulated radiation therapy (IMRT) has been developed, in which radiation energy and aim are adjusted even more precisely, to spare nearby normal cells. As well as X-rays, other forms of radiotherapy include proton therapy. This uses beams of protons (positively charged atomic particles), but prohibitively expensive and complicated equipment is needed to generate the protons – a particle accelerator in effect – so the treatment is not widely available, even now.

The third mainstay of cancer treatment is chemotherapy (treatment with chemicals). Historically, the term was applied to drug treatment for a variety of diseases. In 1909, German scientist Paul Ehrlich developed the anti-syphilitic drug arsphenamine (sold under the name of Salvarsan) – the first modern chemotherapeutic drug. Today, the term chemotherapy applies to anti-cancer agents that are cytotoxic – meaning that they harm, disable, and even kill cells. Methods include disrupting the cells' DNA, latching on to their membranes (outer coverings), and tricking the cells into undergoing a process known as apoptosis (programmed cell death) – in effect, making them commit suicide. Chemotherapy has to tread a fine line between damaging rapidly dividing cancer cells and leaving normal cells as undamaged as possible. Cancer chemotherapy had a curious beginning. Over the course of two world wars it was noted that the devastating chemical warfare agent mustard gas reduced blood cell production in bone marrow – cells that otherwise multiplied at a rate of several million per second (see pp.364–73). By 1943, scientists were investigating mustard-gas-type compounds, both for use as chemical weapons and as defences against them, and had begun looking into their potential use against rapidly multiplying cancer cells. Work at Yale University in the US produced the substance nitrogen mustard (mustine or mechlorethamine). In 1943, it was tested by injecting it into a patient suffering from the white blood cell cancer Hodgkin's lymphoma, with promising results.

After World War II, medical research continued into nitrogen mustard compounds. These stop DNA from being able to copy itself for cell division. Studies have yielded several nitrogen mustard chemotherapies over the past 50 years, including bendamustine, busulphan, chlorambucil, cyclophosphamide, ifosfamide, and melphalan. Another group is the platinum derivatives, first studied in the 1960s. Platinum is more usually associated with vehicle exhaust catalytic convertors, but is used in cancer treatment to trigger cell death. Cisplatin was introduced in the 1970s and carboplatin, a widely used, second-generation platinum anti-cancer drug, in the 1980s.

At Harvard Medical School in the US, American paediatric pathologist Sidney Farber pursued another line of chemotherapy research. In 1947 and 1948, he was looking at treatments for acute lymphoblastic leukaemia – a cancer that affects white blood cells. Concentrates of the newly discovered folic acid (a B-group vitamin) had reduced mammary tumours in mice but Farber noticed that they accelerated the leukaemia process. A diet low in folic acid, on the other hand, seemed to reduce proliferation of cancer cells. So Farber tried aminopterin, a drug that interferes with the action of folic acid, then another, amethopterin, hoping that the drug might inhibit the multiplication of the abnormal leukaemia cells. The results were encouraging. Farber's reasoning led not

FATHER OF MODERN CHEMOTHERAPY
In 1947, pathologist Sidney Farber gave children the first drug – aminopterin – to prove effective against acute leukaemia, earning some temporary remissions.

only to a new line of chemotherapeutic drugs, but also to a logical way of looking for them. Modern chemotherapy was up and running. Amethopterin, now called methotrexate, remains a key drug against cancers and autoimmune disorders, among other diseases. In the second half of the 20th century, chemotherapy itself mushroomed into a vast business. Advances include targeting chemotherapy specifically at cancer cells, rather than indiscriminately destroying body tissues in general.

Biological (bio-) therapy uses substances produced naturally by the body, or similar synthetic varieties. Better targeting have led to it being used to sabotage cancer cells. One bio-therapy is immunotherapy – exploiting the tricks of the body's own immune system. Certain white blood cells make antibodies that adhere to and disrupt "foreign" substances called antigens, on germs for example (see pp.222–27). Some cancer cells have distinctive antigens not found in other body cells. Monoclonal antibodies, produced by cloned (genetically identical) cells all obtained from a single original white cell, can be manufactured to target these specific antigens. They were first made in the 1970s, using a white blood cell which was itself created from multiple myeloma, a cancer. Their role is to bind onto and destroy cancerous cells, or to mark them for attack by the immune system, while ignoring all the normal cells. In each tailor-made batch, all the monoclonal antibodies are the same, so they are very accurate in selecting their targets. As well as counteracting cancers, they are used against autoimmune disorders, both for diagnosis and in research.

Hormonal therapy for cancer is another expanding field. Tamoxifen, a compound first produced in the 1960s, has become a major treatment for breast cancers that need the hormone oestrogen in order to grow and multiply. Tamoxifen latches onto the oestrogen-receiving units on cell surfaces, which prevents oestrogen itself from attaching, so the cancer cells cannot grow.

As cancer specialists (oncologists) increase their research and knowledge, the list of carcinogens grows ever longer, from those in tobacco smoke to industrial pollutants.

TOBACCO USE CAUSES OVER

20%

OF ALL CANCER DEATHS
WORLDWIDE

EXPENSIVE BUT EFFECTIVE
The bio-pharmaceuticals industry is
researching the growth of monoclonal
antibodies — protein drugs — in algae
to lower the cost of drug production.

Lifestyle, diet, obesity, and
occupation are all now implicated
in cancerous changes, as are
genetics. Oncogenes — a term that
dates from 1969 — are genes that are
involved in causing or facilitating
cancerous changes. Another set of
genes, the tumour-suppressors,
make substances that prevent cells
from becoming cancerous, so if a
tumour suppressor gene in a cell is
faulty or fails to work, the cell may
mutate and become cancerous.

The first human oncovirus
(a virus that causes cancer) discovered was the Epstein-Barr virus,
which was identified in the 1960s in Burkitt's lymphoma. In the early
to mid-1980s, German virus researcher Harald zur Hausen discovered
the role of human papilloma virus (HPV) in cervical cancer and duly
received the 2008 Nobel Prize in Physiology or Medicine. HPV is
thought to cause perhaps three-quarters of cervical cancer cases and
is now the target of a major vaccination campaign in the UK that
began in 2008. The vaccine is also widely available in the US.

Tracking down the many causes of cancer, and the biological
mechanisms in its development, in the hope that this will lead to
better prevention, diagnosis, and treatment, is a major thrust of
cancer research today. This is all the more important as people in
developed countries live for longer. As age is one of the major risk
factors, this is making cancer occur with increasing frequency.

Deadly Cells

Cancer is on the increase worldwide. It is the second largest cause of death after cardiovascular disease, and can begin anywhere in the body, caused by cells spreading out of control in tissues such as skin, bone, and muscle. Cancer cells may cluster together to cause tumours, which can be malignant – this occurs when a tumour invades surrounding tissue and replaces it with more cancer cells, as they replicate out of control.

BREAST CANCER
Breast cancer often originates in the milk ducts, and is a carcinoma (cancer of lining tissues). It was one of the earliest forms of cancer to be studied, and is one of the more easily treatable cancers.

BRAIN CANCER STEM CELLS
Cancers have stem cells, just as ordinary tissues do (see pp.364–73). These trigger the growth of cancerous cells and can make cancers appear again after apparently successful therapy.

LYOMYOSARCOMA CELLS
A rare form of cancer, lyomyosarcoma affects smooth muscles – those that work involuntarily, such as the muscles found in the heart and blood vessels.

BLOOD VESSEL AND MELANOMA
Cancer cells send out messages encouraging blood vessels to grow into tumours. Seen in cross-section, here a blood vessel (centre) has grown into a melanoma (a form of skin tumour).

CANCER CELLS UNDER ATTACK
T-cells (above, white) are a type of white blood cell that attacks germs. They can also take on cancer cells (above, grey), but struggle to identify them. Gene therapy (see pp.338–47) can improve their detection abilities.

SKIN CANCER CELL SPLIT OPEN
The structure of cancer cells is varied: this one is frozen and spilt open to display an enlarged nucleus. Cancer cells can also be irregularly shaped or folded. The nucleus holds the DNA, which dictates how the cell grows.

PANCREATIC CANCER CELL
Cancers that grow deep in the body, such as those that occur in the pancreas, are hard to spot. As a result, they sometimes reach an advanced stage before detection and treatment.

CERVICAL CANCER CELL DIVISION
HPV (human papilloma virus) is a relatively common virus. In a small proportion of women it may cause changes in cervical cells, which then ignore messages to stop multiplying and become cancerous.

New Parts for Old

REPLACEMENT HIPS, ARTIFICIAL HEARTS, and other implants have come a long way from ancient Egyptian artificial hands and toes, Etruscan bone or ivory false teeth, Greek wooden and metal noses, and Roman iron hands, metal feet, and carved ears. Many a medieval warrior had a custom-made arm, hand, leg, or foot. Eminent 16th-century astronomer Tycho Brahe even had a selection of brass, copper, silver, and gold noses to wear after part of his own was sliced off in a duel. And in the 18th century, first US President George Washington commissioned several sets of dentures, some carved from hippopotamus ivory and incorporating human teeth.

These pre-20th-century artefacts were all early prostheses – substitutes to replace a missing part – that were worn externally. Today, a prosthetic hand could be an advanced robot, bristling with mechanics and electronics, able to detect the user's nerve signals and move its fingers separately with graduated force (see pp.350–55). Prostheses are not necessarily worn externally. For example, an artificial heart valve or plastic blood vessel can be implanted into the body, but not all implants are prosthetic (replacements). Non-prosthetic implants range from surgically imlanted cosmetic "eye jewels" to pacemakers and contraceptive or other hormone inserts. Each year, up to one million people around the world have their mobility and lives transformed by a new hip. Total hip arthroplasty (THA) or replacement is usually carried out for hip joints that have been degraded and roughened by osteoarthritis. The earliest attempts at hip-repair surgery date back to 1890s Germany, after anaesthesia came into use. First, surgeons

ARTIFICIAL IRON ARM
This forerunner of 20th-century prosthetic limbs dates from the late 16th century. It was made by an armourer for a knight who had lost an arm in combat.

exposed the ball-and-socket joint, then they smoothed off the roughened surfaces of the ball-shaped upper end – the head of the femur (thigh bone) – and the bowl-shaped socket in the hip bone, and closed the incisions. In some cases, a polished ball of ivory replaced the head of the femur, but the risky procedure did not catch on.

Finding suitable materials was a challenge. In the 1920s, Norwegian-born US surgeon Marius Smith-Peterson fitted a cup-shaped glass liner into the socket, into which the natural head of the femur fitted. Twenty years later, in Columbia, South Carolina, Austin T. Moore tried the opposite approach – leaving the natural socket and replacing the femoral head, this time with a newly developed cobalt-chromium metal alloy, Vitallium. Meanwhile, in Paris, French brothers Robert and Jean Judet tested a new acrylic-type plastic material for the ball. They mounted the femoral head on a long spike-like stem that fitted into the bone-marrow cavity along the shaft of the femur. They had some successes, but failures too, when the prosthesis came loose, wore away too fast, or fragmented.

War injuries have provided the impetus for improving prosthetic limbs through the ages. During World War II, British doctor John Charnley, who had been elected a Fellow of the Royal College of Surgeons at the age of 25, travelled in the British Royal Army Medical Corps to Northern Ireland, Egypt, and the English county of Kent – where he attended wounded soldiers from the Dunkerque evacuation. He was fascinated by the engineering skills of his army colleagues. They made not only weapons and military equipment, but also artificial arms, hands, legs, and feet for the war-wounded, and surgical equipment for the doctors. Charnley himself invented several devices, including walking calipers (leg braces). Throughout his career, he worked closely with engineers, lathe-operators, machinists, and materials technicians.

After the war, Charnley gained experience in orthopaedics – the branch of surgery concerned with the spine and joints. He studied bone structure and the roles of the different layers of bone in disease and repair. In one daring but ill-advised experiment, he persuaded a colleague to transplant some shards of bone from his own tibia (thigh bone) into different positions, under the skin and next to the bone, to track how they healed. Bone inflammation ensued and he was incapacitated for weeks. In the early 1950s, Charnley, now Consultant

PERCENTAGE OF TOTAL HIP REPLACEMENTS STILL FUNCTIONING AFTER 10 YEARS

90–95%

Orthopaedic Surgeon at Manchester Royal Infirmary, encountered a male patient whose artificial acrylic hip squeaked loudly. This set Charnley thinking about biomechanics – where machines meet living tissues – and factors such as friction, bearing surfaces, and lubrication. "The cart has been put before the horse; the artificial joint has been made and used, and now we are trying to find out how and why it fails," he said. To ease arthritic hips, Charnley experimented with the low-friction material polytetrafluoroethylene (PTFE, better known by the trade name Teflon) and with cement formulations borrowed from dentistry. He tried a metal ball and stem for the femur, fitting it into a PTFE lining in the socket, but the PTFE wore quickly, and its tiny rubbed-off particles caused severe irritation and reaction. More than 200 patients had repeat surgery to limit the damage, and again Charnley experimented on himself, by injecting himself with some of the worn particles so that he could experience the problem at first hand.

Down but not out, Charnley and his team searched for a better and more slippery material to line the hip socket. Salespeople visited with their latest products. In May 1960, supplier V. C. Binns demonstrated gears and other items made from a possible new material – ultra high molecular weight polyethylene (UHMWP). Charnley thought it a waste of time, but biomechanic Harry Craven saw something in it. When Charnley went on a skiing holiday, Craven tested the UHMWP in laboratory wear rigs. The results were impressive. Meanwhile, with characteristic energy, innovation, and desire to help patients, Charnley established a centre to improve hip replacements. The Centre for Hip Surgery, situated in a former tuberculosis hospital at Wrightington, near Manchester, was formally opened in 1961.

In 1962, Charnley began the first trial hip replacements with the metal ball-and-spike head for the femur and a UHMWP socket lining, both cemented in place. Recalling the PTFE disappointments, he was cautious at first. After about five years, promising outcomes spelled the beginning of modern total hip replacement. Charnley devised

X-RAY OF PROSTHETIC HIP
The metal implant stands out
from the surrounding bone.
Modern hard-wearing metals
used include titanium, stainless
steel, and cobalt chrome.

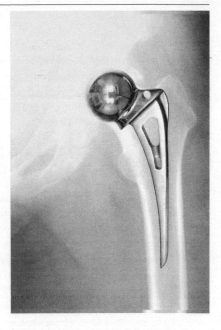

not just hip hardware but the total
package. He devised a type of tent
or air enclosure with filtered air, a
surgeon's whole-body gown or
suit, and a better way of handling
instruments, all to minimize the
risk of infection. He encouraged
post-mortem study of prostheses
for joint wear and tear, and other
imperfections, and he urged
surgeons to record each tiny detail
of every operation and its effect on
their patient, saying: "A few
observations on the human body are often of more value than a large
series of experiments on animals... It has rightly been said that every
surgical operation is a biological experiment." Charnley was honoured
as a Fellow of the Royal Society in 1975, received a knighthood in 1977,
and the Gold Medal of the British Medical Association in 1978.

Progress in hip prostheses continues today with stronger, more
biocompatible (acceptable to living tissue) materials, ball-and-socket
designs that dislocate less easily, improved cements, and "bone-
friendly" surfaces, such as micromeshes, foamed metal, or tiny beads
that encourage bone tissue to grow into them, creating a stronger
bond. This work has benefitted not just artificial hips but the wide
range of modern joint prostheses, from finger knuckles, elbows, and
shoulders to knees and ankles.

In April 1969, as Charnley hips were marching around the world, a
rather more newsworthy prosthetic implant made an entrance. This
was the first total artificial heart replacement in a human, for heart-
failure patient Haskell Karp in Houston, Texas, inserted by US
surgeon Denton Cooley. The device was developed by Argentine
heart surgeon and researcher Domingo Liotta. The mechanical heart

was intended as a temporary "bridge-to-transplant" — it bought time until a suitable donor heart was found, in this case about 64 hours later. The artificial heart did its job, although the patient died around 30 hours after the natural heart transplant, due to complications including kidney failure and lung infection.

The Liotta heart was, like the real thing, a double pump. The left side received blood low in oxygen from the body and sent it to the lungs; the right side received re-oxygenated blood back from the lungs and pumped it around the body. As in the real heart, valves controlled the blood flow. The heart's pushing power came from air pressure forced along tubes from the external power-control unit. The size of a large washing machine, the unit contained pneumatic pumps, and its console controls altered pressure and rate.

Blood that flows in unusual ways, especially over uneven surfaces, runs the risk of clotting. Even if a clot does not affect the heart, bits of it can sweep into the circulation to block a brain artery (a cerebral embolism), for example, and thus cause a stroke. A major challenge for prostheses that deal with moving blood is to minimize this danger. The original Liotta heart had tubes made from the synthetic plastic-like polymer polyethylene terephthalate (PET, also known as Dacron), which is still used for certain implants such as blood vessels. The polymer has good biocompatibility — the body is unlikely to react against it or reject it. The Liotta heart's chambers were made from Dacron and a silicone-based synthetic rubber called Silastic.

Artificial hearts had been in development for years. Liotta had been researching mechanical pumps to assist the heart since the late 1950s. The focus was on the left ventricle — the most muscular, powerful chamber, which ejects blood into the aorta (the largest artery in the body) to circulate around the body. In July 1963, Liotta and

INTERNAL PACEMAKER
At St George's Hospital in the UK, a senior cardiac technician, Geoffrey Davies, designed this implant in the early 1960s because of problems with infection using external pacemakers.

cardiovascular surgeon E. Stanley Crawford implanted the first left ventricular assist device (LVAD), worked by air pressure. It did not succeed, but work continued and electrically driven VADs have improved greatly since then, with power transmitted wirelessly through the intact skin, rather than along tubes or wires through it. Alongside artificial heart development, the first implantable pacemakers were invented in the early 1960s. A pacemaker regulates the beating of the heart in patients who have a heart block or a malfunctioning sinoatrial node (the part of the heart that initiates the heartbeat). It sends low-energy electrical impulses to stimulate a heartbeat at a suitable rate and rhythm, either on demand or all the time, depending upon the patient's condition.

In 1982, there was a second high-profile heart implant – the Jarvik-7 artificial heart, named after bio-researcher Robert Jarvik. Recipient Barney Clarke survived for 112 days after the operation. Like the Liotta design, the Jarvik-7 was powered by air. The pump-and-control unit – the size of a shopping trolley – accompanied Clarke everywhere. Further designs of artificial hearts followed, and several were approved through the years for temporary and permanent implantation. Several types of implantable heart valves were designed too, including ball-and-cage, leaflet, and tilting disc valves. Animal valves were used too – typically from pigs – and hybrid ones with a metal frame and flexible animal tissue leaflets (animal tissues were treated before use to minimize the risk of rejection).

Human tragedy continues to stimulate the advance of technology and understanding of implants. Injuries from war and terrorim still motivate doctors and scientists to improve prosthetic limbs. Other reasons for implants include replacing body parts that are missing at birth, accidentally damaged or detached, or removed by surgery because of trauma, or diseases such as cancer and arthritis. Modern implants range from the purely cosmetic, such as breast enhancements, to the functional, such as plates that strengthen bones or experimental electronic retinal eye implants that could help people who were born blind or lost their eyesight to see again – a far cry from the earliest, albeit ingenious, false body parts of the ancient world.

Implants and Prostheses

Accident, disease, or other medical conditions can take their toll on the body, and many people have depended on false body parts for thousands of years – and, latterly, on devices implanted within the body (see pp.270–75). Today, developments in materials have increased the durability and comfort of prostheses. Computer technology has since led to greater control and precision in devices as diverse as heart pacemakers and "bionic" hands.

ARTIFICIAL LEG (c.1928)
Before the development of synthetic materials, a lightweight metal alloy such as duralumin was the best material available for a full artificial leg. This example has a mechanism to control the knee and a hand-operated knee lock.

STEEL HAND (c.1890)
Attached to a steel forearm, this artificial hand was designed for someone with a lower-arm amputation. Brass mounts made it possible to move the wrist.

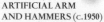

ARTIFICIAL ARM AND HAMMERS (c.1950)
This prosthetic arm was made for a metalworker who had an arm amputated below the elbow. It has a range of hammer attachments that he used in his work.

POWERED LIMBS (c.1964)
Canisters of carbon dioxide gas, triggered by
the user's upper-body movements, powered
artificial limbs manufactured in the 1960s.
A series of cables controlled the movements.

PACEMAKER (c.1970)
A pacemaker sends out
electrical impulses to make
the heart beat regularly.
External pacemakers
appeared in the 1930s, and
implanted ones in the
1950s. They became more
practical with the arrival
of long lasting lithium
batteries in the 1970s.

ARTIFICIAL HEART (c.2005)
Often used as a temporary measure before a
donor heart is transplanted, artificial hearts
are typically made of titanium and fitted with
batteries that can be charged through the skin.

BIONIC HAND (c.2007)
Bionic hands pick up electrical signals
from the user's arm muscles, and
processors in the hand turn these
signals into precise movements.

Medicine and Care for the Elderly

SIXTY-THREE BECAME THE NEW THIRTY-ONE in the 20th century. In 1900, the global average lifespan was around 31 years; by 2000, it had more than doubled to over 63, and in some wealthier developed nations it exceeded 80 years. The medical advances in that century included safer surgery (see pp.206–213); improved care during pregnancy and childbirth (see pp.214–21); the discovery of antibiotics (see pp.252–59); mass vaccination (see pp.286–93); and new generation medicines. Health threats such as carcinogens, pollutants, and occupational hazards became widely recognized – making it possible to take preventive measures – along with risk factors for heart disease, stroke, and other major killers.

Looked at another way, however, the 20th century was the era when, as a result of increased life expectancy combined with changing diets and lifestyles, age-related diseases came to the fore. Prominent among these are heart and vascular (blood vessel) problems and strokes, cancers, and arthritis, as well as degenerative diseases that include neurological (brain and nerve) conditions such as Alzheimer's (see p.283). In 1900, for example, heart disease was scarce among the general population; by the early 21st century, cardiovascular problems accounted for one in three deaths worldwide. As a result, medicine and care for the elderly have developed into a specialized field.

Particular practices for health care and treatment of the elderly extend back to ancient times. They are mentioned in early Ayurvedic texts in India (see pp.74–81), described in traditional Chinese medicine (see pp.64–73), and recorded in Ancient Greece (see pp.30–39), where Hippocrates noted the way illness affected older patients: "In old persons the heat is feeble, and therefore they require little fuel, as it were, to the flame, for it would be extinguished by much. On this account, also, fevers in old persons are not equally acute, because their bodies are cold". Medieval Arab physicians such as Ibn Al Jazzar and Ibn Sina (see pp.100–105) also documented how disease in the older body differed from that in younger adults. Ibn Sina recommended small meals and certain foods such as fruit and ginger for older people to keep the body "warm and moist".

In 1627, François Ranchin, Professor of Medicine and Chancellor of the University of Montpellier, published *Opuscula Medica*, in which he tackled the question, itself age-old: is ageing a natural progression of the human body, or itself a form of disease or illness? Ranchin proposed that old age was an intermediate condition of decreasing health, in which the body was increasingly prone to disease: "Not only physicians, but everybody else attending old people... realize how noble and important, how serious and difficult, how useful and even indispensable is that part of practical Medicine called Gerocomica, which deals with the conservation of old people and the healing of their diseases". In the same century, Thomas Sydenham, known as the "English Hippocrates", declared "a man is as old as his arteries". Like his Ancient Greek namesake, Sydenham put his patients — young and old — first, encouraging the body's innate healing powers and engendering new attitudes and innovative treatments.

A century later, in 1793, US physician Benjamin Rush stated: "Few persons appear to die of old age. Some of the diseases generally cut the last thread of life". The debate continued about whether ageing was part of the human condition, or a disease in itself. In 1892, however, Heinrich Rosin, a professor at the Albert Ludwigs University in Freiburg, Germany, wrote: "... Extreme old age, with its natural degeneration of resources and the natural decline of organs, is a condition of development of the human body; old-age infirmity is no illness". Interestingly, Rosin was not a medical professor but a lawyer specializing in employment insurance.

While the nature of ageing was still under consideration, in 1849, George Day, Professor of Medicine and Anatomy at the University of St Andrews, Scotland, adopted a more pragmatic approach, publishing *A Practical Treatise on the Domestic Management and Most Important Diseases of Advanced Life*. He described two of what would become known as "geriatric giants": incontinence and impaired intellect-memory (dementia), as well as immobility and instability.

THOMAS SYDENHAM
An English physician, Sydenham championed observation and empathy, believing a doctor should be "diligent and tender in relieving his suffering patients".

Elsewhere, eminent French physician Jean-Martin Charcot was part of a movement in 19th-century France to care for and treat older people in specialized facilities – early versions of what later became geriatric hospitals. He described specific conditions of old age such as senile osteomalacia (softening of the bones), and how the symptoms of disease differ between young and old. On a practical level, he observed that the rectal thermometer gave the most accurate measure of core body temperature in the elderly, whose extremities tended to be cooler due to reduced circulation.

The term "geriatrics" was coined in 1909 by American doctor Ignatz Leo Nascher, writing in the *New York Medical Journal*. "Geriatrics, from [the Greek] *geras*, old age, and *iatrikos*, relating to the physician, is a term I would suggest as an addition to our vocabulary to cover the same field, in old age, that is covered by the term "paediatrics" in childhood". In 1914, he published *Geriatrics: The Diseases of Old Age and Their Treatment*, but little change was made to the care of elderly people for another 30 years.

In Europe, the elderly were still not receiving specialist medical attention either. While hospital and nursing care for other groups improved, older patients – regarded as beyond help – were often relegated to survival conditions, a situation inherited from the old "poorhouse" structures. These abandoned inmates found a champion in Marjory Warren, a Londoner who trained at the Royal Free Hospital School of Medicine, and became Deputy Medical Director of the West Middlesex County Hospital in 1931. Four years later, the neighbouring Poor Law Infirmary and former workhouse, Warkworth House, was incorporated into the hospital. Warren became responsible for more than 700 aged patients, most of whom had no diagnosis or treatment and were regarded as incurable.

With characteristic enthusiasm, Warren took on the patients, their carers, and the system. She recorded how patients underwent a gradual physical and mental decline into institutionalized apathy, with wasted muscles, stiff joints, incontinence, and immobility: "… In this miserable state, dull, apathetic, helpless and hopeless, life lingers on sometimes for years, while those around them whisper arguments in favour of euthanasia".

Warren saw that geriatrics should be its own specialism, and yet ought to be integrated into other branches of medicine and nursing care. She arranged visits from general physicians, surgeons,

WORLD POPULATION AGED OVER 60 IN 2000	ESTIMATED POPULATION AGED OVER 60 BY 2050
11%	**22**%

pharmacists, and other practitioners; set up multidisciplinary teams of expert nurses, rehabilitation specialists, physiotherapists, occupational therapists, social workers, and chaplains; and brightened the wards. Importantly, in order to gain recognition from the medical establishment, she gathered evidence that all of this worked. Former incurables rallied and many became well enough to leave the wards for less intensive care in family or residential homes: "Whenever possible, they should be retained in, or returned to, their own homes, provided there is sufficient help for their comfort and welfare, and that the home conditions are suitable ... Home nursing is therefore an absolutely essential part of the health scheme".

In the US, the American Geriatrics Society was set up in 1942. Founder members included Nascher and Malford W. Thewlis, a New England neuropsychiatrist. (Thewlis was also a renowned conjuror and escape artist who funded his passage through medical college by performing magic shows.) Encouraged by this US development, Marjory Warren stepped up her crusade for geriatrics: she wrote pivotal articles in the *British Medical Journal*, in 1943, and *The Lancet*, in 1946, and, in 1947, she became a founding member of the Medical Society for the Care of the Elderly, which later became the British Geriatrics Society. In the 1950s, geriatric medicine acquired specialty status within Britain's National Health Service. Sadly, Warren herself died in a car accident in 1960, at the age of 62.

To this day, standards and practices of care for the elderly vary throughout the world, often driven by a mixture of tradition and available resources. Many Eastern cultures emphasize respect for the elderly as part of the importance of family life; in these cases, families may be more likely to care for their elderly relatives within the household. Indeed, in some developing countries where healthcare and facilities are limited, there may be little alternative.

DAME CICELY SAUNDERS
A great reformer, Saunders launched the modern hospice movement. She received 25 honorary degrees and a BMA Gold Medal before dying in the hospice she founded.

Hospital care of the chronically sick had been dispensed sporadically through the centuries, often by religious orders such as the Knights Hospitaller. In more recent times, France led the way, establishing specialized institutions in the 1800s, and, in 1879, Our Lady's Hospice opened in Dublin, Ireland, bringing new philosophies and standards of care for the seriously and terminally ill patients – many of whom suffered from tuberculosis.

Nearly a century later, in 1967, an innovative new hospice opened in London, England. St Christopher's Hospice was established by Cicely Saunders, a former nurse, social worker, and reformer who launched the modern hospice movement. At the time, many terminally ill patients were left to die on hospital wards or in the care of family at home. Once these patients were deemed incurable, little attention was given to their needs and comfort. Pain relief in particular was inadequate. Saunders had studied pain control in a clinical setting and demonstrated that small, regular doses of morphine and other opioids by mouth could give relief with tolerable side-effects. Far from accepting that there was no more that could be done for the dying patients, she always insisted, "there is so much more to be done".

At St Christopher's, Saunders assembled skilled teams that brought together a range of disciplines, from consultants and researchers to pharmacologists and nurses. Her aim was to bring the highest medical standards to compassionate care of the seriously ill and dying, in a holistic way. One of the early pain relief projects at St Christopher's involved comparing the effectiveness of opioids such as diamorphine for pain relief – most staff had their own opinions about which one produced better control and fewer side-effects such as drowsiness and nausea. The small pilot study, followed by a two-year trial involving 700 patients, provided a clinical basis for future use. Saunders also extended the pain concept to "total pain", which included emotional, psychological, and spiritual, as well as physical, sensations.

St Christopher's became the model for the modern hospice movement. Saunders toured, lectured and wrote extensively. She also inspired others, such as Florence Wald, Dean of the Yale School of Nursing, Connecticut, who established hospice care in the US. Saunders, who qualified as a surgeon in the 1950s, received more than 25 honorary degrees and the British Medical Association Gold Medal. She was a Fellow of three Royal Colleges (Nursing, Physicians, and Surgeons) and was made a Dame of the British Empire in 1979. She died in 2005 – at St Christopher's.

Much of the emphasis in hospice care today is on care within the family at home, supported by hospice workers. In the 1980s, the hospice movement also developed the modern concept of palliative care – actions that prevent or relieve patient suffering – which may also be applied to patients who are not terminally ill, in a hospital setting. In a similar way to hospice care, it employs multidisciplinary teams, from pharmacists expert in pain relief to counsellors and faith workers, to ease distress and bring comfort to patients.

Despite the huge progress made in geriatric medicine and care of the dying, new challenges are constantly emerging. In 1906, German psychiatrist and neurologist Alois Alzheimer described the disease that bears his name. It is now the most commonly diagnosed form of dementia, involving memory loss, confusion, mood swings, failing confidence, disorganized thought processes, language difficulties, and social withdrawal. In pathology, Alzheimer's disease is characterized by structures known as plaques and tangles in the brain, involving proteins. The underlying causes are not well understood, and the risk factors are many and varied, from smoking and high blood pressure to whiplash injury.

A century after Alzheimer's description of the disease, more than 25 million people worldwide had been diagnosed with it. By 2012, this number had increased to 40 million; it is rising by 8 million annually, and this rate is itself increasing, with a predicted doubling every 20 years. After the great strides of the 20th century, the "dementia epidemic" and how to care for its sufferers is just one of the new challenges facing the medical profession in the 21st century.

MEDIEVAL HOSPITAL CARE
Nuns care for patients at the Hospital of
Hôtel Dieu in Paris in this 1492 illustrated
manuscript from *Le Livre de Vie Active de
l'Hôtel-Dieu*. In the crowded ward, many of
the emaciated, elderly patients lie two abed.

Vaccination Comes of Age

ALTHOUGH THEY WERE KNOWN TO EXIST, no one had actually seen a virus before 1939 – the year they were first revealed under an electron microscope. Before then, researchers had relied on the light microscope (see pp.150–51), which was not powerful enough to make these tiniest of microbes visible. Bacteria had been observed, but as far as viral infections were concerned – smallpox, rabies, measles, mumps, hepatitis, and influenza, for example – researchers had effectively been working blind. To get some idea of what they were up against, it is worth noting that the average body cell is 25 micrometres (μm) wide, so 15 cells in a row would stretch half of one millimetre – about the width of this "i". The single-celled *Entamoeba histolytica*, which causes a form of dysentery, is approximately this size too. Among the smallest body cells are red blood cells, which are only 7–8 μm across, approximately the size of the adult stage of the *Plasmodium* that causes malaria (see pp.388–89). One of the smallest bacteria, *Mycoplasma pneumoniae*, which is responsible for a form of pneumonia, is just 0.2 μm long, and the largest viruses are of a similar size.

The first viruses to be observed were tobacco mosaic viruses, which infect tobacco plants (see p.228), but people had long known that viruses affect animals and humans too. Pasteur's work with rabies (see pp.196–

205) had already shown that samples, smears, and scrapes of infected tissue could transfer diseases to others. In the mid-1880s, Pasteur's assistant Charles Chamberland made a porcelain filter that had microscopic holes small enough to trap bacteria, but not small enough to stop something else that was passing through and spreading certain diseases. Over the next decade,

SEEING WITH ELECTRONS
A scientist studies a specimen under an electron microscope in the 1930s. The new technology enabled researchers to see viruses by the end of that decade.

extracts of these "filterable agents" were crystallized, but their detailed structure remained a mystery until the 1940s, when studies of crystallized viruses, using X-ray crystallography combined with early electron microscope images, began to shed light on the structure of individual viruses. These revealed the vital differences between viruses and bacteria. Not only did bacteria live in between cells, but most, given suitable nutrients and conditions, could live and multiply independently of other life forms – unlike viruses, which had to invade living cells to replicate. Also, viruses, unlike bacteria, seemed barely to count as "living", since they spent most of their time inactive and only became active to replicate. Crucially, it also became clear that viruses were rarely affected by the antibiotics that killed bacteria (see pp.252–59).

Viruses, bacteria, unmatched transfused blood, transplanted organs, and other items that are foreign to the body have substances called antigens on their surfaces. The body's immune system is constantly on the lookout for these antigens, detecting them with B-cells, a subgroup of the white blood cells called lymphocytes. B-cells produce large, Y-shaped protein molecules known as antibodies. There are millions of antibodies floating in a person's blood, and most of these differ in the chemical structure of their tips, so that when a virus or bacterium invades, some of the antibodies can bind with its antigens. This makes certain B-cells turn into plasma cells – hard-working antibody factories – which rapidly make armies of antibodies that attack the invader or tag it for destruction. Other B-cells become memory cells and remain in the body for years. If the same microbes reappear later, the B-cells recognize them and destroy them before they cause any harm. Immunity means being resistant to an infection. It can occur naturally, or be induced by means of a vaccine (see pp.292–93). Vaccination introduces harmful antigens into the body, so the immune system fights and destroys them, making a person actively immune to the disease. Passive immunity is conferred by injecting ready-made antibodies into the body. This provides rapid protection, but the effects only last for weeks or months, as the antibodies degrade and cannot be replaced.

In the first half of the 20th century, following the pioneering vaccines for smallpox (see pp.152–61) and rabies (see pp.196–205), researchers worked feverishly to develop vaccines for diphtheria, tuberculosis,

ERADICATING SMALLPOX
A Soviet poster of 1931 urges people to take up vaccination
against smallpox. As suggested by the bar chart at the bottom,
the authorities aimed to eradicate the disease by 1932.

tetanus, polio, whooping cough, yellow fever, and other major infections. Their findings helped to understand antigen-antibody mechanisms and the profound complexities of immunity, which still throw up surprises today.

Diphtheria, the "strangling angel", is a devastating infection that particularly affects children. A tough membrane forms in the throat, causing breathing problems and leading to many fatalities. Diphtheria used to kill millions of people, but by the early 21st century, the number of deaths worldwide had been reduced to a few thousand annually. The bacterium that causes it, *Corynebacterium diphtheriae*, discovered in 1890 by German physiologist Emile von Behring, produces a harmful substance known as diphtheria toxin that gets into healthy body cells and interferes with how they work. The immune system reacts by neutralizing the toxin with a special kind of antibody known as an antitoxin. In the 1890s, early treatment for diphtheria was a ready-made antitoxin extracted from horses. For prevention, there was diphtheria TAT – toxin-and-antitoxin – a combination injection that contained just enough toxin to stimulate immunity, but also enough ready-made antitoxin to prevent the toxin causing the disease. In 1914, the French newspaper *Le Matin* reported that Emile von Behring's latest version of TAT was one of "the Seven Wonders of the modern world [the others being] the aeroplane, wireless, radium, the locomotive, human grafting and the dynamo." Somewhat out of the blue, in 1923, Ramon Gaston, a French vet, then discovered that the preserving chemical formalin altered diphtheria toxin so that it was harmless when injected without the antitoxin, but still triggered immunity. Ramon applied the same chemical to tetanus, establishing the group of vaccines that are correctly called toxoids, as they are based on toxins rather than the microbes, such as *Corynebacterium diphtheriae* in the case of diphtheria, that produce them.

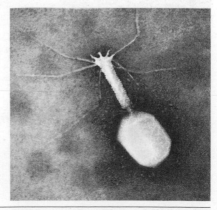

INVISIBLE KILLER
This electron microscope image of a virus shows its 20-sided head, its tail, and tail fibres. The head contains the virus's DNA, which is injected into a host cell during replication.

Another key development in vaccination was the treatment of the poliovirus, a microbe that was first photographed in 1952, the year that the US endured a terrible outbreak of this paralysing infection. As far back as 1905, Swedish physician Ivar Wickman had published the first in a series of studies claiming – controversially at the time – that polio was a contagious disease, spread by physical contact or close proximity. Just three years later, Karl Landsteiner (see pp.242–49) and another Austrian physician, Erwin Popper, had identified the contagion as being viral rather than bacterial; infected material from the spinal cord of a deceased sufferer, filtered to remove bacteria, still transmitted the disease to laboratory monkeys. By 1910, Simon Flexner, Director at the Rockefeller Institute for Medical Research in New York City, had demonstrated that monkeys who recovered from polio had "germicidal substances" (antibodies) in their blood. This suggested that a vaccine of disabled polio viruses might trigger natural antibody production, and thereby lead to immunity.

Although this finding paved the way for research into polio vaccines, early trials did not go well – partly because, in the early 1930s, Australian investigators showed that there was more than one kind of poliovirus. Disaster struck in the mid-1930s when two US projects testing vaccines on more than 20,000 children failed, leaving many dead, paralysed, or suffering from allergic reactions. However, great strides were made in growing polioviruses in the laboratory. It was found that they could grow in human embryonic tissue, thereby reducing the need to use so many monkeys as experimental animals for incubation and testing. The 1954 Nobel Prize in Physiology or Medicine was later awarded to American medical scientist John Enders, and virologists Thomas Weller and Frederick Robbins "for their discovery of the ability of poliomyelitis viruses to grow in cultures of various types of tissue". However, there was a further setback to

THE SALK VACCINE
Medical researcher Jonas Salk developed the first successful polio vaccine, in the 1950s. At the time, the US was suffering its worst ever polio epidemic.

polio research in the early 1950s when work at Johns Hopkins University School of Medicine, Baltimore, by American medical researcher David Bodian and virologist Isabel Morgan, revealed that

DEATHS PREVENTED BY VACCINES EACH YEAR

2,500,000

there were three kinds of poliovirus, which meant that a vaccine had to work against all three.

In 1951, Jonas Salk, Director of the Virus Research Laboratory at the University of Pittsburgh Medical School, began growing polioviruses in monkey kidney tissue. The following year, during the US polio epidemic, Salk and his team began human trials of an injected polio vaccine (IPV) based on killed polioviruses. The following year, 1953, Salk tried the vaccine on his wife and three sons, and the year after that, a huge US trial began, involving almost two million children, doctors, nurses, and public health officials. In April 1955, results showed that the Salk vaccine was up to 90 per cent effective against paralytic polio. Russian-born American medical research scientist Albert Sabin and his team at the University of Cincinnati, Ohio, had also been researching a polio vaccine based on weakened viruses, which could be swallowed rather than injected. In the 1950s, the team began trials on millions of children in the Soviet Union, and by 1963, the Sabin vaccine against all three types of poliovirus was in production.

In 1988, an ambitious target was declared by the World Health Organization – the worldwide eradication of polio by the year 2000. The deadline has since been extended, but the impact of the Salk and Sabin vaccines suggests that polio may well become the next disease (after smallpox) to be successfully eradicated. Yet just as smallpox became extinct, with polio and perhaps also diphtheria hopefully to follow, infections such as HIV/AIDS (see pp.328–35) and new, potentially pandemic strains of influenza have entered the stage, opening new battlegrounds in the age-old war between medicine and germs.

How Immunization Works

The most common medical way to immunize people – stop them getting a disease – is by vaccination. A vaccine contains foreign molecules called antigens that trigger the primary immune response, in which the body releases antibodies to kill the infection. The body also produces memory cells that will recognize the invader and leap into action if it strikes again, fighting off any future infection of the disease – the secondary immune response.

PRIMARY IMMUNE RESPONSE
Vaccines contain antigens either in isolation or attached to germs (bacteria or viruses). The germs are weakened or have their living material removed to make them harmless.

Antigen attached to weakened germ

Antibody (protective substance that coats blood cells)

Antigen attached to the empty shell of a germ

White blood cell

Isolated antigens

Detached antibody

2 Plasma cell releases antibodies to kill infection – the first immune response

1 Antigens bind to antibodies on white blood cells, making them divide to form either plasma cells or memory cells

3 Memory cells live for a long time and remember the germ. If it invades again, memory cells turn into plasma cells and attack the germ vigorously, before it is able to cause much harm

Vaccination

French scientist Louis Pasteur's vaccines for rabies and anthrax, and Spanish physician Jaime Ferrán's cholera vaccine, made a huge impact on human health in the late 19th century. Programmes for vaccinating children have been in place since the mid-20th century.

CHILDREN QUEUE UP FOR VACCINES IN WYOMING, US, IN 1955

Inoculation

While vaccination introduces an antigen to trigger immunity, inoculation administers a mild dose of the germ responsible for a disease. Memory cells in the recipient's body will remember the disease if it tries to enter the body subsequently, and produce plasma cells that release antibodies to destroy the germ, just as by vaccination. Inoculation can also be used to produce a disease for research.

THE MED-E-JET INOCULATION KIT MADE IN OHIO, US, IN 1980, USED A GUN TO FORCE MEDICATION THROUGH THE SKIN AT HIGH PRESSURE WITHOUT THE NEED FOR A NEEDLE

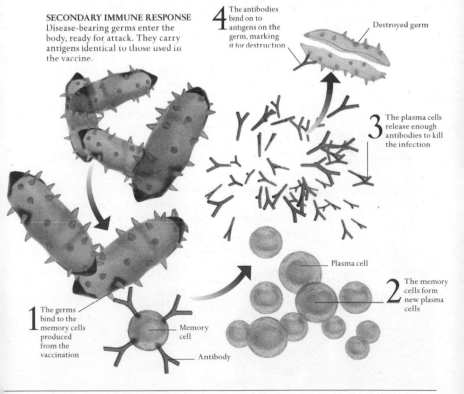

SECONDARY IMMUNE RESPONSE
Disease-bearing germs enter the body, ready for attack. They carry antigens identical to those used in the vaccine.

4 The antibodies bind on to antigens on the germ, marking it for destruction

Destroyed germ

3 The plasma cells release enough antibodies to kill the infection

Plasma cell

2 The memory cells form new plasma cells

1 The germs bind to the memory cells produced from the vaccination

Memory cell

Antibody

The First Transplants

GOOD NEWS RARELY MAKES HEADLINES, but on 3 December 1967, a medical breakthrough – the world's first heart transplant – took the world by storm. Cardiac surgeon Christiaan Barnard and his 30-strong team at Groote Schuur Hospital, Cape Town, South Africa, had spent nine hours on a pioneering operation and saved the life of a 54-year-old patient by giving him the heart of a 25-year-old female donor. In the following days, bulletins on the condition of the patient, Louis Washkansky, dominated world news. Washkansky rallied, but then succumbed to pneumonia because of his suppressed immune system and died 18 days later.

Although the heart transplant was a bolt from the blue to the general public, many medical centres were poised to perform such an operation. The first in the US, for instance, took place just days after Washkansky's. But poor results, mainly from problems linked to rejection, dampened the initial enthusiasm. The following year, 1968, more than 100 procedures were attempted, but the failure rate was unacceptably high. As anti-rejection drugs improved, however, transplant numbers slowly rose again. Today, a heart is transplanted about every two hours somewhere around the world. At some centres, two out of every three recipients are alive ten years later, and one in three after 20 years.

The first human-to-human heart transplant was by no means the first organ transplant. Success with kidneys dated back to 1954, and tissue transplants much earlier. Barnard himself had carried out other transplants, including South Africa's first kidney transplant, just six months before the heart procedure. This taught him how to cope with

CELEBRITY SURGEON
A mere 45 years old, good-looking, and happy in the media spotlight, South African Christiaan Barnard became an overnight sensation for his pioneering heart transplant.

"On Saturday, I was a surgeon in South Africa, little known. On Monday, I was world renowned"

CHRISTIAAN BARNARD

organ rejection, and the recipient, Edith Black, went on to live for more than 20 years. An emboldened Barnard stated: "Everything is ready for a heart transplant. We have the team and we know how to do it." The donor and recipient had to be a perfect match, especially as this first attempt would be closely scrutinized from all angles. The fact that the organ was a heart – the symbol of life – posed new medical, ethical, and social questions about the dividing line between life and death.

When Washkansky arrived at Groote Schuur suffering from congestive heart failure, and was swiftly followed by a car-crash victim, Barnard saw his opportunity. The car accident involved a drunk driver and the donor's mother had been killed. The donor herself had suffered severe head injuries. By modern criteria, she would have been classed as brain-dead, but no such guidelines had been developed at the time (see pp.374–79). She was otherwise fit and healthy, and her heart was still beating. After discussion, the family agreed with Barnard's proposal to donate her heart. A helping injection of potassium hastened the inevitable, stopping the heart while it was still in good condition; the operation began; and the following day, the world learned the astonishing news.

Born in 1922 in Beaufort West, southern South Africa, Christiaan Barnard had graduated from the University of Cape Town Medical School in 1945. He worked in general practice and was so deeply affected by the death of a young boy from a heart-valve defect that he went on to specialize in cardiothoracic (heart-chest) medicine. During a two-year stint in the US, Barnard worked with Professor Owen Wangensteen, Chairman of Surgery at the University of Minnesota, Minneapolis. He watched and learned from Wangensteen and other foremost heart surgeons of the day, including C. Walton Lillehei and Vince Gott. Barnard also came across Norman Shumway of Stanford University, California, who was raising the profile of cardiothoracic surgery and investigating heart-transplant potential.

The first open-heart surgery was carried out with the aid of a mechanical cardiopulmonary bypass (CPB) device, or heart-lung machine (see pp.300–301). CPB dated back to the 1920s, and American John Heysham Gibbon had tested working versions on cats in the 1930s, but no-one used a CPB device during a human operation until 1951, at the University of Minnesota, where Barnard was studying. The heart-lung machine was plumbed into the patient to take deoxygenated blood – from a main vein or the right atrium (smaller upper chamber) – add oxygen to it, and return it to the circulation, via the aorta (the main artery leading away from the heart). There had to be enough force to keep the blood moving through the system. Among the numerous precautions needed were anticoagulants to prevent the blood from clotting as it passed through the tubes and mechanical pump. Although the first open-heart patient did not pull through, success came two years later in Philadelphia, under the auspices of the heart-lung machine's pioneer, Gibbon.

Barnard returned to South Africa in 1958 with a CPB machine. The device was soon in regular use at Groote Schuur Hospital, where Barnard assembled a team capable of the long, complex open-heart procedures he had seen in the US. Barnard himself rose rapidly through the surgical hierarchies. Fascinated by Russian surgeon Vladimir Demikhov's experiments with transplants, including the heart, lungs, and even – horrific to modern eyes – the head, to create two-headed dogs, Barnard developed his own cardiothoracic skills by transplanting dog hearts. Whether dog or human, the existing organ is usually accessed by dividing the sternum (breastbone) in two lengthwise; this saves damaging the ribs, the rib joints and underlying membranes, and the lungs. Sometimes, parts of the atria (the two small upper chambers) are left intact where the main veins join them. The donor heart has these areas removed, then it is fixed in position with sutures along the cut atrial edges.

Barnard's career forged ahead after the epochal operation and he undertook more heart and other transplants. One of his patients from 1971 lived for another 23 years, but this was very much the exception at the time. Despite suffering from rheumatoid arthritis, Barnard continued to operate, and in 1972 he accepted the post of Professor of Surgical Science at his hospital. His personal life was equally eventful. Unlike the staid lifestyle of many senior medical men, Barnard enjoyed jet-setting glamour. With six children by three marriages, he also generated rumours of liaisons with prominent movie stars and other famous women. Barnard retired from surgery in 1983, but continued to act as a consultant and advocate of heart transplants. Controversially, he fronted a campaign to promote a range of anti-ageing skin care products, called Glycel. Countering criticism that he was acting simply for financial gain, Barnard responded: "My father always told me: 'The highest trees get the most wind.' This is something you have to accept." The costly product did not subsequently live up to its claims.

Barnard pioneered not only transplants in which the recipient heart is removed to make way for the donor's, but also procedures where the donor heart "piggybacks" on the recipient's. Throughout his career, he devised many new operations and techniques. Some, especially for children suffering from intestinal and heart conditions, are still practised today. He died in 2001. The Charles Saint Theatre at Groote Schuur Hospital, where Barnard's heart-transplant operation took place, is now the Heart of Cape Town Museum, laid out exactly as it was on 3 December 1967.

While Barnard was preparing for retirement, a quieter revolution in transplant medicine was gaining momentum. From work conducted on vaccinations (see pp.286–93), it was known that the immune system defended the body against material "foreign" to itself, especially invading germs. Transplanted organs or tissues came into this invader category. The transplant was attacked directly by white blood cells, specifically the

CANINE PATIENT
After successful trial operations on dogs, Norman Shumway (left) of Stanford University, California, performed many heart transplants in the US. He persevered when other surgeons gave up amid post-surgical deaths and issues on defining "brain-dead" donors.

CORNEAL TRANSPLANT
If the cornea (the transparent front of the eye) is
damaged, vision is impaired. The stitches are visible
around this recently replaced cornea, where it
projects like a dome beyond the white of the eye.

recipient's T-cells, and by antibodies manufactured by plasma
cells. For a successful transplant, the answer was therefore to
dampen or weaken the immune response using drugs called
immunosuppressants. Medication had to tread a fine line between
quelling the rejection process enough to allow the transplant to
survive and disabling immunity so much that the body was left wide
open to infection. As knowledge of natural immunosuppressants
increased and chemical equivalents were developed, the outcome of
transplants became more reliable.

In around 1930, the steroid cortisone, a natural body hormone
produced by the adrenal glands, was discovered. Along with another
adrenal hormone, adrenaline, it is part of the body's natural "fight-
or-flight" reaction to stress. Cortisone works as an
immunosuppressant partly by affecting the white cells that produce
antibodies, and in 1949 extracts of the hormoe were first used
successfully to treat the disease rheumatoid arthritis. In 1955, a
related but synthetically manufactured medication, prednisone,
came onto the market. It was followed in 1957 by azathioprine,
which was developed primarily to fight cancers. This drug works by

interfering with cell multiplication, which cancer cells do in an uncontrolled manner (see pp.260–69). White blood cells also multiply rapidly as they mount their immune response.

British surgeon Roy Calne achieved many firsts in transplantation, including the first combined liver-heart-lung transplant in 1987. He was active in testing drugs to counter rejection, and he helped to introduce azathioprine. In the late 1970s, he trialled another promising substance, ciclosporin. Like the antibiotic penicillin (see pp.252–57), it had been discovered in a soil fungus, in this case *Tolypocladium* in Norway. It works primarily by reducing the activity of T-cells, thus diminishing the body's immune response. Ciclosporin was a great advance in anti-rejection therapy and, with several drugs to choose from, heart and other transplant success rates climbed.

The first heart transplant may have grabbed the headlines, but many other organs, especially kidneys, but also the liver, lungs (often done as a combined heart-lung transplant), and pancreatic glands are regularly transplanted too. Tissue transplants are far more common than whole organ changes. They include the cornea (the transparent front of the eye), blood (as transfusions, see pp.242–51), bone marrow, skin, blood vessels, and heart valves. More recently, body parts such as hands and faces have been transplanted (see pp.270–75).

There remain many challenges, especially donor shortages, matching a donor and recipient (identical twins are best, close relatives good, and unrelated strangers problematic), taking organs from living rather than dead donors, obtaining permission in the case of deceased donors, and the hazards of transferring infections such as HIV. Lurking among all these considerations are lucrative organ trafficking and "transplant tourism", in which recipients travel to places where operations are readily available with few questions asked. For all that, the future looks promising. Stem cell research, tissue engineering, and implant technologies (see pp.270–75) may combine to grow healthy versions of diseased organs from the patient's own cells. These could then be inserted back into the patient's body with little or no fear of rejection – perhaps prompting the next dramatic headlines in the transplant story.

A New Heart

The first successful human heart
surgery took place in 1895, to treat
a stab wound, but it was not until
World War II that heart surgery made
real advances, when US Army surgeon
Dwight Harken removed shrapnel from
soldiers' hearts. However, since lack of
blood circulation caused brain damage,
operations that stopped the heart for
more than four minutes were impossible.
In the 1950s, the heart-lung machine
enabled longer procedures, including heart
transplants, pioneered by Christiaan
Barnard in 1967 (see pp.294–99). Initially,
the recipient's immune system often rejected
a new heart. Immunosuppressant drugs were
developed from the 1970s to counteract this.

Norman Shumway

Chief heart surgeon at Stanford
University's School of Medicine, Norman
Shumway performed the first successful
heart transplant in the US in 1968. At
first, few patients survived for long, but
Shumway persisted with the procedure.
He found ways of anticipating rejection
and adopted new immunosuppressant
drugs, notably ciclosporin
(derived from a Norwegian
soil fungus). His success
encouraged other
transplant surgeons.

NORMAN
SHUMWAY WITH
A MODEL HEART

Oxygen-poor blood
leaves the patient's
heart and enters the
machine via a tube

Oxygen-rich blood
returns to the body
via another tube that
leads directly into the
aorta, bypassing the
heart and lungs

HEART-LUNG MACHINE
ENGLAND, c.1958

Developed by physiologist Denis
Melrose in the 1950s, the heart-lung
machine takes over both the pumping
action of the heart and oxygenation
by the lungs, allowing the heart
to be stopped during surgery.

The patient's blood
is passed through a large
plastic cylinder, where it flows
over rotating discs, while a
stream of oxygen is blown over it

Blood is spread in thin
films over a large surface,
which exposes the red cells
to oxygen for uptake

Transplanting a heart

The surgeon opens the patient's chest
and pericardium (the membrane
around the heart) and attaches the
patient to a heart-lung machine.
The heart is removed by cutting the
great blood vessels (large blood vessels
that carry blood to and from the heart),
leaving only the pulmonary veins in
place, along with part of the left atrium
(the chamber through which blood
enters the heart from the lungs). The
surgeon attaches the donor heart to
the great vessels and the intact part
of the left atrium, starts the heart, and
deactivates the bypass system.

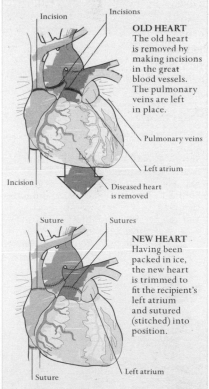

Incision   Incisions

OLD HEART
The old heart
is removed by
making incisions
in the great
blood vessels.
The pulmonary
veins are left
in place.

Pulmonary veins

Left atrium

Incision

Diseased heart
is removed

Suture   Sutures

NEW HEART
Having been
packed in ice,
the new heart
is trimmed to
fit the recipient's
left atrium
and sutured
(stitched) into
position.

Suture

Left atrium

Imaging the Body

MOST BRANCHES OF MEDICINE have been around since Hippocrates of Ancient Greece, Zhang Zhongjing in China, and Charaka of India. How these ancients would marvel at the modern miracle of medical imaging – seeing inside the body without cutting it open. Radiology is the medical specialism that uses imaging to diagnose disease, monitor progress, and carry out therapies. It is a province that mixes biology, biochemistry, and medicine with physics and technology. Its innovators have garnered more than a sprinkling of Nobel Prizes and other accolades, and it is notorious for its dizzying arrays of acronyms – CT, MRI, PET, SPECT, US, and so on.

Imaging technologies have existed for just over a century. First came X-rays, the story of which is well documented. On 8 November 1895, German physicist Wilhelm Röntgen was experimenting with the fashionable electrical gadget of his time – the high-voltage vacuum or Crookes tube. This used electricity to produce "cathode rays", later discovered to be beams of particles called electrons. Röntgen noticed that, although his tube was shielded by cardboard, it made a nearby screen glow – a screen that was coated with a chemical called barium plantinocyanide in preparation for another experiment on cathode rays. Other investigators had noticed this phenomenon with high-voltage tubes, but had not pursued it. Röntgen decided to investigate fully. For several weeks, he feverishly studied the "mysterious rays" coming from the tube, and found that they passed through less dense materials such as paper and card, but not through dense, heavy substances such as metals. Also, as he held objects in their path to see if they cast shadows, he saw that the bones of his hands were projected onto the screen – a phenomenon that had huge medical potential.

WILHELM RÖNTGEN
Known as the father of diagnostic radiology, German physicist Wilhelm Röntgen pioneered the use of X-rays for medical imaging.

MRS RÖNTGEN'S HAND
In 1895–96, Röntgen took several
X-ray photographs of his wife's
hand, this one complete with two
rings and a pair of drawing dividers.

On December 22, Röntgen placed
a sheet of photographic film on
the screen and took a photograph
of his wife's hand to reveal its
bones – prompting her to say:
"I have seen my own death!"
Röntgen named the rays "X rays",
since their nature was unknown,
and published his results later that
month. In 1901, he was duly
awarded the first-ever Nobel Prize
in Physics "in recognition of the
extraordinary services he has
rendered by the discovery of the remarkable rays subsequently named
after him" – although the name "Röntgen rays" was soon superseded
by that of "X-rays". Soon after Röntgen's discovery, doctors were
making the most of the new technology. On January 11, 1896, in
Birmingham, UK, surgeon John Hall-Edwards X-rayed a needle
embedded in a patient's hand, and on February 3, in Connecticut, US,
Professor of Medicine Gilman Frost made an X-ray photograph of the
wrist of 14-year-old Eddie McCarthy, who had fractured it two weeks
previously. On February 14, back in Birmingham, Hall-Edwards X-rayed
a patient before surgery to help guide the operation.

By the start of the 20th century, the use of X-rays had become
widespread, and it was noted that the denser a body tissue is, the more
it reduces (attenuates) the rays, meaning that bones and cartilage
show up best, while softer tissues are hard to see. It was some years
before the damaging effects of such radiation became clear, and still
more before radiotherapy turned this to an advantage (see pp.260–67).
In 1908, Hall-Edwards had to have his left arm amputated due to
radiation damage. Nevertheless, radiation doses were reduced and
equipment gradually improved, providing images that could be
recorded on photographic film or viewed "live", moving on a
fluorescent screen. The images on these "fluoroscopy" screens were

extremely pale and dim, which meant that light levels in the examination room had to be kept to a minimum. In the 1950s, electronic image intensifiers and new kinds of cameras made fluorescent screen pictures bright enough to be viewed in normal light and recorded for later study.

Other X-ray techniques had also been developed. As early as 1906, contrast or radio-opaque agents, or "dyes", were in use. These block (are opaque to) X-rays, so they show up clearly on an X-ray image. They can be introduced into the body as liquids, to show the details of hollow structures such as the stomach and intestines. By the 1920s, barium-based compounds were being ingested or introduced via an enema to show the outline of the gut. The same technique was also applied to blood vessels, using iodine-based dyes. Its developer, Portuguese neurologist António Egas Moniz, pioneered cerebral angiography to visualize the blood vessels of the brain, for which he received a Nobel Prize in Physiology or Medicine in 1949.

In 1913, American physicist William David Coolidge invented the "hot cathode" or thermionic X-ray tube to replace the old "cold" Crookes type. Its X-rays yielded clearer, sharper images than those of the Crookes tube, especially of areas deep within the body. In the same year, German surgeon-pathologist Albert Salomon examined 3,000 mastectomy (breast removal) specimens minutely, took X-ray images of them for comparison, and showed how spots on the images correlated with breast cancer growths. His work formed the foundation for mammography, the branch of medicine dedicated to the detection of early signs of breast cancer.

Two other Nobel recipients for medical imaging were Godfrey Hounsfield and Allan Cormack, who received the honour jointly in 1979 "for the development of computer assisted tomography –

commonly known as the CAT or CT scan", a scan being an image that is built up as a series of tiny light units, line upon line. Hounsfield grew up on a farm in Nottinghamshire, England, and from an early age, he invented, tinkered with, and adapted toys and machines, even leaping from haystacks to try out a home-made glider. He continued to pursue his interest in aircraft during World War II, moved into radio and radar, worked in West London for EMI (Electrical and Musical Industries – then an industrial research company as well as a record label). Looking for future projects, he noted: "It was while exploring various aspects of pattern recognition and their potential, in 1967, that the idea occurred to me which was eventually to become the EMI-Scanner and the technique of computed tomography".

Scanning required computers to process the raw data into images, so it did not became a part of mainstream medical procedure until the 1970s. A CT scanner's beam of weak X-rays passes through the patient's body to a detector on the other side, as the whole unit pivots around the patient. The unit then moves along to the next section of the patient's body and repeats the process, and so on. The computer analyses the results and then generates a series of cross-sectional images of the body. This technique is known as "tomography", derived from the term for "drawing slices" in Greek. The cross sections are then compiled to create a full 3D representation of the body that reveals not just the bones and cartilage, but also the full range of soft tissues. Unlike traditional X-ray images, each point of the scan is encoded digitally, which means it can be magnified and manipulated as never before, and communicated electronically far and wide.

Hounsfield's early CT trials in the late 1960s focused on the brain, which could not be seen in ordinary X-rays because it was shielded within the skull. Initially, Hounsfield scanned animal organs with gamma rays, a process that took days to carry out on a large mainframe computer. Switching to X-rays and better scanners greatly reduced this time it took to produce a scan. Hounsfield's team went public on preliminary CTs in 1968, carried out clinical CT head scans in 1971, launched the first EMI scanners in 1972, and moved on to whole-body scans in 1974. Hounsfield volunteered to be the guinea pig for the brain and body scans himself, claiming that he could see his pub lunch of ale and crisps in the latter. At a conference in Bermuda in 1975, he showed off whole-body CT scans of himself – after which, the new scanning technique was accepted by the establishment.

Hounsfield's Nobel co-recipient was South African physicist Allan Cormack, who had published the theoretical basis of CT scanning early in the 1960s. The two men had never met, however, before the Nobel ceremony in Stockholm.

X-rays are a form of electromagnetic radiation, which has a broad spectrum of wavelengths. These wavelengths range from the relatively long radio waves to the ever-shorter microwaves, infrared light, visible light, ultraviolet light, X-rays, and gamma rays. These last, shortest rays are used in what is called nuclear imaging, which is an "inside out" style of medical scanning ("nuclear" deriving from "nucleus" – the central part of the smallest particle of ordinary matter, the atom). Unlike most imaging technologies, which fire radiation into and through the body, nuclear imaging works by introducing substances that emit gamma rays or similar radiation within the body and using external detectors to track their movements. These substances are variously known as radionuclides, radioactive isotopes, radioisotopes, radiotracers, radiotags, and radiolabels.

Radionuclides have unstable nuclei that give off electromagnetic waves (and sometimes particles) as they change into more stable forms. They are incorporated into substances that are introduced into the body by ingestion, injection, or inhalation, and are monitored in specific places. Their first detectors were gamma (or "scintillation") cameras, also known as Anger cameras, after the American physicist Hal Anger who developed them in 1957. One of the most commonly used radionuclide substances is technetium-99m. Discovered in 1938, it became readily available in the 1960s, after a generator to make it was invented by Powell Richards, Walter Tucker, and a team at the US Department of Energy's Brookhaven National Laboratory, Long Island. Technetium-99m reduces by half every six hours, so patient exposure is low, although its radiation is readily detectable by diagnostic equipment. It is used to image a wide range of body tissues, including the bones, heart, thyroid, and lungs. Technetium-99m is usually used as part of a SPECT (single photon emission computed tomography) scan, which, like a CT scan, builds a slice-by-slice 3D image as detectors rotate around the body.

Another electromagnetic imaging technique is MRI (magnetic resonance imaging). MRI too yields a series of slices that disclose soft tissues as well as harder bone and cartilage. It works by magnetically aligning the nuclei of hydrogen atoms in the patient's body – nuclei that otherwise spin and wobble in all directions – and then releasing them to emit radio pulses that are then detected by sensors around the patient's body. Since hydrogen atoms account for two thirds of the body – as a constituent of water (H_2O), carbohydrates, and fats – MRI can picture most parts of the body, including the brain, muscles, connective tissues, nerves, blood vessels, and various types of tumour.

MRI was first investigated in 1946 by Swiss-born American physicist Felix Bloch at Stanford University and American physicist Edward Purcell at Harvard. Early on, they thought of using MRI to image the body's interior, but their main concern was to study the structural make-up of chemicals. In the 1960s and 1970s, American chemist Paul Lauterbur adapted the technique for medical imaging, and used the MRI machine at Stony Brook University, New York, for tests. At the same time, British physicist Peter Mansfield was also working on MRI, establishing how to make images out of the radio pulses emitted by hydrogen nuclei. By the late 1970s, he had produced scans of entire human bodies. Lauterbur and Mansfield shared the Nobel Prize in Physiology or Medicine in 2003 "for their discoveries concerning magnetic resonance imaging". Mansfield went on to develop MRI further with a technique called echo-planar imaging, which allowed images to be taken even faster.

More recently, scanners that combine two or more technologies have been devised. The PET/CT scanner, for instance, reveals both tissue structure – via CT (computerized tomography) – and tissue function – via PET (positron emission tomography). PET has a long history, including advances made in the early 1970s at Brookhaven National Laboratory, US, by James Roberston and Sy Rankowitz, and in Montreal, Canada, by Chris Thompson, Ernst Myer, and Lucas Yamato. Michael Phelps and his colleagues at Washington University, US, constructed the first tomography machines in 1973–74. One of

"Great discoveries are made accidentally less often than the populace likes to think"

EDWARD PURCELL

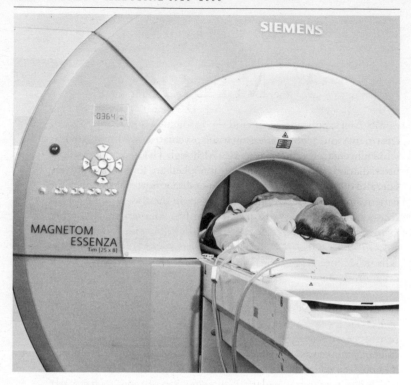

MRI SCAN
A patient lies inside an MRI scanner. The machine is effectively a
large, powerful magnet that acts on various atomic nuclei in the body
to produce images that can be used to assess the patient's condition.

these, PET III, produced the first scans of today's quality, and in 1978,
the first commercial PET scanner, ECAT II (Emission Computed
Axial Tomograph II) went on the market.

Like radionuclide scanning, PET scans require an unstable
radiotracer substance to be introduced into the body, a common
example being a form of glucose. This shoots out particles called
positrons – the opposites of the electrons that "orbit" the atomic
nucleus – and as each positron collides with an opposite electron,
the two annihilate each other in a burst of gamma rays that are
detected by sensors. The most active cells and tissues burn glucose
the fastest, so appear as hot spots on the resulting image. PET scans
reveal how the organs and tissues are functioning, and have a large

ESTIMATED NUMBER OF MRI SCANS
PERFORMED WORLDWIDE ANNUALLY

30 MILLION

number of applications, including cardiology, oncology (cancer treatment), and even in assessing some psychiatric conditions such as schizophrenia or substance abuse. Although PET scans necessarily use radiation, the levels at which it is applied are low, comparatively safe, and do not cause the patient pain or discomfort – although some patients may feel claustrophobic as they lie in the close confines of the scanner. PET scans are also often used in conjunction with other forms of imaging, such as CT and MRI, which illuminate tissue structure. PET is particularly useful for identifying the busily dividing cells in tumours, and a variant of MRI scanning, called fMRI (f for functional), shows brain activity in a similar way.

PET/CT scanners were *TIME Magazine*'s medical invention of the year in 2000. The development of scanning technology has been of huge benefit to patients all over the world, both in terms of diagnosis and in being non-invasive, relatively safe, and comfortable procedures. Radiologists today choose from a wide range of imagers, each of which has its own particular advantages. Ultrasound (US; see p.311), for example, uses sound waves rather than electromagnetic waves to produce an image – this is an extremely safe form of imaging, and is commonly used to examine babies in the womb. The digital pictures of modern scans can be greatly magnified and distributed electronically around the globe for any number of second opinions. Every day, millions of scans identify or rule out problems, help to plan surgery, monitor treatment, and generally save lives – all from outside the body, and without a scalpel in sight.

Seeing Inside the Body

The discovery of X-rays at the end of the 19th century made it possible to see images of the body's interior for the first time, transforming our understanding of its structure, how it works, and how it is affected by illness (see pp.302–309). Increasingly sophisticated types of scan have been developed since then – some for specific organs or tissues, and others for the whole body. They are all invaluable aids to diagnosis, surgery, and treatment.

X-RAY
Passing through soft body tissues such as muscle easily, X-rays are blocked by denser tissues such as bones, which therefore show up clearly on the resulting image.

3D CT SCAN
CT (computerized tomography) or CAT scans take X-rays from several different angles at a time. As in this scan of a heart, this builds up three-dimensional images of organs rather than the simple outlines of standard X-ray images.

ANGIOGRAM
This type of X-ray uses a special injected dye to highlight a patient's blood vessels, so that doctors can check if they are narrow, blocked, enlarged, or malformed.

LAYERED CT SCAN
The layered, cross-sectional images produced by a CT scan show all body tissues and can be compiled into a 3D image on a computer. This picture reveals the interior of a narrowed artery.

AREA ACTIVE
WHEN LISTENING

AREA ACTIVE
WHEN SPEAKING

MRI SCAN
Magnetic resonance imaging (MRI)
is a versatile electromagnetic imaging
technique. It creates detailed images of
soft tissues, such as the brain (above),
and is well suited to detecting
cancerous tumours.

PET SCAN
Using a tracer introduced into the body,
a PET (positron emission tomography)
scan shows which areas of an organ are
the most active (the lighter parts of the
brain scans above). It is an effective scan
for diagnosing cancer.

RADIONUCLIDE BONE SCAN
Before a bone scan, radioactive tracer
is injected into a patient and enters the
bones. As the tracer wears off, it gives
off radiation picked up by a camera as
it scans the patient's body.

ULTRASOUND SCAN
Often used to scan foetuses in the
womb, an ultrasound (US) scan
uses high-frequency sound waves
to create images of organs and
structures inside the body.

The Birth of IVF

IVF BABIES ARE CONCEIVED OUTSIDE THE BODY, then the fertilized egg is returned to the mother's womb to develop and grow as usual. The first such baby, born in 1959, hardly rocked the world – no doubt because it was a rabbit. However the first human baby born as a result of IVF – Louise Brown, delivered in Oldham, England, on 25 July 1978 – generated global headlines. The event gave hope to millions of couples around the world who were having problems conceiving. It also stirred up a huge ethical debate. Doctors were accused of "playing God" by creating life where there would otherwise be none. Their response was that they did not in fact originate that life; medicine was simply aiding a natural biological process, hence the term "assisted reproduction".

A newborn baby is the end result of a series of complex, delicate processes that take some nine months to complete. These processes start in the female body with the release (ovulation) of a ripe egg cell (mature ovum) from its follicle in one of the two egg-making ovaries. The egg then moves along the fallopian tube towards the womb (uterus). Meanwhile, in the male body, millions of sperm cells (spermatozoa) mature daily in the testicles. During sex, about 250–500 million sperm in their nutrient liquid (seminal fluid) are released into the women's vagina, and some make their way through the cervix into the womb, and onwards into the two fallopian tubes. If there is a ripe egg in one of the tubes, a sperm may fertilize the egg. The fertilized egg (zygote) then continues along the tube into the womb, dividing as it goes – into two cells, four cells, eight cells, and so on, until several days later there is a blackberry-like ball of cells – the early embryo, or morula (see pp. 364–66). The cells of the morula carry on multiplying until they form a hollow cluster of cells called a blastocyst, which then beds down into the lining of the uterus to continue its development. This whole sequence is carefully timed, and each stage relies on the previous one being successfully completed, so a problem anywhere along the line can prevent conception.

IVF, or *in vitro* fertilization, helps an egg and sperm to meet – "*in vitro*" literally meaning "in glass", or laboratory glassware, as opposed to *in vivo*, in the "living tissue" of the mother. In 1978, the original IVF birth was touted as the first "test tube baby", although the actual fertilization can occur in various types of container, such as a beaker, a flask, or a Petri dish (as it was for Louise Brown). After fertilization, development is monitored under the microscope, and, three to five days later, the early embryo, still less than half a millimetre in size, is inserted into the womb – a process that is called embryo transfer.

In up to half of all infertility cases, failure to conceive naturally is caused by deficiencies in the male sperm. It may also be the result of a disrupted female menstrual cycle, which can prevent or limit egg release. This may in turn be due to a lack of, or imbalance between, the hormones that regulate the cycle – in particular oestrogen, progesterone, and follicle-stimulating hormone. Irregularity or absence of ovulation due to hormonal problems may be treated by so-called fertility drugs. One of the first of these was clomifene (trademarked as Clomid and Omifin), which appeared in the 1960s. It works by making the brain think that the body is not producing enough oestrogen, encouraging the body to increase hormone levels, which usually results in ovulation. Another group of fertility boosters are menotropins, which were introduced in the 1970s. These are extracted from the urine of post-menopausal women and contain natural follicle-stimulating and luteinizing hormones, both of which stimulate the growth of eggs in their follicles. One of the menotropins,

THE FIRST IVF BABY
Robert Edwards holds Louise Brown, the first IVF baby. Beside him are the midwife and Patrick Steptoe.

Pergonal, was pioneered by physiologist Robert Edwards and gynaecologist-obstetrician Patrick Steptoe, the duo who achieved the first IVF birth, that of Louise Brown.

Patrick Steptoe grew up near Oxford, trained in medicine in London, and took up a post at Oldham General Hospital in Lancashire, northwest England, where he headed a human reproduction unit. Robert Edwards spent his youth in Yorkshire and Manchester, then studied and furthered his work in various locations around the UK, including Bangor, Edinburgh, London, and Glasgow, and at the California Institute of Technology, before settling at Cambridge University in 1963 to work on developmental biology. Throughout his long alliance with Steptoe, Edwards provided the laboratory and physiological know-how, trying to create conditions that would enable egg and sperm to unite outside the body, while Steptoe developed methods of collecting eggs from women. The pair met in 1968 and began working with patients in 1970. Edwards had already been successful in fertilizing an egg in the laboratory, a process that involved producing a liquid or culture medium in which the eggs and sperm could mingle. This medium had to mimic the temperature and the mixture

PETRI DISH BABIES
Human embryos in a Petri dish at an IVF laboratory in the US. Fertilization of "test tube babies" can occur equally well in Petri dishes, beakers, or flasks.

"We had a lot of critics but we fought like hell for our patients"

ROBERT EDWARDS

of the nutrients, body minerals, and other substances found in the fallopian tube, and had to activate sperm cells – the second major challenge for IVF. This involves weakening the "cap" at the front end of the sperm cell so that the sperm can fuse with the egg – a process that happens naturally in the body when the sperm comes into contact with the fluids in the vagina and the uterus.

Steptoe was gaining experience with the laparoscope – a long, slim device inserted through a small incision in the abdominal wall (see pp.350–55) – and developed expertise in removing ripe egg cells from their follicles. He also made use of ultrasound (see p.311), which could be used to display a scanned image of the ovaries, to facilitate egg harvesting. In 1969, he began to offer volunteer women Pergonal and other fertility drugs. This resulted in superovulation – producing several mature eggs. Edwards tried various fertilization media and methods, using sperm donated by each woman's partner. When fertilization was successful, the early balls of cells were examined closely for any abnormalities.

At around this time, there was increasing controversy about the ethics of IVF research in the UK, not only among the public, but also within the medical community, religious bodies, the British parliament, and the establishment generally. Edwards and Steptoe were refused grants and found funding difficult to attract. The team eventually moved to the small Dr Kershaw's Cottage Hospital in Oldham, where they set up clinics and laboratories and moved on to the next phase – transferring an early embryo into the womb. However, failures of various kinds continued to blight the programme, and Steptoe and Edwards reasoned that the fertility treatments given to prospective mothers to bring on controlled superovulation were interfering with the womb, so that it was unable to accept the early embryo several days later. They tried injections of another hormone to help the womb lining maintain its readiness, but this produced mixed results and growing frustration for everyone concerned.

In 1977, after more than 70 failed pregnancies, Edwards and Steptoe reverted to a policy of minimal interference – collecting a single egg that had ripened naturally for ovulation, fertilizing it *in vitro*, monitoring its early development, and transferring it back into the mother, whose womb would be ready as normal. To ensure success, the mothers had to provide a urine sample every few hours to test it for luteinizing hormone, levels of which rose about 36 hours before ovulation. The team also decided to transfer embryos at an earlier stage – when they were only eight cells in size. In November 1977, Lesley Brown, the second patient on the new trial, arrived at Kershaw's. Her menstrual cycle and ovulation were normal, but her fallopian tubes were blocked. Steptoe used his laparoscope to obtain a ripe egg, which was then fertilized with her husband John's sperm. The eight-cell embryo was then transferred back into the womb – and nine months later baby Louise was born.

In 1980, Steptoe and Edwards established Bourn Hall Clinic, near Cambridge – the world's first clinic specializing in IVF. In 2010, Edwards received the Nobel Prize in Physiology or Medicine "for the development of *in vitro* fertilization" (Steptoe was not awarded as he had died in 1988).

The birth of Louise Brown was soon followed by live IVF births around the world: in Australia in 1980, in the US in 1981, and in Sweden and France in 1982. Research teams in these countries began working on diverse ways to improve the process. IVF would still be a time-consuming procedure if it had remained reliant on the single egg ovulated by the mother during each menstrual cycle. During the 1980s, however, better fertility drugs and regimes were produced, enabling more eggs to be released with greater predictability, greatly improving IVF success rates. By the 2010s, these reached one live birth per three treatment sessions for women under 35 years old. Ways of freezing an early embryo for later thaw and transfer to the mother were also established, which meant that a woman could conceive after undergoing treatment that might interfere with her reproductive system. GIFT (gamete intrafallopian transfer) was also developed – a process by which eggs and sperm are put together into the fallopian tube, so that fertilization can take place in the body, as if conception had occurred naturally. By 1990, screening also became available. Properly known as preimplantation genetic diagnosis (P(I)GD, or PGS), screening is a process in which one or more cells of an IVF early embryo are isolated before the embryo is transferred to the womb. These cells are analysed for genetic or chromosomal problems, such as Down's Syndrome, and if they are faulty, the embryo is not

SPERM BANK
A technician removes frozen sperm cells from a tank of
liquid nitrogen. After the sample has thawed, the healthiest
cells are selected, using a computer imaging system, and
are each injected into an egg to form an embryo.

transferred. Another innovation was intracytoplasmic sperm injection
(ICSI). Instead of letting eggs and sperm mingle freely, a single sperm
is selected under the microscope and sucked into an incredibly thin
glass tube, which is then pushed through the outer layers of the egg
cell to insert the sperm. ICSI is useful for men with a very low sperm
count, or when many sperm are malformed or otherwise abnormal.

Meanwhile, the ethical debates continued. In 1984, the Government
of Victoria, Australia, introduced the first legislation to regulate IVF
and associated human embryo research, following a review of the
new practices. As a result of advances in assisted reproduction and
stem cell research (see pp.364–73), most countries have legislated to
regulate related activities. In the UK, the Human Fertilisation and
Embryology Authority (HFEA) was established in 1991 to do this.

In the 35 years since Louise Brown made headlines, some five
million babies around the world have been born thanks to assisted
conception. Who knows what the number will be in another 30 years?
Theoretically, a baby could have four "mothers" (and a "father"): a
same-sex female couple could adopt a baby from a donated egg that
(with help from a sperm) merged to form an embryo that was then
implanted into a surrogate mother.

THE MOMENT OF CONCEPTION
In a process called intracytoplasmic sperm injection (ICSI), a doctor guides a needle (left) containing a sperm cell towards an egg cell. The successful joining of the two marks the beginning of a human life.

Complementary and Alternative Medicines

IN MANY AREAS OF LIFE, such as music, food, and fashion, one person's "mainstream" is another's "alternative", or yet another's "complementary" – and the same is true of health and medicine. Alternative and complementary therapies include almost any system or philosophy that aims to improve health and wellbeing but is not part of conventional Western medicine. "Alternative" therapies are exactly that – a different, independent option to the mainstream, while "complementary" implies a supplement or aid working alongside established medical practice. A related term is "holistic" medicine, which is directed at the whole patient, taking biological, psychological, and spiritual factors into account, rather than just the "machinery" of the body.

As Western nations recovered after the austerity of World War II, a new era of freedom and prosperity dawned – and by the 1960s, countercultures were blossoming in the arts, religion, and medicine. Newly affordable televisions and air travel exposed people to medical approaches from around the world. Coupled with dissatisfaction with the "production line" philosophy of conventional medicine, with its high-tech machines, invasive surgery, synthetic drugs, and ever-busy practitioners, there was an upsurge of interest in other forms of therapy, especially those of Eastern cultures. During the late 20th century, these attitudes continued to permeate Western society, and the first World Congress of Alternative Medicines was hosted in Rome, Italy, in 1973. The third, held in Sri Lanka, in 1982, announced its goal of providing "Holistic Medicine for all by the year 2000". In 1992, the US National Institutes of Health (NIH) set up the National Center for Complementary and Alternative Medicine (NCCAM), one of its long-term goals being to "enable better evidence-based decision making regarding complementary and alternative medicine use and its integration into health care and health promotion." Perhaps unsurprisingly, by the early 21st century, surveys in Europe and North America showed that half or more of adults consulting conventional general practitioners had also tried some form of complementary or alternative medicine (CAM).

From a conventional Western viewpoint, up to a hundred and fifty therapies have been listed as complementary, alternative, or holistic. Some, such as acupuncture, Ayurvedic medicine, herbalism, kampo, massage, and yoga, have long-standing traditions (see pp.64–97), but many, such as those discussed here, are later, modern inventions. Laser therapy, for instance, was not possible until American physicist Theodore Maiman invented the laser in 1960. Since 1968, lasers have been used conventionally as "light scalpels" that can be aimed with incredible precision to sear through tissues and seal blood vessels to reduce bleeding. Laser treatment to reshape the cornea began in the late 1980s, and laser atherectomy, which unblocks arteries clogged with fatty plaques, was developed around the same time. Lasers are also used for hair removal, lipo/fat reduction, and minor cosmetic procedures such as eye lifts. More controversial, however, is low-level laser therapy (LLLT), a complementary therapy in which specially designed lasers are used to produce deeply penetrating light that is said to stimulate unhealthy tissues and cells to increase their metabolism and to re-energize them. This is said to help healing after surgery or injury, ease pain by releasing endorphins (the body's natural

LASER THERAPY
A patient receives low-level laser therapy for rheumatoid arthritis. The treatment, which reportedly reduces pain, is also used for osteoarthritis, back pain, and chronic joint disorders.

painkillers), improve mobility and function, and even stimulate specific acupoint-type locations to reduce withdrawal symptoms when giving up drugs such as nicotine and alcohol.

Homoeopathy, a technique developed by German physician Samuel Hahnemann in the 19th century, is even more controversial. The guiding principle of homeopathy, which means "same suffering" in Greek, is "like heals like", or the "law of similars". Dating back to Ancient Greece, Rome, and Asia, this doctrine holds that a substance that causes certain effects or symptoms in the healthy body can, in lesser quantities, cure a disease with the same symptoms. For example, a powerful emetic (which brings on vomiting), given in small doses, can be used to treat an illness whose principal symptoms include vomiting. In *Organon der rationellen Heilkunde* (*The Organon of the Healing Art*), Hahnemann argued that sickness was caused by the body being invaded by "miasms" – disease entities that were attracted by negative states of mind – and claimed that many diseases were exacerbated by conventional medicine. This was, in his view, because doctors tended to treat the symptoms of diseases with their opposites, rather than treating the underlying causes (or miasms) with something similar. To counter this, Hahnemann produced a *materia medica* of substances that could be used to combat miasms. He tested hundreds of plant and animal extracts, minerals, and other substances on healthy people, and came to the conculsion, that, counterintuitively, the more a substance was diluted, the more powerful its effects apparently became. He called this process "potentization", and found that it was encouraged by shaking, banging, and vibrating a solution at each stage of its dilution. The end result was often a mixture so weak

HOMEOPATHIST'S MEDICINE CHEST
This French medicine chest, complete with over a hundred homeopathic medicines, dates from the late 19th century.

that only a few molecules of the original curative substance were left. After much experimentation, Hahnemann produced remedies for all kinds of highly specific conditions. For instance, if a headache was made worse by lying down, then Gelsemium was prescribed – if it eased, then Bryonia was recommended.

APPROXIMATE NUMBER OF HOMEOPATHIC MEDICINES

4,000

Another influential therapy, known as the Alexander Technique, was developed in the late 19th and early 20th centuries. This was pioneered by Australian actor Frederick Matthias Alexander, who, experiencing breathing problems that affected his stage work, underwent an intense period of self-analysis. During the course of this, he discovered patterns of stress and tension in his face, neck, back, and elsewhere that affected his ability to move freely and speak well. He extended the concept to his mind, and developed patterns of thought, posture, and movement that were designed to bring balance to all aspects of his mind and body. When others consulted Alexander, he devised ways of using his hands to help them relax their muscles, joints, and bones, and taught them about body awareness and coordination, and how to improve their breathing, speech, and general health – all of which he described in his 1932 book *The Use of the Self*.

Around the same time, Daniel David Palmer of Davenport, Iowa, US, was developing the chiropractic discipline. Palmer was a complex character who had had a variety of jobs, including spiritual counsellor and magnetic healer (see p.236), but he had received no formal medical training. In 1895, he manipulated the neck bones of a local patient with long-term hearing problems, and the man regained his hearing. As a manual treatment, chiropractic involves pushing, pulling, levering, and generally manipulating the spinal vertebrae and joints to restore their natural positions and function, thereby helping the nerve and muscle systems and a variety of associated health problems. He conjectured that misaligned spinal joints affected nerves and the general flow of energy around the body, thereby causing a wide range of health problems. Modern chiropractic has refined Palmer's techniques, but its main attention is still on the manipulation of the spine and musculoskeletal system, particularly to relieve lower back and neck pain. Chiropractic is similar to osteopathy, which was founded slightly earlier by US physician and political activist Andrew Taylor Still. The goal of osteopathy is also to activate the body's innate self-healing mechanisms to overcome health problems, by manipulation of muscles and joints.

Another way of balancing the body's energies emerged with the technique of reflexology, which uses "reflexes", or responsive zones on the feet and hands that are believed to correspond to regions and organs of the body. Like many complementary and alternative therapies, this technique has ancient origins and was Westernized only recently, in this case by US ear, nose, and throat surgeon William Fitzgerald, whose work of the 1910s was developed by US physiotherapist Eunice Ingham in the 1930s. At the same time, in Germany, psychiatrist Johannes Schultz developed autogenics (meaning "created by self") – a series of six mental exercises designed to free the individual of stress and worries, so they can focus on their inner being, or spirit. Schultz borrowed elements from Eastern traditions, such as Zen and certain forms of yoga, to help overcome the fight-or-flight instinct encouraged by modern life, and to foster a state of "relax and restore", in which the body can cope better with anxiety, mood swings, insomnia, high blood pressure, muscle tensions, and stress-related health problems.

Two other therapies developed in the 1930s were Bach flower remedies – named after British bacteriologist Edward Bach – and aromatherapy. Bach flower remedies aim to reduce the negative thoughts and feelings that are believed to underlie so many physical disorders. Bach devised a system in which 12 types of negative mental and emotional states – such as fear, uncertainty, lack of interest, loneliness, and depression – could be overcome by the effects of water-based extracts from certain flowers or buds. He called these extracts the 12 Healers, and later supplemented them with the 26 Helpers. Rock Rose, for example, is recommended for states of terror, and Agrimony for concealed worry. Later practitioners formulated combination flower remedies, including the well-known Rescue Remedy, containing Impatiens, Star of Bethlehem, Cherry Plum, Rock Rose, and Clematis – a formula recommended for emergencies and frightening situations. The term "aromatherapy" was coined in 1937 by French cosmetic chemist Professor René-Maurice Gattefossé, although the effects of scents and aromas on the mind and emotions have been appreciated for millennia. Gattefossé developed the use of

LAVENDER OIL
This electron microscope image shows lavender oil droplets
on the surface of a lavender leaf. Practitioners of alternative
medicine use lavender oil as an antiseptic, an analgesic, and a
chest rub for asthma.

essential oils extracted from flowers, leaves, bark, sap, resins, roots,
and other plant parts, which could be inhaled, massaged into the
skin, or added to bathwater. Garlic oil rubbed onto the abdomen, for
instance, is recommended for digestive problems, chamomile or
rosemary for joint aches, and cinnamon for toothache.

Aside from the dangers of misdiagnosis (which dog all types of
medicine), the question is, do these treatments actually work? Anecdotal
evidence suggests that millions of people have been helped, and all of
the therapies described above now have expert practitioners and official
organizations around the world. What tends to be lacking, from a
conventional point-of-view, is accountable peer-reviewed evidence
derived from controlled trials, and an underlying scientific hypothesis.
The placebo effect does suggest that belief in a cure can effect a cure,
raising the possibility that homeopathy patients, for instance, are
elaborately healing themselves. However, the question of "why" will
always come second to "whether" — and it is likely to be academic to
anyone who benefits from these hitherto mysterious arts.

REVISITING THE APOTHECARY
A 15th-century French apothecary turns plants into medicines. Alternative practitioners in the 20th century sought to reinvigorate the natural remedies of their forefathers, as modern medicine grew ever more reliant on chemicals.

Potential Pandemics

BUBONIC PLAGUE, SMALLPOX, CHOLERA – infections have menaced humankind down the centuries. At their worst, they are pandemics: outbreaks on continental, even global, scales (see pp.180–87). The first and worst pandemic of the 20th century was the three-wave spread of influenza from 1918–19, known as Spanish flu; estimated fatalities ranged from 30 million to more than 100 million people, nearly one in 20 of the world population at the time.

The body's immune system naturally tries to destroy invading microbes and protect the body against future attacks (see pp.286–93). Infecting microorganisms, however, have a nasty habit of mutating (changing) their genes and structures. Different strains can also interact in the body, sharing their existing genes. This means that the immune system may not recognize a new strain as the previous intruder, allowing the infection to take hold. The common cold and influenza viruses are masters of this art, constantly mutating to adapt and evade the defences of the immune system. On a wider scale, microbes that infect one group or species, such as birds or monkeys, may change so that they can transfer to another – such as humans.

Around 1981, US medical establishments recognized that some rare diseases and conditions, such as Kaposi's sarcoma, a skin cancer, and *Pneumocystis carinii* pneumonia (PCP, now called *P. jirovecii*), were

DISCOVERY OF HIV
French scientists Luc Montagnier and Françoise Barré-Sinoussi (left and right) received the Nobel Prize in 2008 for their 1983 discovery of the virus later called HIV. Jean-Claude Chermann (centre) was head of the retrovirology laboratory.

unexpectedly occurring together in certain patients – the first sufferers of what was being referred to by 1982 as Acquired Immunodeficiency Syndrome (AIDS). At that point, the cause was unknown. Then, in May 1983, an article in the journal *Science* reported the discovery of a new virus. It was identified at the Institut Pasteur in Paris by French virologists Luc Montagnier and Françoise Barré-Sinoussi, and called Lymphadenopathy-Associated Virus (LAV). Lymphadenopathy means any disease affecting the lymph nodes (the familiar swollen glands of so many infections), which are part of the immune system, and the virus had been isolated from this source. In April 1984, a related announcement came from a US research team headed by Robert Gallo at the National Cancer Institute, Bethesda. Called Human T-Lymphotropic Virus Type III (HTLV III), Gallo's virus seemed to be related to Types I and II, which had already been discovered and linked to T-cell lymphoma, a type of white blood cell cancer (see pp.260–69). It was suspected, and soon confirmed, that LAV and HTLV III were the same. In 1986, they were renamed Human Immunodeficiency Virus (HIV), the cause of AIDS.

Perceived as a modern plague that could spread like wildfire, AIDS was global news. Its origins were a mystery and it had no cure. It appeared to be linked to certain lifestyles and behaviours, in particular, homosexuality and intravenous drug use. Myths and misconceptions were rife. Governments set up national campaigns to correct fallacies about HIV/AIDS, communicate impartial facts, and encourage precautions to prevent the spread of the disease.

HIV is a retrovirus. Most viruses contain genetic material, DNA (see pp.338–49), inside a protective covering. The virus invades a host cell and tricks it into building more viruses (see pp.228–29). A retrovirus adds a retro (backward) step to this process: it codes its genetic information in a different form and employs a distinctive enzyme to convert it to DNA, which then behaves in the same way as in an ordinary virus. Robert Gallo detected the first evidence of retroviruses in humans in the early 1970s. What HIV does is target the very parts and processes of the body that are designed to repel invaders – the immune system. In particular, it infects and destroys a type of white blood cell crucial to the body's ability to fight germs and make antibodies. As HIV reduces the number of these cells, the immune system is robbed of vital forces. The body's defences weaken, leaving it vulnerable to opportunistic infections and cancerous changes.

HIV UNDER THE MICROSCOPE
The RNA (which encodes genes) appears as a dark oblong shape in this cross-section of HIV. Its outer coat (the dark-edged outline) contains a protein that attaches to a T-helper cell (a type of white blood cell).

Retroviruses infect many animals, including birds, cattle, mice, cats, monkeys, and apes. Herein lie clues to the origins of HIV. Researchers began to check through stored samples of blood and other tissues from people whose symptoms and diagnoses matched the HIV/AIDS profile. From 1985, they identified a similar group of viruses known as SIVs (Simian Immunodeficiency Viruses; "simian" meaning monkeys and apes). These occurred in African monkeys and in apes, a group that includes humans and our closest living relatives, chimpanzees and gorillas. By the mid-2000s, intense analysis concluded that HIV had jumped from chimpanzees to humans, probably in West Africa as a result of bushmeat butchering. The jump may have happened in the first half of the 20th century, as the earliest preserved tissue samples testing positive for HIV dated back to 1959 and 1960. From West Africa, the virus travelled in human hosts to Haiti and thence to North America, where sophisticated health care made identification possible. HIV/AIDS has since been detected in every country. By 2010, more than 30 million people had died of it.

In the decade before AIDS emerged, two other significant infections were newly identified. The first recognized case of Legionnaire's disease was in 1976 in the US. It is one of a group of pneumonias – infections that affect primarily the lungs, and especially the millions of alveoli (microscopic air sacs), where essential oxygen passes from air into the blood and carbon dioxide passes out of the blood into the lungs. Pneumonia has many causes, mainly numerous viruses and

ESTIMATE OF PEOPLE LIVING WITH HIV/AIDS

30 MILLION

bacteria. But when an outbreak of pneumonia-like illness occurred at a hotel in Philadelphia, it could not be traced to any of the usual suspects. Delegates at the convention were members of the American Legion, hence the name given to the disease. Eventually, the cause was traced to the bacterium *Legionella pneumophila*. Unlike HIV, this is not a newly evolved germ, but an established, common inhabitant of watery and damp environments. The hotel's air-conditioning system and cooling towers just happened to provide the ideal temperature and humidity for the bacteria to multiply and spread in tiny mist-like water droplets, which were easily breathed in. Most of the convention delegates were middle-aged or older – a group now known to be prone to the infection. Their symptoms appeared a few days later, and local Philadelphia doctor Ernie Campbell noted that several patients had attended the convention. This first outbreak resulted in 220 cases and 34 deaths, so systems were put in place to identify future outbreaks much more quickly. New regulations were also introduced to minimize the risks in equipment such as air-conditioning, heaters, humidifiers, saunas, misting machines, and whirlpool tubs.

Legionnaire's disease is potentially serious but rare, and continues to rumble on at the rate of a few reported outbreaks each year – since its discovery, it has caused small numbers of fatalities in various regions, including Norway, Australia, Spain, and North America. Probably many more cases go unrecognized, especially in areas with less developed health care. Important limiting factors are that Legionnaire's disease tends to occur in certain types of "unnatural" indoor settings and does not spread directly from person to person.

The second infection that was newly identified, also in around 1976, was Ebola virus disease. It was first noted in Sudan and in the Ebola River region of the Democratic Republic of Congo in Central Africa. Extremely serious, it starts, like so many other diseases, with flu-type symptoms, but then progresses to the digestive system, where it causes nausea, vomiting, and diarrhoea; to the nervous system with severe headache, confusion, agitation, seizures, and sometimes coma; and to the respiratory system with breathing difficulties. Haemorrhage or bleeding in the skin and other organs is a characteristic symptom. It is deadly in about two-thirds of cases.

Ebola virus disease is spread primarily by contact with blood and other body fluids, either directly or through contaminated objects. In health centres and hospitals, it can rapidly spread among staff from a patient whose Ebola infection has not been diagnosed. This is why isolation, infection control, and barrier nursing – goggles, masks, gloves, gowns, and thorough equipment sterilization – are paramount.

As with HIV and other viruses, Ebola virus disease probably came from animals, which constitute a reservoir of infection, so that even if all human cases were eliminated at once, people could still be infected in future from close contact with animals. Certain species of fruit bat are the primary and continuing source of the virus. Gorillas, chimpanzees, monkeys, forest antelopes, and porcupines are also recognized sources. Since these creatures are found in few places other than West and Central Africa, and human-to-human transmission can be prevented with intensive precautions, Ebola virus disease is unlikely to be a potential pandemic.

In the mid-1990s, a new strain of avian influenza ("bird flu") was identified in China. It was a subtype of the influenza A virus designated H5N1. At the time, and like its predecessors, it infected only birds, mainly chickens and waterfowl such as geese and ducks. Culling flocks helped to limit these early outbreaks. In the early 2000s, more bird and then human outbreaks spread through China and Southeast Asia, and occasionally elsewhere. By 2012, there were more than 580 cases of bird flu in humans across 15 countries, and almost 350 deaths.

Bird flu moves from infected birds to humans through close contact with feathers, skin, organs, fluids, and droppings (which dry and disperse as dust). Properly handled, cooked food and eggs do not spread the disease. As with other infections, the fear is that the genetic make-up of the virus may alter so that it passes more easily from person to person, triggering a pandemic. In 2013, a different strain, H7N9, was reported to spread more easily from birds to humans, but so far there is no evidence of human-to-human transmission.

Another recent infectious disease is Severe Acute Respiratory Syndrome (SARS). Caused by a type of coronavirus (under the microscope, it looks like a halo or crown – *corona* in Latin), it was named for its effects on the body, which at first resemble influenza. The SARS outbreak in southern China from 2002 to 2003 was both helped and hindered by 21st-century technology, with the internet and electronic communications playing important roles. The disease spread at once via international air travel and global media quickly alerted the world, likening it to Spanish flu. Its cause was rapidly

POLICE PROTECTION FROM SARS
In an effort to contain a SARS outbreak in 2003, a military policeman, masked for protection, stands guard outside a 102-ward hospital in Taiwan, the first to be used solely for SARS sufferers.

identified by the cooperative efforts of several nations, using the most advanced medical methods. Precautions and prevention soon followed. As a result, the SARS outbreak was contained to fewer than 9,000 recorded cases and 800 fatalities, and did not graduate from epidemic to pandemic.

All these infections continue to cause concern, as do resurgent old enemies such as new strains of drug-resistant tuberculosis. Another area for concern is the pox group. Smallpox has gone, declared extinct in 1980 (see pp.160–61). Since then, smallpox vaccination has ceased, but it may be that the immunization programme had helped to protect against the related *Orthopoxvirus* strains, such as mousepox, monkeypox, and cowpox, which are carried by rats and other rodents. Just a small change in one of these strains could enable it to pass from animal to human, and then from one human to another – the ideal requisites for a pandemic.

Battling HIV and AIDS

HIV (human immunodeficiency virus) is one of the fastest-evolving entities known to medicine – it reproduces lightning-fast, spawning millions of copies of itself in the space of just one day. Producing flu-like symptoms, it leads to a breakdown of its victims' immune system, leaving them vulnerable to life-threatening infection. A recent disease, it probably originated in Africa early in the 20th century, but has nonetheless caused over 30 million deaths, and is still spreading rapidly. There is currently no cure, but antiviral drugs can slow the progress of the disease.

AIDS AWARENESS RIBBON

1986 Research in France and in the US identifies the virus that **causes AIDS**; it is confirmed that the retroviruses **LAV** and **HTLV-III** are in fact the same, and the virus is renamed HIV.

1985 Experiments using the antiviral drug **zidovudine** (AZT) reduce replication of HIV, slowing the disease.

1959 The earliest documented case of AIDs occurs in **the Belgian Congo** (Democratic Republic of Congo).

1983 Scientists at the Institut Pasteur in Paris isolate a retrovirus, LAV, that is the **likely cause of AIDS**.

1987 The antiviral drug AZT is made widely available as the **first treatment** for HIV.

1969 The HIV virus is probably **brought to the US** (possibly by a sufferer who travelled from Haiti).

1981 The first cases of the **immunodeficiency syndrome** are identified in New York and California.

1984 A team led by American scientist Robert Gallo **identifies a retrovirus** and calls it HTLV-III.

1982 The disease becomes known as **AIDS**.

RATIO OF THE POPULATION OF SUB-SAHARAN AFRICA WITH HIV

1 IN 20

1990S HIV prevention campaigns around the world encourage safe sex and responsible drug use. This poster, showing the figure of death marked "AIDS", and wielding a scythe and a syringe labelled "heroin", is part of a campaign in Vietnam.

2013 Researchers in the US work on a vaccine that helps the immune system **recognize and attack** HIV.

1990 The Ryan White Care Act provides funds in the US to care for **HIV patients**.

1992 A new drug, Hivid, becomes available for use **in combination** with AZT.

1997 AZT is increasingly prescribed for HIV-positive **pregnant mothers** and reduces transmission to the child.

1998 Human trials of an HIV/AIDS **vaccine** begin.

2004 The US approves the first generic **HIV drug**, paving the way for less expensive medication.

1996 Powerful new drugs called **protease inhibitors** are used against HIV in combination with other drugs.

2000 In response to **widespread ignorance**, 5,000 scientists sign a declaration that AIDS and HIV are linked.

2009 American scientists complete their project to **decode** the entire HIV genome.

2001 US drug companies drop patent claims, enabling European manufacturers to make cheaper, **generic drugs** for use in hard-hit areas of the developing world, especially Africa.

Genes and
Future Dreams

2000–PRESENT

Welcome to a brave new world. Stem cells grow into any tissue or organ for rejection-free implant into their original owner's body. Cloned cells aid them. So does tissue-engineering, with bio-friendly scaffolds that give cells 3D frameworks to help them build spare parts. Nanotechnology delivers molecule-sized machines that melt blood clots with lasers, invade and destroy tumour cells, and attach powerful anti-germ drugs directly on to microscopic invaders. Tailor-made genetic profiling allows doctors to identify detailed risk factors, disease likelihood, and the perfect drug mix for each individual. Gene therapy corrects all manner of inherited defects and treats cell mutations that could lead to cancer. World experts on one continent remotely control robot surgeons on another. The internet gives instant expert diagnosis and prescription. Advanced life-support technologies nurse ailing bodies through the most difficult of disease crises. Anti-ageing treatments, anti-obesity pills, tablets to increase brainpower, even proper cures for baldness and wrinkles – they all work.

Some of these advances are on the way now; some are hopefully not more than a few decades away; others will fall at one hurdle or another. But the 21st century harbours threats, too – the spread of antibiotic-resistant germs; plague pandemics of new infections that have spread from animals; a colossal increase in dementias; more illnesses caused by affluence and old age; spiralling costs and struggles for funding and resources. For medicine, the 2000s may be the century of the greatest extremes and inequalities yet.

Genetics and Medicine

IN JUNE 2000, THE HUMAN GENOME PROJECT announced a breakthrough. For the first time, it had successfully mapped a "rough draft" of the human genome – the entire set of DNA (deoxyribonucleic acid), the genetic material that forms the instructions for building, running, and maintaining a human body. The draft was a phenomenal achievement with immense implications for human biology, health, and medicine, but it was widely misunderstood. It did not identify every gene in the body, explaining how it worked and what it did. To appreciate the relevance of the genome, and the relationship between genetics and medicine, it helps to go back a couple of centuries and explore thebackground of genes and DNA.

Children resemble their parents. Not in all respects, but in general likeness and personality, plus a few very similar family features such as nose shape. The principles of this process, called inheritance or heredity, were laid down by Austrian monk Gregor Mendel, who experimented with pea plants rather than people, and published his results in 1866. He had interbred some 29,000 pea plants that had various contrasting features, such as flowers that were different colours, and had discovered that many parental features were not blended together like some kind of hybrid soup in the offspring, but were passed on in discrete particles or units – now known as genes – that kept their integrity and were inherited in specific patterns over succeeding generations.

In the early 1900s, several biologists rediscovered Mendel's work and quickly brought it to the attention of the scientific community. German biologist Theodor Boveri, who was doing research with sea urchins, and American physician Walter Sutton, who was experimenting on grasshoppers, both independently reached the conclusion that a dividing cell passes sets of chromosomes to each of the new cells, and this is what makes them inherit features and characteristics. Chromosomes had first been identified in the mid-19th century, and were formally described in 1878 by another German biologist, Walther Flemming. Through the light microscope, they appear as thread-like, X-shaped objects when cells prepare to divide. By 1915, American biologist Thomas Hunt Morgan, using fruit flies for experiments, had demonstrated that chromosomes carry

CELL DIVISION
This light-microscope image shows a single cell
dividing into two separate cells. The two sets of
chromosomes can be seen in the centre in light grey.

hereditary information, and in 1933, he was duly awarded the Nobel
Prize in Physiology or Medicine for "discoveries concerning the role
played by the chromosome in heredity".

What are chromosomes made of? In the 1920s, the answer became
clearer – proteins called histones, as well as the substance we know as
DNA (see pp.348–49). The latter had first been isolated and studied as
"nuclein" by Swiss physician-researcher Friedrich Miescher in around
1870. During the early decades of the 20th century, the building-block
components of DNA were identified in more detail as deoxyribose
sugars, phosphate groups, and four types of component called
nucleotide bases, or simply bases. By the 1940s, investigators had shown
that DNA is a giant molecule and the carrier of genetic information, a
fact that was further confirmed in 1952 by experiments with viruses.
DNA's precise physical structure, however, was still unclear. In 1953,
came the momentous discovery of DNA's double-helix arrangement by
English scientist Francis Crick and US biologist James Watson, aided by
English biophysicist Rosalind Franklin and New Zealand-born Maurice
Wilkins. The finding explained how genetic information in DNA is
carried in the sequence of its bases, which are copied when the cell

divides and then pass to both new cells, including egg and sperm cells, and thus to the fertilized egg and the next generation. It was shown that DNA works in the same way in bacteria, moulds, plants, fruit flies, and other animals, including humans.

At the same time, medical researchers were also studying chromosomes. In the 1920s, research scientists suggested that there were 24 pairs of chromosomes in each human body cell – one of each pair inherited from the mother, and the other from the father. In 1956, with much improved technology, Indonesian-born American cellular geneticist Joe Hin Tjio, working in Sweden, was able to revise this number to the now-accepted 23 pairs, making 46 chromosomes altogether in each body cell. Before long, scientists were discovering that chromosomal abnormalities were responsible for various congenital (present at birth) conditions. In 1958, it was found that people with Down's syndrome have three chromosomes instead of

BUILDING BLOCKS OF LIFE
Geneticists James Watson (left) and Francis Crick
with a model of DNA – the molecule in which
genetic information is encoded.

two on the 21st of the 23 pairs. They are therefore sometimes referred to as "having an extra chromosome".

Despite these discoveries, pinpointing the mechanics of individual genetic abnormalities and understanding how to mend them, or even knowing how many genes the human body has, was still

PROPORTION OF GENES SHARED BETWEEN A HUMAN AND A TREE

50%

some way off. What was known for certain, however, was that a gene was a length of DNA that contained the information necessary to make proteins. Some proteins are the structural building blocks of cells and tissues – such as collagen in skin and keratin in fingernails – whereas others are involved in control and coordination: insulin, for example, manages blood glucose, and antibodies counteract microbes. The substances called enzymes that break down food during digestion are also proteins, as are other enzymes that synchronize the mass of chemical changes occurring every second within cells.

Proteins are built from smaller units known as amino acids, which are linked together in sequence. A genetic fault can cause the body to use the wrong amino acid when a protein is made, resulting in a malformed protein. An example of this is an inherited condition called sickle-cell anaemia, in which red blood cells are not the usual doughnut-like shape, but sickle-shaped, which reduces their ability to carry oxygen. In 1949, US scientists Linus Pauling, Harvey Itano, Seymour Jonathan Singer, and Ibert C. Wells published evidence that sickle-cell patients' haemoglobin – the component of red blood cells that transports oxygen and carbon-dioxide around the body – differs from normal haemoglobin. In 1956, the root cause of this condition was pinpointed to a tiny part of the amino acid sequence, in which a different amino acid from usual was present. This was the first discovery of the molecular basis for a genetic disorder.

The Human Genome Project's rough draft was not a catalogue of all the genes and what they did – what it provided was a list of DNA's chemical subunits, or bases. These bases are strung out along the immense length of every coiled DNA molecule, each of which forms one of the 46 chromosomes. DNA has four different types of chemical base : A (adenine), T (thymine), G (guanine), and C (cytosine).

These bases form pairs, and the sequence the pairs form along the double helix carries genetic information that is written out as strings of the four letters: A-T-C-C-G-T-T-, and so on. Crucially, the base on one strand of the double helix can only attach to one other base, which is its partner on the second helix: A always pairs up with T, and G always pairs up with C.

When a cell divides, the double helix splits lengthwise to form two single helices, then each helix builds a new partner strand (see p.348). An A on the existing helix therefore attaches to a T for the new strand. If the next base is C, this links to a new G, and so on. This results in two new double helices, each consisting of one strand of the original double helix plus a new complementary partner strand. Because of base pairing, these two double helices are identical both to each other and to the parent double helix. The genetic information has been copied from the original cell to its two offspring cells. As we have seen, there are only four different kinds of base in DNA, but their numbers are astronomical – more than three billion base pairs are strung out along all the DNA molecules in all the chromosomes of the human genome. And this genetic information is economically packaged. Joined end to end, the set of DNA molecules would stretch over 2m (6ft), yet they are tightly coiled and folded into a cell so small that 500 of them could fit on a pinhead.

The Human Genome Project began in 1990 and aimed to sequence all the DNA bases in the main parts of the genome. It was declared complete in April 2003, and the information was made freely available online to the public, including research scientists, doctors, drug companies, biotechnologists, life insurance companies, mortgage lenders, and lawyers. There would be other far-reaching effects – understanding in greater detail how genes actually work, unravelling what happens in genetic or inherited diseases and conditions, and finding out how and why the DNA in some cells in the body changes or mutates to produce tumours, for example. The project's Ethical, Legal, and Social Implications (ELSI) programme considered the consequences of this knowledge, especially its application to human health and medicine. The "rough draft" published in June 2000 listed sequences for

THE HUMAN GENOME
A scientist working on the Human Genome Project in 1998 at Washington University in the US uses ultraviolet light to study strands of human DNA.

SCANNING THE GENOME
A technician working at the California Institute of Technology uses a circular scanner to read sections of DNA radiograms for computer analysis.

about 85 per cent of the bases – 25 per cent to such a high degree of accuracy that they were regarded as finished, and more than another 50 per cent very nearly so.

One particular area of genome study is that of SNPs (single-nucleotide polymorphisms), pronounced "snips". These are variations in the location of a particular base. For example, one person may have base A at a certain location on a particular chromosome, while another person might have base C. In fact, SNPs occur on average once every 100–300 bases along the whole human genome. They are part of what makes each human genetically unique (apart from identical twins). Many SNPs have no effect on health, but some do. One SNP results in sickle-cell disease, as mentioned above, and we now know that the change or mutation occurs within a gene called HBB, which contains instructions for a part of haemoglobin. The chromosome on which it occurs is about 134 million base pairs long, has around 1,500 genes, and is involved in more than 150 genetic disorders and other health problems. As details such as these become known for genetic disorders, the hope is that they will lead to better treatment and possible cures.

SNPs help to track inherited disorders through family lines, even if the SNPs themselves are not directly responsible for the disorder. Those that are located near or among the mutated sequences can act as "markers" to determine patterns of heredity. SNPs and similar changes in genes are also linked to more general phenomena, such as reaction to environmental factors such as inhaled toxins; response to certain drugs and foods; and the chances of developing particular diseases – even complex diseases such as cancers. For instance, in 2010, the gene APCDD1 was linked to a form of hereditary hair loss. In 2011, the loss of a group, or cluster, of 27 genes was linked to autism-like features. In 2013, a research consortium reported finding another seven positions, or loci, in the genome linked to age-related macular degeneration, which is the main cause of sight loss in the elderly.

As we learn more about genes, what they do, and how they go wrong, the question arises: can we treat genetic conditions by introducing normal DNA into the body to enable it to produce a substance, such as an enzyme or a hormone, that is otherwise missing or abnormal? Introducing normal DNA into body cells is known as "delivery", and one such method exploits viruses (see p.228–29). When a virus invades a cell, it hijacks the cell's production machinery, then uses its own genes to make more viruses. In gene therapy, the virus is used to deliver normal human genes into the cell. A virus used in this way is known as a "virus vector". The vector technique has been widely used in other areas of biological sciences since the 1970s, to make genetically modified bacteria and crops, for example. Another form of gene therapy is to insert the correct genes as "naked" lengths of DNA. One such technique, electroporation, involves applying an electric field to a cell in short, sharp bursts, to create pores in the cell's outer skin through which much larger molecules or substances than usual can be admitted – including drugs to destroy a tumour, or lengths of DNA to repair a genetic condition. Electroporation has been performed both on cells floating in laboratory liquid (*in vitro*) and on living tissue that is accessed by tiny probes inserted into the body (*in vivo*). Inserting genes into cells like this is known as gene electrotransfer. Another way of delivering the DNA is to wrap it in fatty substances to form artificial bubbles, or vesicles, known as liposomes, which are then injected into the cell. This method is used to treat cancers. The healthy DNA stimulates the natural cancer-

"What more powerful form of study of mankind could there be than to read our own instruction book?"

FRANCIS S. COLLINS, US GENETICIST

suppressing genes already present in the genome, which for some reason are not working. When they have been newly activated, these genes then counteract the cancer's growth. Liposome delivery has also been researched for the inherited condition of cystic fibrosis. Whichever method is used, the aim is to get as many normal genes into as many cells as possible, and to ensure that they remain active for as long as possible.

In 1990, gene therapy came of age when a four-year-old girl was treated for a rare enzyme disorder known as ADA deficiency (adenosine deaminase deficiency). However, faith in the new treatment was damaged in 1999, when Jesse Gelsinger died in Philadelphia, US. Gelsinger, who was only 18 years old, was participating in clinical research for a genetic disorder that renders the liver unable to deal with ammonia, a waste product created when proteins are broken down. Virus vectors were used to introduce normal copies of the gene, but Gelsinger's immune system reacted in a catastrophic manner. He developed brain damage, went into a coma, and died four days later. Subsequent investigations revealed that the organizers of the trial had not informed Gelsinger and his family about previous reactions to the treatment. This was followed by news that other gene therapy trials had failed, with more than 600 reports of "adverse events", including deaths. These tragedies were severe blows to gene therapy, but as time has gone by, the numbers of clinical trials have increased.

One area in which gene therapy is flourishing is vaccination – the introduction of harmless versions of a disease-causing microbe or its products into the body (see

LIPOSOME CLUSTER
This scanning electron micrograph shows liposomes – bubbles made from the same material as cell membranes – used to deliver DNA into patients.

pp.286–93). The body's immune system recognizes the foreign substances, called antigens, and mobilizes defences against them. DNA vaccination goes a step further and introduces artificially made genes that carry instructions to make the antigens. When the antigens are produced, the body's defence mechanisms swing into action. Such vaccines have been under trial since the 1990s, and their targets include tuberculosis, HIV (see pp.334–35), and malaria (see pp.388–89). DNA vaccination could help in eradicating these diseases, as could genetic studies such as those investigating why sickle-cell disease protects people against malaria.

During the 1980s, estimates of the total number of genes in the human genome usually exceeded 100,000. As the Human Genome Project progressed, scientific consensus reduced this total to 60,000–70,000, then to 40,000–50,000. In 2013, around ten years after the project finished, most estimates were in the area of 20,000–25,000 – a number that, 20 years earlier, would have seemed impossibly small for an organism as complex and sophisticated as a human being. Furthermore, most of the DNA in the human genome does not actually represent the genetic code as such. The base sequences that we call genes, known as coding DNA, account for less than two per cent of the genome. The rest, non-coding DNA, was assumed to be an array of harmless leftovers or accidental copies – what is sometimes labelled "junk DNA". Recently, it has become clear that large portions of this DNA are in fact not "junk"at all and contain instructions for making substances and molecules that control if, when, and how genes work (see pp.364–73).

After decades of promises but failed delivery, 2017 saw major advances in this area of medicine, especially in the field of haematology where a number of new therapies were approved by the US Food and Drug Administration (FDA). Significant progress has also been made using gene therapy to cure devastating genetic disorders and in 2018 the FDA also approved the first gene therapy to target mutated DNA for patients with a rare form of inherited blindness. All of this has huge implications for the study of genetic disease and designing gene therapies for the future.

The Genetic Code

All living beings are made of complex chemicals called proteins. The substance in a cell's nucleus that controls how these proteins are produced – and therefore determines the similarities and differences between individuals – is DNA (deoxyribonucleic acid). DNA has a regular structure. It was identified as a double helix – like two intertwined coil springs – by James Watson and Francis Crick in 1953.

DNA is present in every living cell, and contains a set of instructions – genes – that control inherited characteristics. As an organism grows, its cells divide in such a way that every cell has a copy of the DNA instructions for making protein. So, genes are consistent within an individual, but vary from one individual of the same species to another. Unravelling the genetic code – how genes influence the body's chemical make-up – continues to occupy scientists (see pp.338–47), and is leading to a greater understanding of diseases and genetic disorders.

Friedrich Miescher

Swiss scientist Friedrich Miescher began studying the proteins in white blood cells soon after qualifying as a physician in 1868–69. In the nuclei of the cells, he found a substance that contained phosphates and other elements that are not usually found in proteins. Miescher named this mysterious substance "nuclein", because it occurred in the cells' nuclei, and this term is still part of the substance's modern name: deoxyribonucleic acid (DNA).

FRIEDRICH MIESCHER BECAME PROFESSOR OF PHYSIOLOGY AT THE UNIVERSITY OF BASEL IN 1871

DOUBLE HELIX
DNA is a long-chain molecule made up of repeated building blocks called nucleotides (see top right). How the nucleotides are arranged influences the composition of proteins.

Complementary base pairs of nucleotides are arranged in a specific order that is replicated before cells divide

Structure of DNA

Nucleotides – the building blocks of DNA – are each made up of one sugar, one phosphate, and one base. There are four types of base (see p.342), which pair up in only two combinations because of their shape and size. Each pair consists of one large and one small base.

Three bonds join C and G

Phosphate

C — G

T — A

G — C

A — T

Sugar

Base

Two bonds join A and T

The nucleus is the cell's control centre and contains DNA in the form of chromosomes

DNA coils around proteins called histones

Adenine-thymine link (A-T base pair)

Histone protein acts as a scaffold for the huge quantity of DNA to coil around

Guanine-cytosine link (G-C base pair)

A double helix of DNA consists of two chains of nucleotides. These chains are made up of units of sugar and phosphates either side of a core of base pairs

Robots and Telemedicine

O N A FUTURE BATTLEFIELD, an armoured truck arrives near the front line – a military surgical unit, ready for action. Inside is a miniature operating theatre packed with diagnostic and surgical equipment. Each wounded patient brought in is hooked up to monitors for detailed assessment – then fast, expert treatment, including surgery, is delivered to almost any part of the body by top consultants in virtually every branch of medicine. Yet the unit carries only a few, albeit highly trained, personnel. The medical experts are far away, providing their services remotely via super-fast satellite communications and robotic operating technology. This is one scenario for telesurgery, itself a branch of telemedicine – medical care from a distance. Telemedicine is just a tiny part of a revolution in medicine that is being powered by computing and information technology – a revolution that began in the early 20th century and is still gaining momentum.

In 2001, telesurgery was carried out for the first time across the Atlantic. Surgeons in New York joined the patient and operating team in Strasbourg, France, by fast fibre-optic link. Guided by cameras showing close-ups of the operating area, along with patient monitor read-outs and two-way audio, surgeons in New York operated a remote surgical console, the movements of which were copied in Strasbourg by robotic effector arms and equipment. The 68-year-old female patient underwent laparoscopic cholecystectomy – removal of the gall bladder through a minimal incision. Since this was chiefly a pioneering trial to demonstrate telesurgery's potential, a highly experienced medical team stood by in France in case of problems. Among the challenges facing the telesurgeons was making the robotic manipulators copy the surgeon's movements in almost real time across a distance of nearly 7,000km (4,350 miles). Tests had shown that a time lag of more than 250–300 milliseconds (about one quarter of a second) from the operator's movement to the robot arm/camera and back to the operator's visual display could make the surgeon feel detached and disorientated. The NY–Strasbourg–NY lag was an acceptable 155 milliseconds. Also vital was an isolated communications link that, unlike usual worldwide web traffic, would not slow down or be interrupted, and which could also carry the amounts of data needed for robot control, medical monitoring, and two-way audio and visual communication. The whole operation took less than an hour, and the patient went home two days later. The milestone event was dubbed the "Lindbergh Operation", after the first solo, non-stop transatlantic flight in 1927 by Charles Lindbergh. Director of the European Institute of Telesurgery Professor Jacques Marescaux, who conducted the operation remotely from New York, said: "It lays the foundations for the globalization of surgical procedures, making it possible to imagine that a surgeon could perform an operation on a patient anywhere in the world".

The Lindbergh Operation employed a remote three-arm robotic system called ZEUS, which was controlled by the motions of the surgeon's hands. Two of ZEUS's arms held surgical instruments, including a laparoscope, while another held a laparoscope positioner called AESOP (Automated Endoscopic System for Optimal Positioning). A laparoscope is a long, slender tube that can carry a light, a camera, and various surgical tools – including forceps, grabs, crushers, blades, and cautery tips. It is inserted into the patient through a small incision made in the abdominal wall. A laparoscopy is an example of minimally invasive surgery, or MIS – otherwise known as "keyhole surgery" – which, compared to the traditional method of making a large incision, greatly reduces tissue disruption, blood loss, post-operative pain, recovery time, and scarring. AESOP was designed primarily to help the surgeon guide the laparoscope, and as such, it was an early stage of computer-assisted robotic surgery. Following AESOP and ZEUS came the da Vinci system in 2000. Using NASA's space technology adapted initially for battlefield conditions, the da Vinci system has three or four robotic arms. One carries a laparoscope and

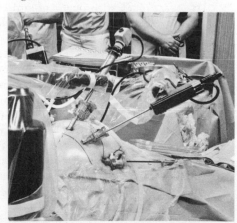

THE LINDBERGH OPERATION
Doctors stand by as the remotely controlled arms of the ZEUS surgical robot perform a laparoscopic cholecystectomy during the historic Lindbergh Operation of 2001.

REMOTE HEART SURGERY
A surgeon operates the arms of
a da Vinci robot during the first
organ transplant performed using
such a system. The operation took
place at Guy's and St Thomas'
Hospital, London, in 2004.

twin cameras for 3D visual display, while the others hold various surgical instruments. Its arms and wrists exploit so many pivots and swivels that they have a greater range of movements than those of any human. The surgeon uses hands, feet, head, and voice to control the laparoscope, instruments, visual display, lighting, and other features.

Hundreds of thousands of procedures are carried out yearly by da Vinci, although most of these are not conducted over vast distances – the operator and console are usually next to the patient's bedside. This computer/robot interface is prohibitively expensive for many medical centres, but is said to have benefits over direct manual manipulation. For instance, it helps to reduce the normal small hand vibrations of even the most experienced surgeon. It can "gear down" motion so that a large hand movement produces a much smaller robot version, thereby improving precision for microsurgery. The system helps to detect and negate rare accidental slips, and the surgeon can sit in a comfortable, efficient position that minimizes fatigue. It also allows the surgeon to trial manoeuvres on the console; the system takes details from the actual patient and adapts them using a database to display predicted results on a virtual patient. If all is well, the surgeon then orders the manipulators to perform the manoeuvre.

During the 2000s, telesurgery reached a new level of sophistication – touch sensitivity, or haptic feedback. Arrays of sensors detect the smallest of vibrations passing through the operating instruments, yielding information such as tissue resistance and fluid slipperiness. This is fed back in the form of resistance in the surgeon's controls, effectively allowing the surgeon to feel what is happening.

Computerized robot-assisted surgery has a growing list of applications. Hysterectomy (womb removal) and other gynaeological procedures, heart valve and coronary artery bypass, the removal of tumours, and neurosurgery have all been carried out in this way and forms of telesurgery in which patient and surgeon are far apart are on the increase. Telementoring and teleteaching allow experienced surgeons to advise, monitor, and even assist trainees around the world as they practise on animals or computer-simulated virtual patients, or even (given all the safeguards) with real-life patients. Surgeons can also watch and support each other, discuss individual cases, and pool their knowledge.

Telesurgery is the high-tech end of the increasing use of computers in medicine. In many places around the world, computers work away in the background helping physicians and patients. They analyse and visualize molecules and compounds that have potential as new drugs, and coordinate data on drug effectiveness and side-effects. They crunch numbers to track outbreaks of infection, and link cause and effect for epidemiologists (see pp.180–87). They sharpen, colour, and interpret images from scanners that also rely on computer power, and suggest diagnoses based on these. Computer-automated medical history questionnaires help doctors use their time more efficiently, and evidence shows that patients answer a machine more honestly than they do a human doctor, especially on sensitive topics, such as alcohol or drug intake and sexual relationships. From alerting the family doctor to the side-effects a medicine might have on a particular patient, to performing a life-saving operation on an astronaut via a telesurgeon here on Earth, these electronic devices may one day supplant human doctors. In the meantime, medicine – certainly surgery – is becoming hard to imagine without them.

ROBOTIC SURGERY
A surgeon (left) performs minimally invasive
surgery (MIS, or "keyhole" surgery), on a patient's
heart using a remotely controlled da Vinci robot.
The surgeon views a three-dimensional image of
the operation site on his screen.

Emergency Medicine

"**I**T'S A MAJOR INCIDENT. Alert all first responders, paramedics, and other EMTs. Scramble the air ambulance. Contact ER, A&E, ICU, CCU, HDU. Make ready for triage, SCA, MI, CAB, CPR, defib, and AED. We'll do BP and other vital signs, sats..." Medicine is full of acronyms, abbreviations, and jargon. One of the branches richest in these is emergency medicine, or EM – partly, it is said, to shorten speaking, reading, and writing in this area of medical care where time is most precious.

It has been a long journey from the emergency procedures carried out on the battlefields of Ancient Rome, Persia, and China (tightening tourniquets near wounds, or roughly sewing gashes with a dagger and threads ripped from clothing) to today's sophisticated EMS (emergency medical services). Progress in emergency medicine has accelerated rapidly, especially since the 1980s, thanks to instant communications via mobile phones and the internet, the increasingly rapid transport of patients and personnel by fast cars, helicopters, planes, and speedboats, and the use of computers in diagnosis and treatment plans. There has also been an increasing move towards professionalization, away from panicky amateurs trying out partly forgotten first-aid techniques, to the latest highly trained and qualified, constantly updated experts in the field. The precise terminology varies among countries and regions, but there is now a wide spectrum of authorized emergency medical personnel, ranging from casual, licensed first-aiders to first responders, basic and

BATTLEFIELD SURGEON
Baron Dominique Jean
Larrey, surgeon-in-chief
of Napoleon's army, gives
emergency aid to a soldier at
the Battle of Hanau in 1813.

advanced EMTs (emergency medical technicians), and paramedics. It also includes medical centre and hospital ED (emergency department) and ER (emergency room) staff, such as nurses, junior doctors, and senior consultants.

As an official branch of the medical system, emergency medicine is relatively young. Its first hospital specialists were appointed in the 1950s. Prior to this, staff from other specialisms did their rota duties in Casualty or A&E (Accident and Emergency). Fully recognized emergency medicine departments were established in major hospitals in the US, Europe, Canada, Australia, and Japan from the 1970s. The US's *American Journal of Emergency Medicine* began in 1983; issue 1 of the UK's *Emergency Medicine Journal* was published in 1984; and by 2010 a major survey showed that around one third of the world's nations recognized emergency medicine as a formal speciality.

Where did it all begin? During the First Crusade (1096–99), European armies organized groups such as the Knights of the Order of St John of Jerusalem (Knights Hospitaller), who specialized in giving first aid to soldiers wounded in battle and helping pilgrims in need of medical treatment. One of the UK's leading first-aid organizations, St John Ambulance, traces its origins to this time. Such orders continued through the Late Middle Ages and into the Renaissance, especially across Europe (see pp.126–31). In the early 19th century, battlefield surgeon Baron Dominique Jean Larrey and his advisors pioneered the concept of the ambulance in the form of rapid horse-drawn transport for the wounded in Napoleon's armies. They arranged for medically trained personnel to man front-line units, and set up early versions of combat medical care facilities or field hospitals. Larrey's teams refined the idea of triage – the process of quickly assessing and prioritizing patients in the face of overwhelming casualties. Those who could probably be saved by treatment were prioritized, ahead of those who would probably recover without treatment, and those who were likely to die even with treatment. Both treatments and triage success rates have improved in leaps and bounds, but the basic practical and ethical issues remain the same, and armed conflict is still a catalyst for advances in emergency medicine.

Today, one of the most common treatments in emergency medicine is mouth-to-mouth ventilation, or rescue breathing. The practice has a long history, being mentioned in antiquity and the Middle Ages, but it was only in the 18th century that it became commonplace. In 1744, Scottish surgeon William Tossach recorded

RESUSCITATION KIT
This 19th-century apparatus for blowing tobacco smoke into the lungs of a patient was used to revive people whose hearts had ceased beating and who had stopped breathing.

one such instance when he had revived a comatose coal miner: "There was not the least pulse in either heart or arteries, and not the least breathing could be observed... I applied my mouth close to his, and blowed my breath strong as I could; but having neglected to stop his nostrils all the air came out at them; wherefore taking hold of them with one hand... I blew again... raising his chest fully with it... immediately I felt six or seven very quick beats of the heart". The practice spread across Europe and North America in the 1760s and 1770s as "rescue organizations" were established – largely in response to the number of people who died falling through ice on frozen rivers in winter. Ventilation was sometimes performed using a bellows (which might be used to blow tobacco smoke rather than air), but the mouth-to-mouth method proved to be more effective.

This is how one of emergency medicine's best-known, most high-profile techniques evolved – CPR (cardiopulmonary resuscitation). In the early 1900s, the "cardio" part of the process – ECC (external chest compression) – was added to the "pulmonary" component of assisted breathing. Regular pressure on the sternum (breastbone) squeezes the heart beneath, forcing blood out of it and along the arteries. Valves in the heart and main veins (see p.134–43) maintain some kind of one-way circulatory flow and distribute at least some oxygen to the vital organs – critically, to the brain. By the 1960s, CPR was on a more scientific footing and was recommended not only for victims of drowning, but also for medical emergencies such as SCA (sudden cardiac arrest), in which the heart suddenly stops beating. SCA has a variety of causes, including the common form of heart attack – when a piece of fatty deposit called atheroma inside an artery detaches and causes a blood clot in the arteries supplying the heart muscle, leading to myocardial infarction (MI), death of the heart muscle. SCA is one of the main reasons that emergency medicine is summoned.

CPR is part of a protocol called "ABC" for the treatment of an unconscious casualty who has no detectable breathing or pulse. The acronym ABC stands for airway, breathing, circulation: A, ensure that the airways down into the lungs are unobstructed; B, assist breathing by mouth-to-mouth; C, encourage circulation by chest compressions. Each step is needed for the next to succeed – there is no point in giving assisted breathing, for instance, if the airway is blocked, such as by vomit. ABC was developed during the 1950s by physicians Peter Safar and James Elam in the US. Safar wrote *ABC of Resuscitation* (1957) and Elam produced *Rescue Breathing* (1959). In 2018, the American Heart Association (AHA) and other US experts recommended changing ABC to CAB (except for new babies), and upping the compression rate from 100 to 120 per minute. This shifted the very first casualty-side task away from checking the airway and assisted breathing to compressions and maintaining circulation. The AHA explained: "In the A-B-C sequence chest compressions are often delayed while the responder opens the airway to give mouth-to-mouth breaths or retrieves a barrier device or other ventilation equipment. By changing the sequence to C-A-B, chest compressions will be initiated sooner and ventilation only minimally delayed until completion of the first cycle of chest compressions (30 compressions)". Applying compressions first delays the start of assisted breathing by less than 20 seconds, and most people can hold their breath for longer than this. Another recent trend is to ignore assisted breathing and to concentrate on chest compression once the airway is clear, since the compressions give some air movement into and out of the lungs.

A variant of CAB/ABC adds D for "defib", or defibrillation – administering carefully controlled electric shocks through the chest and heart, in an attempt to jolt the heart's electrical control system back into action (see pp.362–63). Cardiac defibrillators have existed for more

"For the service of mankind"

ST JOHN AMBULANCE MOTTO

than a century, although they were initially intended for animal research only. The first hospital use of defibrillators took place in 1947, on hearts exposed during open-chest surgery. Defibrillation was applied to closed chests from the mid-1950s, using electrode "paddles" that were pressed against the skin. Over the following decade, portable defibrillators appeared and were soon being carried by most ambulances and emergency medical transports. In the 1970s, in Portland, Oregon, US, physician Archibald Warren "Arch" Diack and his collaborators devised the first of the devices now known as AEDs, or automated external defibrillators. In Britain, early versions, trialled in the 1980s, were known as Heart Aid. Electronics made AEDs smaller and easier to use, so that after they were connected to the patient, emergency diagnosis could be made and suitable treatment applied. AEDs can now be used with minimal or even no training, and are installed in all manner of premises, from offices and factories to shopping malls, swimming centres, and gyms.

As well as defibs and other hardware, many drugs are available for emergency patients. For example, a thrombolytic, or "clot-buster", drug can dissolve and disperse a thrombus, or blood clot, to restore blood supply. Clots are involved in many medical emergencies, including myocardial infarction, stroke, and deep-vein thrombosis. As far back as 1933, William Smith Tillett at Johns Hopkins University, Baltimore, USA, discovered that certain bacteria make a clot-dissolving substance, which he called streptokinase. In the late 1950s, this was given to patients with sudden or acute MI, though due to unclear data on its side effects it only came into restricted use in the 1970s, and general use in the late 1980s. Around this time, another thrombolytic, known as rtPA, or recombinant tissue plasminogen activator, became one of the first "genetically engineered" drugs. It was derived from a natural clot-dissolver in the body, tPA, discovered in the 1940s. Administered as soon as possible, these and other clot-busters now save lives and reduce lasting damage in untold numbers of people each year.

Hospital emergency assessment is well rehearsed and rapid. Traditionally, the four main vital signs that are checked are body temperature, heart rate (pulse), BP (blood pressure), and breathing or respiratory rate. Some assessment schemes add pupil response, pain experience, and "sats" – blood oxygen saturation, or the percentage of oxygen carried by the blood. Along with pulse rate, sats is non-invasively, conveniently, and continuously measured by a pulse oximeter; a small

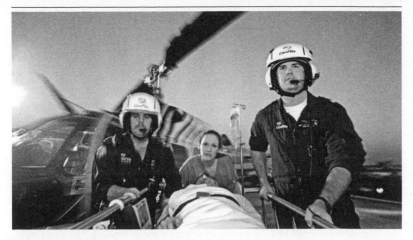

THE GOLDEN HOUR
Paramedics rush to an emergency room, having
spent the transportation time assessing the patient's
condition and delivering preliminary treatment.

clip-on sensor on a fingertip or ear lobe uses light of specific wavelengths
to detect how much of the haemoglobin in red blood cells is in the form
of oxyhaemoglobin, which contains oxygen. Emergency patients in
most need may be cared for in an ICU (intensive care unit), a CCU
(critical care unit), or a similar department – the exact names for them
vary from one place to another. For example, a life-threatening heart
condition may demand the Cardiac Intensive Care Unit, CICU, while
new babies are in units for Neonatal Intensive Care, NICU.

Lodged in popular consciousness is the notion of the "Golden
Hour" – the theory that emergency treatment will have the greatest
chance of success if it is administered within the first 60 minutes after
a trauma. This has since led to the Platinum Ten Minutes – the time
it should take for EMTs or paramedics to assess, treat, and instigate
transport of an emergency patient. In a sense, this is the paramedic's
share of the Golden Hour. As ambulance crews become more highly
trained, and their equipment becomes increasingly extensive and
sophisticated, the chance to save life and improve eventual outcome
shifts to the very first minutes of emergency medical care.

A Shock to the System

When a person has a heart attack, the muscles of the heart often contract randomly, a symptom known as ventricular fibrillation. In the late 19th century, scientists discovered that they could stop fibrillation and resuscitate their subject – a dog – by applying an electric shock to its heart. In 1947, this technique was first used on a human. American surgeon Claude Beck successfully used a combination of electrical current and internal cardiac massage to resuscitate a child who had gone into cardiac arrest during an operation. In the 1950s, external defibrillators became available, which worked without the need to open up the patient's chest. Some modern units are able to calculate the patient's heart rhythm automatically, so can be used in emergencies by people with little or no training.

Trial and error

Before the 20th century, doctors tried many methods of getting a patient's heart to start beating again, from bloodletting to tickling the throat. Breathing into the mouth and pressing the abdomen were advocated in the 18th century, but not widely used. This was the forerunner of modern cardiopulmonary resuscitation (CPR), used from the early 1960s, which keeps the brain alive with artificial blood circulation using mouth-to-mouth ventilation and chest compression.

FRENCH COUNT GASTON DE FOIX DYING OF A CARDIAC ARREST IN 1391

type 180

④

defibrillate

DANGER HIGH VOLTAGE

① patient

⚡

The electrodes are held in paddles with insulated plastic handles to protect the operator

DEFIBRILLATOR
1970–80
By the 1970s, portable defibrillators with a
rechargeable power pack were available.
Their compact size made them useful to
emergency services and hospitals.

Voltage and battery indicator

Battery test and capacitor
charge switch

lator
ated

CARDIAC RECORDERS LTD
LONDON ENGLAND

test battery

charge capacitor

external
battery
12V

00

TYPE 1R2
Rechargeable
Power Pack
MAINS

UNNEL

Output dial

Mains plug to
recharge battery

How it works

The heart's regular beat is controlled
by electrical impulses in the body. In a
cardiac arrest, these electrical impulses
go haywire. The defibrillator stores a
powerful electric current and contains
a transformer that enables the operator
to control the amount of current
it administers. When the current
is applied to the patient via two
electrodes, the electric shock "resets"
the heart's regular electrical rhythm
and the heart starts beating again.

ELECTRODE POSITION
The operator places the
anterior electrode just below
the patient's right collarbone.
The posterior electrode is
placed on the patient's left,
below the pectoral muscle.

Current

Anterior
electrode

Posterior
electrode

Stem Cell Therapy

A PLANT SEED SENDS OUT A SHOOT, which grows into a stem. From this seemingly mundane, unremarkable structure, the sophisticated, specialized parts of the plant gradually develop – buds, side shoots, leaves, and delicate, intricate flowers. The stem analogy works quite well for the so-called stem cells of humans and other animals, and plants. A stem cell is a "general-purpose" cell. It has not yet developed any features for a specialized function – unlike nerve cells (neurons), for example, which typically have branches (dendrites) and a longer axon (a special cellular extension) and are specialized to transmit and receive nerve impulses; or red blood cells (erythrocytes), which are disc-shaped and packed with haemoglobin to carry oxygen. Stem cells do, however, have distinguishing characteristics. They can self-regenerate – keep up their numbers by splitting or dividing to make more cells like themselves – and in certain conditions, they can make many other kinds of specialized cell.

In a sense, the ultimate stem cell is the zygote – an egg cell that has been fertilized by a sperm cell. It divides into two, then four, and so on. At first, its offspring cells all look similar, making a blackberry-like ball known as a morula. The offspring cells continue to multiply and form a hollow ball of cells called a blastocyst. Cell division continues, but now the various cells begin to specialize, so that they no longer look alike and work differently from each other – a process called differentiation. Next, during the embryo stage, thousands of multiplying cells make millions of specialized cells that eventually constitute the body's 200-plus kinds of tissue. By the time cells are fully specialized, and have become nerve cells or red blood cells, for example, they usually cannot change any further, or even renew themselves by dividing to produce more of their kind. They are, as it were, at the "end of the line", and can only carry out their particular jobs and then die. This is because most cells, and specialized cells in particular, have a limited lifespan. A red cell in the blood, for example,

HUMAN STEM CELLS
These early embryonic stem cells all look alike.
As they continue to multiply, they will give rise
to millions of specialized cells that will form every
type of tissue in the human body.

lives for around three months, and a cell in the lining of the intestine lasts for less than a week, so new cells must be made to replace them. New red cells, for instance, are produced at the rate of three million every second. This is the job of stem cells in the adult body. Unlike the original zygote, they are not able to form any kind of cell or tissue, but have a more limited function – to create a set of related cells. The stem cells for blood are known as haematopoietic stem cells. They are found mainly in bone marrow, and they keep dividing, supplying lines of descent for the dozen or more different kinds of blood cell in the circulation – red cells, platelets (which help blood clot), and numerous kinds of white cell in the body's immune system that fight disease and invading microbes. Because haematopoietic stem cells exist throughout a person's life, and not just during the embryo stage, they are known as adult (somatic) stem cells. So there are two broad categories of stem cells: embryonic stem cells, and adult stem cells.

A stem cell's degree of flexibility – the numbers and types of specialized cell it can create – is known as its potency. The fertilized egg cell, and the cells it makes in the morula stage of development, are known as omnipotent stem cells. These can generate all the types of cell in the body, plus the supporting cells and tissues that the embryo needs in order to grow and develop, such as the placenta, the umbilical cord, and the surrounding membranes and fluids in the womb. Next are the so-called pluripotent stem cells, which generate every type of body cell, apart from the tissues in the womb (so a single pluripotent stem cell could not create a human being by development in the womb). Multipotent stem cells are more limited, as they can make a range of related cells, but none that are too dissimilar. Haematopoietic stem cells, for example, create various kinds of blood cell, but cannot make muscle cells, liver cells, etc. Unipotent stem cells, or precursor cells, are even more limited and can only make one kind of specialized cell.

So, stem cells range from those with extensive potential but little differentiation, to those that are very specialized but have almost no potency. Why do some cell lines differentiate, while others remain as stem cells? Nearly all human cells have, in their genetic material or DNA (see pp.348–49), the entire human genome – the full set of 20,000–25,000 genes that form the instructions for building and running a human body (see pp.338–47). Differentiation, or becoming specialized, does not apparently involve losing or destroying some

DIFFERENTIATION
Omnipotent stem cells — those in
a fertilized egg or early embryo
— can develop into multiple types
of cells in the body.

OMNIPOTENT
STEM CELL

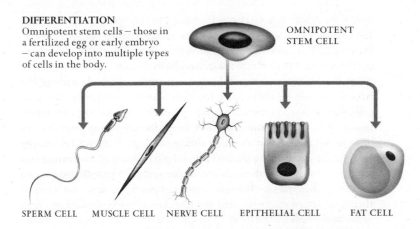

SPERM CELL   MUSCLE CELL   NERVE CELL   EPITHELIAL CELL   FAT CELL

genes and creating or duplicating others. All the genes remain intact,
but only some subgroups of genes in the full set are "switched on". In
a nerve cell, for instance, the genes needed to create nerve cells and
make them work are active but the rest are not; in a bone cell, the
genes that create and maintain bone tissue work, but the others do
not. In a stem cell, these subgroups of specialized genes are not
switched on, but are held ready for activation at a future date. What
are working are the genes that make the cell keep dividing and
making copies of itself. The key to the medical use of stem cells lies
in knowing how to manipulate different subgroups of genes so that
they can be turned on and off as and when they are needed.

After the atomic bomb attacks on the Japanese cities of Hiroshima
and Nagasaki in 1945, it was found that exposure to radiation caused
damage to the blood and immune system. White blood cells were not
renewed, and the numbers of platelets, needed for blood to clot, were
reduced. This led to experiments with mice that traced the source of
new, healthy blood cells to the bone marrow — and to haematopoietic
stem cells. Several medical disorders can also have an affect on
haematopoietic stem cells, disrupting their busy production lines of
new blood cells. These include aplastic anaemia, which damages the
bone marrow and its haematopoietic stem cells, and various forms of
leukaemia — cancers that affect white blood cells, making them either
multiply too fast or fail to do their jobs, crowding out or destroying

other, normal cells. Radiation or drug treatments can destroy these wayward cells, but – like atomic bomb radiation – such treatments also kill off the all-important haematopoietic stem cells.

Could transplanting haematopoietic stem cells treat such problems? If marrow were taken from one person's bone and put into a patient, would the stem cells "take" and replenish the patient's specialized blood cells? This procedure, known as haematopoietic stem cell transplantation (HSCT), or a bone marrow transplant, was first performed in 1956 by Dr E. Donnall Thomas and his team at the Mary Imogene Bassett Hospital, New York. The subjects were identical twins, one of whom had leukaemia. Being identical twins, the problem of rejection – of substances regarded as foreign to the body being attacked by the recipient's immune system – did not occur. This was, in effect, the first successful trial of a new class of treatments called stem cell therapies – and, in 1990, Dr Thomas was duly awarded the Nobel Prize in Physiology or Medicine for "discoveries concerning organ and cell transplantation in the treatment of human disease".

Developing HSCT involved overcoming many obstacles, including rejection, which was countered by a process called immuno-suppression. Thanks to this, the first transplant between non-identical siblings was made in 1968, and between unrelated but tissue-matched donors and recipients in 1973. Today, there are several forms of HSCT, many of which involve giving the patient back his own haematopoietic stem cells that were gathered and stored before a course of chemotherapy or radiotherapy eradicated the diseased cells in the bone marrow. Haematopoietic stem cells are then reintroduced into the marrow and restart blood cell production. HSCT from one person to another follows the same procedure, but involves

"There is no disagreement among scientists over the need to aggressively pursue [stem cell research]"

DR DOUGLAS MELTON,
HARVARD STEM CELL INSTITUTE

NUCLEAR TRANSFER
An adult stem cell is injected into a human egg that has
had its nucleus removed. This creates a new, "cloned"
human embryo from which stem cells can be harvested.

suppressing the immune system to prevent rejection. In both cases, the haematopoietic stem cells can be obtained from the donor's blood by passing it through a device that removes white cells by spinning the blood very fast in a centrifuge, so that the different fluids and cells separate into different layers. The stem cells can also be taken from the donor's marrow, which is drawn out through a wide needle inserted into a big bone, often the hip bone or pelvis. More recently, stem cells have also been sourced from umbilical cord blood.

HSCT is still the most common therapy involving stem cells, but in this fast-moving area of medicine it is hoped that stem cells in general will have many uses. Studying how and why embryonic stem cells work sheds light on the way the early human embryo develops, which in turn provides insights into congenital problems such as spina bifida and certain heart malformations. Serious medical conditions, such as cancer, arise from cells that multiply abnormally, and fail to differentiate as they should. Again, stem cell research may help to identify how and why the "wrong" genes are active in these cells, and so lead to treatments. Stem cell research can also provide more ways of testing potential medicinal drugs and toxic chemicals. For many years, certain types of cell grown in laboratory culture have

NEURAL STEM CELLS
This fluorescent light micrograph shows neural stem cells migrating from the culture in which they are growing. Neural stem cells can develop into nerve cells, or support cells that could be used to replace damaged or lost brain cells.

been exploited to screen drugs for their effects, both wanted and unwanted. Some lines of cancer cells were cultivated like this in the 1950s, and have been central to the development of new anti-tumour drugs. Various kinds of stem cell are being added to this armoury of cultured cell lines, including induced pluripotent stem cells, or iPSCs.

As explained earlier, a pluripotent stem cell in an embryo can proliferate to make any tissue of the body, except those external to the embryo, such as placental tissue. The iPSC is usually a mature, specialized cell taken from an adult body. When subjected to certain conditions and substances in the laboratory, it is persuaded to regress to the pluripotent state, as though it were in an early-stage embryo. Human iPSCs were first obtained in 2007 by processing or "reprogramming" adult cells called fibroblasts, which make a variety of structural components, including fibrous proteins such as collagen for the body's connective tissues. In 2012, Japanese doctor and researcher Shinya Yamanaka and British stem cell researcher John Gurdon received the Nobel Prize in Physiology or Medicine "for the discovery that mature cells can be reprogrammed to become pluripotent". Also in 2012, iPSCs were generated from cells shed from the inner lining of the kidney. Instead of needles, scalpels, or similar invasive techniques, all this required was a urine sample.

The exciting aspect of iPSCs is that they can be manipulated in the laboratory so that they start to develop into specialized cells, much as if they were embryonic stem cells. The cells can be induced to form

the particular types of cell and tissues that are needed to treat disease in the patient, the owner of the originating cells. If specialized cells and tissues came from embryonic stem cells transplanted from someone else, they might be rejected because the embryo would be from a genetically different individual. The solution is to take

COLD STORAGE
Stem cells, which hold the promise of new cell-based therapies for critical medical conditions, can be stored until they are required. This is done by immersing them in liquid nitrogen to freeze them.

adult specialized cells from the patient, make them revert to the embryo-like stem cell condition as iPSCs, then induce them to develop into the cells or tissues required for the patient's treatment and put them back into the patient.

Haematopoietic stem cells are not the only kind of adult stem cell. By the 1960s, mesenchymal stem cells (bone marrow adult stem cells) had been identified. These can generate bone, cartilage, fat, and many other types of tissue. More types of adult stem cell have since been discovered, each able to multiply to replace itself and make lines that can become specialized cells. These stem cells have been found in skin, blood vessels, muscles, heart, teeth, intestines, the liver, ovaries, and testes. Even the adult brain, with its highly specialized nerve cells, is now known to house stem cells that can generate the three main types of cell in its tissues. Many adult stem cells remain dormant until they are needed to divide and replenish cells, both as part of normal cellular renewal and in the event of injury or disease. Like iPSCs, adult stem cells seem to be excellent candidates for stem cell therapies, but they are small in number, are difficult to propagate outside their natural environment, and making them differentiate to order is problematic. There are, however, promising signs of early progress in adult stem cell treatments for skin burns and damage to the cornea (the domed "window" at the front of the eye).

Will stem cell technology lead to growing "spare parts" and even whole organs for implantation? There is a long way to go before a patient can donate a few cells that are then grown into a new heart, liver, eye, or mending patch for the spinal cord, but the technology is already being used to generate cartilage, for example for knee surgery. There are also legal and ethical questions such as who, if anyone, should control patents for manipulating stem cells. Nevertheless, treatments involving iPSCs and adult stem cells are currently being proposed for hundreds of conditions, including Alzheimer's disease, baldness, certain cancers, cerebral palsy, coeliac disease, defects of hearing and sight, diabetes type 1, heart failure, infertility, Parkinson's disease, rheumatoid arthritis, spinal cord injury, stroke, systemic lupus erythematosis, and tooth decay – a lengthening list that already represents a revolution in medical treatment.

Dignity and Death

THE PASSING OF HUMAN LIFE IS INEVITABLE. It is usually coloured with sadness, and sometimes with tragedy. If it happens within the medical care system, it can also be complicated. However, everyday meanings, philosophical concepts, and scientific definitions of death have changed over time, and differ from place to place.

Religious faiths, for example, often incorporate the notion of an afterlife, which renders death a mere transitional stage between this world and the next. According to this idea, the immortal soul adopts a human form at birth, and at death it moves onwards, and perhaps upwards or down, depending on its behaviour on Earth. The Ancient Egyptians regarded death as a temporary state before revival. The deceased first entered the dreaded realm of the underworld, where, overseen by the god Osiris, he or she was assessed by a 42-member judging panel, perhaps aided by Anubis, the jackal-headed god of mummification and the afterlife. In a ritual called "weighing the heart", a set of scales balanced the deceased's heart against a feather, the goddess Maat's symbol of justice and truth. If the scales showed that good prevailed, the deceased was then allowed to move on to the Field of Rushes — a paradise of everlasting bliss. However, if bad deeds predominated, then the heart was fed to Ammit, Devourer of the Dead, and the rest of the body was consigned to Seth, god of doom, gloom, darkness, disorder, and chaos.

The idea that the heart is the essence of a person's life predates Ancient Egypt, and flourished throughout antiquity to the Middle Ages and beyond. In the 11th century, Arab philosopher physician Ibn Sina (see pp.100–105) described the soul as acting via the heart to regulate the body's sensitive, vegetative, and physical "spirits". Regular breathing was also regarded as necessary for life, and when either breathing or heart activity ceased, the individual was declared dead. These criteria for judging the moment of death prevailed in scientific medicine until the early 1920s, yet as far back as the 12th century, Jewish scholar, teacher, and physician Musa ibn Maymun (also known as Maimonides) suggested that there was another element to take into account. He noted that when a person is decapitated, their heart and lungs still work for a short time, but it

WEIGHING THE HEART
Jackal-headed Anubis weighs a dead man's heart on a set of scales in the Egyptian underworld. Ammit, the Devourer of the Dead, waits beneath the scales, while Osiris (right) delivers judgment.

"The boundaries which divide Life from Death are at best shadowy and vague"

EDGAR ALLEN POE

would be wrong to say that they were still alive. Foreshadowing the notion of "brain death" that arose some eight centuries later, he suggested that a central controlling mechanism for movement had been removed, and that this signified death.

During the late Middle Ages, and up to the 19th century, this idea that you could be dead according to your lack of heartbeat and breathing, and yet still alive, became popular as stories arose of people being incorrectly presumed dead and buried alive. This most serious of misdiagnoses became a staple of horror fiction and supposed true-life tales. In 1844, American author Edgar Allen Poe published *The Premature Burial*, in which the central character is obsessed with waking up after being mistakenly entombed while unconscious from catalepsy. This short story fed into contemporary fears and led to safety coffins and crypts being equipped with signals or devices with which the recovered occupant could alert the outside world. In some designs, the unlucky "corpse" pulled a rope attached to a bell or flag.

In 1952, a polio epidemic gripped Denmark. Some patients were so badly affected by the disease that their breathing muscles were paralysed and they died of suffocation. In an attempt to save lives, Danish anaesthetist Bjorn Ibsen adapted existing "iron lung" mechanical ventilation equipment. The iron lung exposed polio sufferers to negative air pressure to stimulate breathing, but Ibsen changed the air pressure to positive, forcing air into a patient's lungs with the assistance of the drug sodium thiopental. Death rates for patients treated with this equipment fell from more than 80 per cent to less than 20 per cent, and Ibsen went on to establish the world's first dedicated medical and surgical intensive care unit (see pp.356–63).

His work was also used to help patients with such severe brain damage that it prevented them from breathing. Physicians studying such comatose patients included Pierre Mollaret and Marcel Goulon of the Claude Bernard Hospital, Paris. A coma is usually defined as a state of unconsciousness, lasting several hours or more, from which a person cannot be roused. In 1959, Mollaret and Goulon devised the term *le coma dépassé*, or "irretrievable coma", to describe deep unconsciousness combined with little or no sign of electrical activity in the brain. In a state of irretrievable coma, the heart might beat – or stop, then be restarted by defibrillation (see pp.362–63) – and the lungs might breathe, but the brain has no hope of recovery. This limbo between life and death, in which the heart and lungs are working, but the brain is not, is known as "brain death" – a state in which, thanks to improved life-support machinery, a body can be kept functioning for hours, days, or even weeks.

Further studies of terminally ill patients led to the convening of an ad hoc committee to examine the definition of death at Harvard Medical School, US, in 1968. Its report discussed not just death, but also the delicate subject of organ donation. Commenting on the condition of irreversible coma, which was recommended to indicate that death had occurred, Chairman Henry Beecher added: "Can society afford to discard the tissues and organs of the hopelessly unconscious patient when he could be used to restore the otherwise hopelessly ill, but still salvageable individual? ... It is best to choose a level where although the brain is dead, usefulness of other organs is still present".

This shifted the criteria for death from cardiorespiratory symptoms (meaning lack of circulation

IRON LUNG
This mechanical ventilator was adapted in the 1950s to provide positive pressure to enable patients with brain damage to breathe. It was later modified to become the first life-support machine.

NUMBER OF YEARS OF THE LONGEST COMA EVER RECORDED

42

or breathing) to symptoms based on the non-functioning of the brain and nervous system.

In 1970, Kansas became the first US state to incorporate brain death into its legal definitions. In Europe, Finland followed in 1971. Within a couple of decades, most nations with advanced medical care routinely used brain-based criteria to declare that a person was officially dead — at which point the "harvesting" of tissues and organs for transplantation could begin. Brain death criteria vary from country to country, but they may include irreversible coma, lack of certain reflexes based in the brainstem (see below), the absence of unassisted breathing or responsive movements, and lack of significant electrical activity as shown by the EEG trace. The cause of all these features is also taken into account and is checked again after a suitable interval. At least two qualified physicians must be involved, and should have the agreement of their nursing and support staff.

Medicine is rarely cut-and-dried. Even when other organs still function on life support, a dead brain can be used as a sign of an individual's demise — but which part of the brain? The whole brain, the brainstem, or the higher brain (the neocortex)? Traditional signs of life include spontaneous breathing, response to stimuli such as spoken words or pain, and automatic reflexes, such as the pupil of the eye constricting in bright light. These indicate that several parts of the brain are functioning, and their absence, along with lack of electrical activity, can be taken as evidence of whole-brain death. Centres for maintaining breathing, heartbeat, and other basic functions are based in the the brainstem, the lowest part of the brain, just above the upper spinal cord. This region is also responsible for consciousness, helps to regulate body temperature and blood pressure, and coordinates actions such as swallowing, coughing, sneezing, and eyeball movement. When the brainstem does not work, many or all of these vital functions cease. The neocortex, or higher brain, includes the familiar, large wrinkled domes at the top, the cerebral hemispheres. This is where most sensation and mental activity occurs. If the higher brain stops functioning, lower parts such as the brainstem may continue to provide breathing, heartbeat, and life-support for the organs – but consciousness, personality, and other attributes that make a human body into an individual person cease.

As medicine adopted the idea of brain death, further grey areas between life and death were identified. These included persistent vegetative state, a term introduced in 1972 by US neurologist Fred Plum and Scottish neurosurgeon Bryan Jennet to describe a hybrid state between full consciousness and coma. Patients in this state are not totally inactive and unresponsive; they may perform reflex actions, such as sleeping and waking, gripping people's hands or objects, and making facial movements, but they remain unaware of their surroundings and bodily sensations. If the condition lasts for more than a certain number of months, the person is said to be in a permanent vegetative state. Another state of limbo, identified in 1966, is locked-in syndrome (LIS), also established by Fred Plum, with US neurologist Jerome Posner, another specialist in impaired consciousness. In this condition, a patient can receive and assimilate stimuli such as sounds, sights, smells, and touch, but has extensive muscle paralysis and cannot speak or make any movements, except perhaps with their eyeballs or eyelids. Posner summarized: "In the locked-in state, patients look unconscious but are conscious".

Fred Plum was an early supporter of the "living will" proposed in 1969 by US lawyer Louis Kutner – a document compiled by a person still of sound mind to instruct how they should be treated if they later become unable to make informed, important decisions about their health. This leads to another extremely complex medico-legal area for physicians and patients: the wish to die, quality of life and maintaining dignity, being allowed to die, DNR (do not resuscitate) and AND (allow natural death) notices, withholding treatment or nutrition, the wishes of partners and close relatives, assisted suicide, when to switch off life-support, euthanasia, and the possibility of tissue and organ donation. Here, clinical considerations become increasingly entangled with ethical, legal, and religious concerns. At the moment, voluntary euthanasia is legal only in Belgium, Luxembourg, the Netherlands, Canada, and Colombia with specific criteria and assisted suicide only in Switzerland and some US states. In most countries, the question of who should have the power to make such life-or-death decisions is part of an ongoing debate that shows little sign of being resolved.

KEEPING PATIENTS ALIVE
In some operations, such as open-heart surgery, the heart has to be stopped. To keep the patient alive, a heart-lung machine is used. Often referred to as the "pump", this does the work of the heart and lungs during the operation.

Medicine in the Third Millennium

LOOKING BACK TO THE PAST shows how tricky it is to predict future challenges. Halfway through the 20th century, no one knew of Ebola (discovered in 1976), the *Helicobacter pylori* microbes of digestive ulcers (1982), HIV/AIDS (1983), or SARS (2002). Until 1977, Alzheimer's disease was a diagnosis reserved for early-onset dementia, and a term unfamiliar to most of the public. IVF (achieved in 1978) was a twinkle in the eyes of a few researchers. With scanners yet to come (1958), the only body-imaging methods were standard X-rays. Kidney transplants had just begun (1950), and antibiotics were prescribed with almost no regard for the possibility that microbes might develop resistance. What will come to pass, either good or bad, in another century?

Among medicine's "ticking time bombs" is increasing antibiotic resistance. Antibiotics revolutionized not only treatment of infectious diseases, but also surgery (see pp.252–57) and other areas of medicine. However, microbes adapted so rapidly that within three years of the first "designer antibiotic", meticillin, being introduced in 1959, MRSA (meticillin-resistant *Staphylococcus aureus*) appeared. Dozens of other new bacterial strains have since joined the ranks of superbugs. In Europe, the number of strains of *Neisseria gonorrhoeae* – the cause of the sexual infection gonorrhoea – that are resistant to the main antibiotic used to treat it doubled between 2009 and 2010. *C. diff* (*Clostridium difficile*), a bacterium in the gut that causes diarrhoea, is another rising demon, with strains resistant to fluoroquinolone antibiotics appearing in the mid-2000s.

INFLUENZA OUTBREAK
A commuter in Tokyo, Japan, wears a surgical mask to help protect herself from infection during an influenza outbreak.

Increasingly resistant strains of microbes are appearing ever more frequently across the globe – a disaster, given that antibiotics are fully integrated into all of our medical systems. Gene manipulation, genetic engineering, and the creation of GMOs (genetically modified organisms) for agriculture, livestock, and even for dispersing oil slicks, are another potential source of new harmful microbes. Scare stories about artificially created "supergerms" that are resistant to any known antibiotics or other drugs occasionally make their way into the news.

Tackling the ominous peril of antibiotic resistance requires action on several fronts. In 2001, the World Health Organization (WHO) published its Global Strategy for Containment of Antimicrobial Resistance, in which it stated: "Many countries have expressed growing concern about the problem of antimicrobial resistance... Despite the mass of literature... there is depressingly little on the true costs of resistance and the effectiveness of interventions. Given this lack of data... actions need to be taken now to avert future disaster". Inventing new, more powerful antibiotics might seem the obvious answer, but developing any new drug is an immense task. For the near future, the estimated overall cost of producing new antibiotics – adjusted to include failures – is in excess of £3 billion (approaching US$5 billion), and some estimates are double this figure. Even if this strategy is successful in the short term, it only delays the inevitable as microbes adapt and become resistant to the new antibiotics. Doctors regularly receive new prescription guidelines that take into account the rise in antibiotic resistance, and WHO emphasizes that better patient education is vital for the future. Take antibiotics or other drugs exactly as prescribed; do not skip doses; complete the course even if you are already feeling better; do not share prescriptions or save leftovers until next time; vitally, do not demand medication when a doctor says it is not needed; and follow the best hygiene and preventative measures such as handwashing, careful food preparation, and the use of insect nets and repellents. This rudimentary advice has been with us for half a century, but somehow it is still not ingrained.

Information technology and communications networks developed during the last few decades continue to bring great changes in medical decision-making. Evidence-based medicine, or EBM, systematically appraises the available clinical research and uses it to help deliver

PHARMACEUTICAL PRODUCTION LINE
Workers package drugs at a pharmaceutical
production line in China – the third-largest
prescription drugs market in the world.

optimum care to patients. The evidence comes from a clinician's personal experience and that of colleagues, from informed reasoning and intuition, and especially from information published in medical and clinical databases. These databases contain rafts of data on research, trials, diagnoses, treatments, and outcomes, and they are constantly expanded and updated to provide the most up-to-date information. EBM helps doctors to weigh up risks and benefits in light of a sound scientific context, and then to propose the most appropriate action for the patient. Woven into EBM are not only statistics for morbidity (incidence of illness and disease) and mortality (death), which are relatively easy to quantify, but also more complex measures, such as quality of life. The basic principle is to treat a patient where on balance there is evidence of benefit, and not treat where there is no such evidence.

Regarding hi-tech future hardware, the smart cellphone – that most ubiquitous of devices – is lined up to take a starring role. From 2012, apps have been available that record heart rate and rhythm (a simple ECG) and send data to a medical centre for expert evaluation. The medical use of smartphones is expected to rise exponentially in the coming decades, with sensors and apps designed to analyse breathing, blood pressure, and oxygen sats (see p.360–61), take images of possible skin cancers, and – by the detailed analysis of vocal sounds – even to alert users to conditions such as Parkinson's, motor neurone disease, and Alzheimer's. However, the biggest advances are expected to come from the science of nanotechnology, which is poised to transform many areas of medicine. The "nano" level is considerably smaller than the "micro" level of body cells, and deals with individual molecules and even atoms at scales of thousandths of one millimetre. In the wondrous new world of nanomedicine, "quantum dot" nanoparticles are already being designed that can be absorbed by particular tissues, such as those of a tumour, and then show up brightly with astonishing detail on a scan tuned to their wavelength. Nanocapsules have also been produced with coatings that break down to release the drug inside them when they reach the appropriate environment inside a damaged body part. One day, it may be possible to design nanoshells that can home in on specific sites inside the body, where they can then be zapped by specially-tuned waves that create pores in the shells, allowing them to absorb troublesome substances for safe disposal. Perhaps the high-point of this technology will be the creation of nanobots (nanoscale robots) that can carry out simple mechanical actions such as reconstructing damaged tissue and removing fat deposits.

Tissue engineering exists at the interface between the living and the non-living. Living cells and artificial bio-friendly materials are put together to produce new tissues and even whole new organs. Cells respond to many features in their environment – not just temperature, chemicals, and nutrient concentration, but also physical factors, such as contact with each other and with a suitable surface or shaped framework. A combination of congenial chemical and physical conditions, specific growth factors and hormones, and a suitable bio-scaffold on which they can crawl and form layers and patterns, allows them to multiply and develop as directed, into a tissue, or several tissues with a 3D architecture, or even a whole new organ. Transplant

YEAR OF THE FIRST STEM CELL-GROWN ORGAN TRANSPLANT

2011

patients suffer from lack of donors (see pp.294–301), so organ engineering could plug this gap, especially using induced pluripotent stem cells, or iPSCs (see pp.364–73). Research on embryonic layers of cells that form an organ as complex as an eye indicates that if cells are treated appropriately, they know what to do: they multiply, move, specialize, or differentiate, and self-arrange. Maybe iPSCs can be coaxed to grow, on bio-scaffolds, into whole organs such as kidneys, livers, and hearts, and then be reintroduced into the bodies from which they came, thereby avoiding the problem of rejection encountered during transplantation from a donor.

Another developing technology is 3D printing. This technique is currently used by engineers to make 3D models, prototypes, customized implants – for example, knee caps – and prostheses, but one day it could be adapted to print living cells rather than inorganic composites. Shaped layers of cells could be built into tissues that could eventually form a whole organ. Currently, researchers are looking into the possibility of fashioning layers of cells over burns or wounds to encourage faster healing. One day, it may even be possible to access the body's interior with an endoscope that can also print cell layers from its tip to build up tissues in situ.

Other frontiers of progress are less concerned with new technology than with extending established medical practices. Immunization research, for example, is working on vaccines against malaria (see pp.388–89), HIV (see pp.334–35), and other diseases, while cloning may have ever more helpful applications. Another great advance is genetic profiling, which may lead to personalized medicine. For example, an individual's genome may be identified as carrying a sequence of genes that predisposes them to a specific cancer – information that allows the person to take preventative measures, such as altering their diet or avoiding exposure to particular carcinogens (cancer-triggering substances). Should the malignancy appear, the anti-cancer drug known to be most effective in such situations could then be prescribed. Ultrasound technology has also been adapted to perform surgery, rather than simply to make diagnoses. The sound waves are focused onto a particular target and are used to disrupt or destroy tissues such as tumours. There is no need to make an incision; the waves come from outside the body and are aimed to come together with maximum power at a precise point. Known as HIFU (high-intensity focused ultrasound), this is one of

BIONIC HAND
Recent technological advances have led
to the i-LIMB ultra revolution – making
it possible to create a prosthetic hand that
has an unparalleled degree of flexibility.

several areas exploring the use of concentrated energy to replace traditional surgery.

As the world and its nations evolve, medicine responds to changing needs. Cutting-edge research flags the possibilities, which are then reduced to what is practicable. Targets shift and fresh innovations leapfrog the previous year's advances, and at each stage politicians, interest groups, and society in general have their say. Medicine is always bound up with ethical issues and the trials and tribulations of legislation and litigation. It is a long, laborious, and costly business, but the current wave of innovation – including gene therapy, tissue engineering, personalized medicine, bloodless and fast-healing surgery, organ culture, and pills for obesity, hair loss, and almost anything else – is set to have an impact similar to that of immunization, anaesthesia, antibiotics, electronic imaging, and fertility control combined. With continued perseverance, we may yet find that the best medicines and therapies are waiting to be discovered.

Mosquito-borne Malaria

Malaria is a dangerous tropical fever, caused by a parasite transmitted by mosquitoes – a person can be infected from a single bite, and if not treated quickly, it can be fatal. Each year, 10 per cent of the global population contracts malaria, and it is still one of the modern world's deadliest killers. Drugs can provide effective treatment, but are not always available in the tropical and subtropical parts of the world that are most badly affected.

MALARIA-CARRYING MOSQUITO

1880 French army surgeon Charles Louis Alphonse Laveran discovers microscopic **parasites** in the blood of a malaria sufferer.

1906–10 The systematic use of mosquito screens and draining standing water reduces malaria cases among workers on the **Panama Canal**.

1632 Jesuit missionary Barnabé de Cobo brings **cinchona bark,** used medicinally, from Peru to Spain.

1820 French chemists Caventou and Pelletier isolate **quinine**, the active ingredient in cinchona bark.

1885–86 Camillo Golgi, an Italian scientist, shows that there are **different forms of malaria**, with varying periods of fever.

1898 A team working in Rome establishes that human malaria is **transmitted** by mosquitoes of the genus *Anopheles*.

1712 Italian physician Francesco Torti announces that cinchona bark is effective against **"intermittent fever"** (malaria).

C.1850 Attempts are made to develop **synthetic quinine** to bring down the cost of anti-malarial treatment.

1897 British medical officer Ronald Ross shows that malaria can be transmitted by **mosquitoes**.

1902 Ross is awarded the **Nobel Prize** for Medicine in recognition of his work.

ESTIMATED ANNUAL DEATHS FROM MALARIA

700,000

1939 A malaria outbreak occurs in Italy; **fumigation** is used in an attempt to curtail it.

1940S
Posters urge British **wartime troops** posted abroad to take precautions against mosquito bites in countries where malaria is a risk.

1946 The US **Communicable Disease Center** (CDC) is founded to work on controlling malaria in the US.

1951 As a result of the CDC's work, malaria is **eliminated** from the US.

1972 DDT is banned in the US because of the **environmental impact** of spraying. Alternative pesticides such as pyrethrins are adopted.

2007 World Malaria Day is instituted every 25 April to encourage investment in malaria containment and even **eradication** of the disease.

1939 Working in Switzerland, Paul Müller discovers the insecticidal property of the chemical **DDT**.

1930S German company I.G. Farben produces a **synthetic substitute** for quinine.

1955 World Health Organization sets out to eliminate malaria **worldwide** using insecticides and drug treatment.

1981 Chinese pharmacologist Tu Youyou presents her findings that **artemisinin** is an effective anti-malarial treatment.

1980S Rapid **diagnostic tests** for malaria are developed.

Glossary

AGONIST DRUG A drug that simulates a natural substance and replicates its effects in the body.

ALTERNATIVE MEDICINE Systems of health, diagnoses, and treatments that are outside the mainstream of science-based medicine.

ANAESTHESIA Drug-induced loss of sensation, including of touch and pain, either in a part of the body (local anaesthesia) or in all of the body (general anaesthesia).

ANALGESIA Pain relief.

ANTAGONIST DRUG A drug that blocks the action of a natural substance in the body.

ANTIBIOTIC A substance that kills, stops the growth of, or somehow neutralizes bacteria and certain other harmful microbes.

ANTIBODY A substance in the blood that kills, neutralizes, or identifies any foreign material, such as microbes and transplanted tissues.

ANTIGEN Foreign material that provokes the production of antibodies.

ANTISEPTIC A substance that kills or renders harmless microbes; especially used on the skin and surgical instruments.

ARTERY A blood vessel that carries blood away from the heart.

BACTERIUM A type of microbe that is too small to see and lacks a nucleus.

BIOPSY The taking of a sample of fluid or tissue for analysis.

BLOOD PRESSURE The pushing force of blood as it flows around the circulatory system.

BLOOD TYPE/GROUP An individual body's specific combination of antigens on red blood cells and antibodies in blood fluid (plasma).

CANCER A group of diseases characterized by cells that multiply fast, out of normal control, and fail to carry out their usual functions.

CARDIOVASCULAR SYSTEM The heart, blood vessels, and blood.

CELL A microscopic living unit, or "building block", of the body. The human body has over 250 different kinds of cells.

CHEMOTHERAPY Drugs used against cancers and certain other disorders.

CHROMOSOME A thread-like strand of DNA that carries the genes in which hereditary information is encoded. The human body is made of 46 chromosomes.

CIRCULATION The passage of blood through the heart and blood vessels.

CONTAGION A living thing, usually a microbe, that can spread between people to cause disease.

CT/CAT SCANNING Computerized (axial) tomography scanning, a form of computerized scanning that uses weak X-rays to visualize thin, 2D, slice-like images through the body and combines them to make 3D images.

DIASTOLIC In the heartbeat cycle, the lowest measure of blood pressure, as the heart relaxes.

DNA Deoxyribonucleic acid. A long, thin, double-helix molecule in which genetic information is encoded.

ELECTROCARDIOGRAM (ECG) A display or recording of the electrical activity of the heart, especially its muscle action.

ELECTROENCEPHALOGRAM (EEG) A display or recording of the electrical activity of the brain, especially its nerve impulses.

ENDOCRINE SYSTEM The body's chemical messengers (hormones), which control the activity of many tissues and organs, and the endocrine glands that produce them.

ENDOSCOPE A viewing instrument inserted into the body through a natural orifice, or a surgical incision that can often also carry out procedures such as sample-taking.

ENZYME A substance that speeds up or slows down the rate of chemical changes in the body, such as when food is digested.

EPIDEMIC An outbreak of a contagious disease that spreads widely and rapidly.

EPIDEMIOLOGY The study of diseases, how common they are, their causes and effects, and how they can be controlled.

GENE An instruction in chemical form for making a substance or controlling a process in the body.

GERM A harmful microbe, such as a virus, bacterium, fungal spore, or protist.

HISTOLOGY The study of cells and tissues, especially under a microscope.

HORMONE A substance produced in an endocrine gland that circulates in the blood and controls a biological process or activity.

IVF In vitro fertilization; the joining together of an egg and a sperm outside the body.

IMMUNE SYSTEM A defence network, including lymph fluid, lymph nodes, thymus, spleen, and white blood cells, which protects the body against infections and other diseases.

IMMUNIZATION Rendering an individual resistant to attack from microbes that would otherwise cause an infectious disease.

IMMUNOSUPPRESSANT A substance that reduces the workings of the immune system.

IMPLANT An item surgically inserted into the body. The implant may be living (e.g. bone marrow cells), mechanical (e.g an artificial hip joint), electronic (e.g. a heart pacemaker), or a combination of all three.

IN VITRO Literally "in glass". In a laboratory container, such as a test tube, as opposed to in living tissue.

IN VIVO Literally "in living tissue". Inside the body, as opposed to in a laboratory container.

INFECTION A disease caused by invading microbes, such as bacteria, viruses, protists, or similar life-forms.

INOCULATION The placement of a vaccine, antigenic substance, or serum into the body, usually for the purposes of immunization.

LAPAROSCOPE A type of endoscope inserted into the abdomen.

LESION An abnormality, such as an ulcer or tumour, in a tissue or organ.

MRI Magnetic resonance imaging – a form of computerized scanning that uses a powerful magnetic field and radio pulses to visualize thin, 2D, slice-like images through the body, and combine them to make 3D images.

METABOLISM The sum of all the chemical processes in the body, from digesting food to using energy for muscle action.

METASTASIS The spread of cancerous cells from one part of the body to another.

MICROBE A tiny life-form visible only under a microscope.

MITOCHONDRIA Sausage-shaped organelles inside cells that make energy available for the cell to live and function.

MUSCULOSKELETAL SYSTEM The body's muscles, bones, and joints.

MYOCARDIAL INFARCTION Loss of blood supply to heart muscle, causing damage or death to the muscle cells; a common form of heart attack.

NERVOUS SYSTEM The brain, spinal cord, and body-wide system of nerves.

NUCLEOTIDES Chemical subunits of DNA and RNA that function as "code letters" for genetic information.

NUCLEUS The part of a cell in which genetic information is stored.

OBSTETRICS The branch of medicine concerned with pregnancy, childbirth, and postnatal care.

ONCOLOGY The branch of medicine concerned with cancers and similar diseases.

PANDEMIC A very large-scale outbreak of a disease, which affects a huge region.

PATHOGEN A harmful microbe, such as a virus, bacterium, fungal spore, or protist.

PET Positron emission tomography, a form of computerized scanning that uses rays given off by substances put into the body to identify very busy (metabolically active) cells and tissues.

PLASMA The liquid part of the blood that holds the blood cells in suspension.

PLATELETS Cells in the blood that are vital to the blood-clotting process.

PROSTHESIS An artificial item used as a substitute or replacement body part.

PROTEINS Chemical substances made from subunits called amino acids that form essential structural and functional parts of the body, from hair and nails to enzymes.

RNA Ribonucleic acid. A long, thin, helical molecule with many functions in the body, including protein production and gene control. Some viruses use RNA to carry genetic information.

RED BLOOD CELLS Doughnut-shaped blood cells that carry oxygen from the lungs to tissues, and carbon dioxide from tissues to the lungs.

RESPIRATORY SYSTEM The parts of the body responsible for breathing: the nose, throat, windpipe (trachea), the main lower airways (bronchi), and the lungs.

STEM CELL A non-specialized cell that is able to specialize, or differentiate, into particular types of cell, such as nerve cells, muscle cells, or skin cells.

STETHOSCOPE A device for listening to body sounds such as breathing, heartbeat, blood flow, and bubbling gases in the intestines.

SUTURE A closure, or "stitch", for holding ruptured tissues together.

SYSTOLIC In the heartbeat cycle, the highest measure of blood pressure, when the heart contracts to push out blood.

TRANSFUSION The transferral of blood, or parts of blood such as plasma or red blood cells, from one body to another.

TRANSPLANT The transferral of cells, tissues, or organs from one body to another, or from one site to another in the same body.

TUMOUR A growth or lump of abnormal cells that may be benign (non-cancerous) or malignant (cancerous).

ULTRASOUND Sound waves of such high frequency that they are inaudible to humans. An imaging technique based on bouncing such waves off living tissue.

VACCINATION Giving a vaccine to cause future immunity, or protection against, infectious diseases.

VACCINE A preparation of weakened or neutralized germs and/or their harmful products that makes the body become immune to those germs.

VARIOLATION An early form of vaccination against smallpox that uses smallpox itself.

VEIN A blood vessel that carries blood towards the heart.

WHITE BLOOD CELLS Blood cells that protect the body by counteracting invading germs and other foreign matter.

VIRUS The smallest type of harmful microbe, consisting of genetic material wrapped in a protective coating. Viruses can only multiply by invading living cells.

X-RAYS Electromagnetic waves that have a very short wavelength and so can penetrate through many materials, including most living matter; images made by the use of such waves.

Bibliography

Many hundreds of information sources and references, both primary and secondary, and printed, digital and online, were used in compiling this book. A very brief selection is included below. For a fuller listing, please contact the author.

GENERAL PRINTED SOURCES

Roberta Bivins, *Alternative Medicine? A History*, Oxford University Press, 2007

William Bynum and Helen Bynum, eds, *Great Discoveries in Medicine*, Thames & Hudson, 2011

James Le Fanu, *The Rise and Fall of Modern Medicine*, Little, Brown Book Group, 2011

Mark Jackson, ed, *The Oxford Handbook of the History of Medicine*, Oxford University Press, 2013

Peter E. Pormann, *Medieval Islamic Medicine*, Georgetown University Press, 2007

Roy Porter, ed, *The Cambridge Illustrated History of Medicine*, Cambridge University Press, 2006

Larry Trivieri, John W. Anderson, Burton Goldberg, eds, *Alternative Medicine: The Definitive Guide* (second edition), Celestial Arts, 2013

GENERAL ONLINE SOURCES

American Association for the History of Medicine
www.histmed.org

Department of History and Philosophy of Science, University of Cambridge
www.hps.cam.ac.uk/medicine

European Association for the History of Medicine and Health (EAHMH)
www.eahmh.net

Traditional Medicines
ca.traditionalmedicinals.comsystems_of_THM

University College London – UCL Centre for the History of Medicine
www.ucl.ac.uk/histmed

US National Library of Medicine, National Institutes of Health
www.nlm.nih.gov/hmd

Wellcome Library, History of Medicine Collection
wellcomelibrary.org/about-us/about-the-collections/history-of-medicine-collection

Wellcome Unit for the History of Medicine, University of Oxford
www.wuhmo.ox.ac.uk

HOSPITAL AND HEALTH CENTRE ARCHIVES AND ARTICLES

Bethlem Royal Hospital Archives and Museum Service
www.bethlemheritage.org.uk

Groote Schuur Hospital
www.gsh.co.za/christiaan-barnard

Johns Hopkins School of Medicine
webapps.jhu.edu/jhuniverse/academics/schools/school_of_medicine

Massachusetts General Hospital
www.massgeneral.org/history

Papworth Hospital
www.papworthhospital.nhs.uk/content.php?/about/history

St Christopher's Hospice
www.stchristophers.org.uk/about/history

Wrightington Hospital
www.wwl.nhs.uk/Internet/Home/wrt/john_charnley.asp

ORGANIZATIONS, MUSEUMS, AND EXHIBITIONS

American Cancer Society (History of Cancer)
www.cancer.org/cancer/cancerbasics/thehistoryofcancer/index

Aphorisms by Hippocrates
classics.mit.edu/Hippocrates/aphorisms.html

Cancer Research UK
www.cancerresearchuk.org/cancer-info/cancerandresearch/progress/a-century-of-progress

Elizabeth Garrett Anderson Hospital for Women
www.english-heritage.org.uk/discover/people-and-places/womens-history/women-and-healthcare/elizabeth-garrett-anderson-hospital-for-women

Florence Nightingale Museum
www.florence-nightingale.co.uk

Galen and Greek Medicine
www.greekmedicine.net/whos_who/Galen.html

Human Fertilisation and Embryology Authority (HFEA)
www.hfea.gov.uk/history-of-ivf.html

Institut Pasteur
www.pasteur-international.org/ip/easysite/pasteur-international-en/institut-pasteur-international-network/history-in-movement

Nobel Prize Foundation
www.nobelprize.org/nobel_prizes/medicine

Robert Koch Institute
www.rki.de/EN/Content/Institute/History/history_node_en.html

Royal College of Midwives
www.rcm.org.uk/midwives/by-subject/midwifery-history

Royal College of Nursing
www.rcn.org.uk/aboutus/our_history

Royal College of Physicians
www.rcplondon.ac.uk/about/history

Royal College of Surgeons
www.rcseng.ac.uk/museums/hunterian/history

Stem Cells (National Institutes of Health)
stemcells.nih.gov/Pages/Default.aspx

World Health Organization (WHO)
www.who.int/research/en

Index

Page numbers for illustrations are in italics.

Acknowledgments

Dorling Kindersley would like to thank the following for their help on this book:

Philip Wilkinson for additional text; Satu Fox for editorial assistance; Katie Cavanagh, Stephen Bere, and Peter Laws for design assistance; Margaret McCormack for indexing.

The publisher would also like to thank the following for their kind permission to reproduce their photographs:

(Key: a-above; b-below/bottom; c-centre; f-far; l-left; r-right; t-top)

2–3 Getty Images: De Agostini . 5 The Bridgeman Art Library: Musée d'Histoire de la Médecine, Paris, France / Archives Charmet. 9 Science & Society Picture Library: Science Museum. 12 Science Photo Library: S. Plailly / E. Daynes. 15 Science Photo Library: Mauricio Anton. 16 akg-images: Florilegius; 17 Getty Images: Gamma-Rapho. 19 Getty Images: The Bridgeman Art Library. 20–21 Science & Society Picture Library: Science Museum (c). 20 Science & Society Picture Library: Science Museum (bc, bl). 21 Alex Peck Medical Antiques: (r). 22 Getty Images: G. Dagli Orti / De Agostini (br). 24 Getty Images: De Agostini. 25 akg-images: Francis Dzikowski. 26 Science & Society Picture Library: Science Museum. 28–29 akg-images: Bildarchiv Steffens (b). 28 Getty Images: Marwan Naamani / AFP (bl). 29 Getty Images: De Agostini. 31 Corbis: Gianni Dagli Orti. 32 Getty Images: De Agostini. 34–35 Scala, Florence: White Images. 37 Getty Images: A. Dagli Orti / De Agostini. 38 Corbis. 40 Corbis: Ken Welsh / Design Pics. 42 akg-images: Nimatallah. 44 Corbis: Araldo de Luca. 45 Getty Images: A. De Gregorio / De Agostini (tr). 46–47 Courtesy of Historical Collections & Services, Claude Moore Health Sciences Library, University of Virginia. 49 akg-images: Erich Lessing. 51 Science Photo Library: Jean-Loup Charmet (t). 53 The Art Archive: Biblioteca Augusta Perugia / Gianni Dagli Orti. 54–55 (background) Getty Images: Photo12 / UIG; Wellcome Library, London: (c). 54 Corbis: (c); Science Photo Library: (cla). 55 Corbis: Dr. Robert Calentine / Visuals Unlimited (cr); 55 Science Photo Library: Eye of Science (c). 57 akg-images: Erich Lessing. 59 Scala, Florence: Ann Ronan / Heritage Images. 60 akg-images: IAM. 62-63 Getty Images: Josef Mensing Gallery, Hamm-Rhynern, Germany / The Bridgeman Art Library. 64 akg-images: R. u. S. Michaud. 67 Wellcome Library, London. 69 Scala, Florence: Digital Image Museum Associates / LACMA / Art Resource NY.

70–71 akg-images: Erich Lessing. 73 Ancient Art & Architecture Collection: Heojun Museum / EuroCreon. 74 Getty Images: Musee Guimet, Paris, France. 76 akg-images: British Library. 79 akg-images: R. u. S. Michaud. 80–81 The Bridgeman Art Library: Luca Tettoni. 83 Getty Images: Universal History Archive / UIG / The Bridgeman Art Library. 84 akg-images: Rabatti Domingie. 85 Getty Images: The Bridgeman Art Library. 87 The Bridgeman Art Library: Collection of the Lowe Art Museum, University of Miami / Gift of the Institute of Maya Studies. 88 The Bridgeman Art Library: Collection of the Lowe Art Museum, University of Miami / Gift of the Estate of Ann M. Grimshawe (cl); Getty Images: UIG via (bl); Science & Society Picture Library: Science Museum (tr). 89 The Bridgeman Art Library: Werner Forman Archive (cr); Corbis: Werner Forman (cl); Getty Images: Werner Forman / UIG (crb); Science & Society Picture Library: Science Museum (clb, tl, tr). 90 Getty Images: Robert Harding World Imagery. 92 Corbis: Bowers Museum (tl). 93 Alamy: Zev Radovan / BibleLand Pictures. 94–95 Getty Images: Hulton Archive. 97 akg-images: africanpictures. 98 Getty Images: M. Seemuller / De Agostini. 100 Wellcome Images. 103 Getty Images: De Agostini. 104 akg-images: Erich Lessing. 106–107 akg-images: British Library (c). 106 The Bridgeman Art Library: Bibliotheque Nationale, Paris, France / Archives Charmet (bl). 107 The Art Archive: Saint Stephen's Cathedral Vienna / Dagli Orti (br, ca, cb,cr). 109 The Art Archive: Bodleian Library Oxford. 110 Getty Images: De Agostini. 112–113 akg-images: Erich Lessing. 114 Scala, Florence: Ann Ronan / Heritage Images. 115 Wellcome Images. 116 Getty Images: Universal History Archive. 118 Corbis. 121 The Bridgeman Art Library: Christie's Images. 124–125 The Bridgeman Art Library: Musee des Beaux-Arts, Marseille, France. 126 akg-images. 129 The Art Archive: Museo del Prado Madrid / Gianni Dagli Orti. 130 The Bridgeman Art Library: British Library, London, UK / © British Library Board. All Rights Reserved. 132–133 Science & Society Picture Library: Science Museum (c). 132 Wellcome Library, London. 133 Getty Images: Visuals Unlimited, Inc. / Scientifica (bl); Science & Society Picture Library: Science Museum (br, ca); Wellcome Library, London. 134 Wellcome Library, London. 137 The Bridgeman Art Library: Bibliothèque des Arts Décoratifs, Paris, France / Archives Charmet. 139 Wellcome Images. 141 Wellcome Images. 142–143 akg-images: Album / Oronoz. 144 Getty Images: Hulton Archive. 145 Getty Images: De Agostini.

149 Corbis: Bettmann. 150 Science & Society Picture Library: Science Museum (br, cr, l, tr); Wellcome Images: (br). 151 Science & Society Picture Library: Science Museum (b, r). 152 Science & Society Picture Library: Science Museum. 153 Science Photo Library: NYPL / Science Source. 154 Wellcome Images. 157 Wellcome Images. 160–161 (background) Corbis: Bettmann. 160 Science Photo Library: NYPL / Science Source (cl); Science Photo Library: CCI Archives (cla); Wellcome Library, London: (cr). 161 Getty Images: Leemage (cl); Getty Images: Lynn Pelham (cr); 162 Corbis: Bettmann. 165 Getty Images: Werner Forman / UIG. 166 The Bridgeman Art Library: Biblioteca Universitaria, Bologna, Italy / Archives Charmet. 168 Getty Images: Time & Life Pictures. 169 Getty Images: Hulton Archive. 170–171 Wellcome Library, London. 173 Wellcome Library, London. 175 Wellcome Library, London. (t); 176 Science & Society Picture Library: Science Museum. 178 Science & Society Picture Library: Science Museum (br, cr, l); Science & Society Picture Library: SCM (cl). 179 Science & Society Picture Library: Science Museum. 181 U.S. National Library of Medicine, History of Medicine Division. 182 Science & Society Picture Library: Science Museum. 184 Alamy: Neil Setchfield. 186–187 Wellcome Library, London. 188 Getty Images: Time & Life Pictures. 190 Getty Images: Universal History Archive. 193 Getty Images: Universal History Archive. 194–195 Science & Society Picture Library: Science Museum (c). 194 Mary Evans Picture Library: INTERFOTO / Bildarchiv Hansmann. 196 Getty Images: Roger Viollet Collection. 199 The Art Archive: Eileen Tweedy (t). 201 Getty Images: BSIP / UIG. 202 The Bridgeman Art Library: Musée Pasteur, Institut Pasteur, Paris, France / Archives Charmet. 204–205 (background) U.S. National Library of Medicine, History of Medicine Division. 204 Wellcome Library, London: (cl); Science Photo Library: Dr P. Marazzi (cla); Corbis: Bettmann (cr). 205 Corbis: Dr. Fred Murphy / Visuals Unlimited (cl); Science Photo Library: Simon Fraser (cr). 206 Science & Society Picture Library: Science Museum. 209 Corbis: Bettmann (t). 210 Science & Society Picture Library: Science Museum. 211 Science & Society Picture Library: Science Museum. 212–213 The Bridgeman Art Library: Deutsches Historisches Museum, Berlin, Germany. 214 U.S. National Library of Medicine, History of Medicine Division. 216 Wellcome Library, London. 217 Wellcome Library, London. 218–219 U.S. National Library of Medicine, History of Medicine Division. 221 Wellcome Library,

London. 222 Corbis: Bettmann. 224 Getty Images: Universal History Archive. 227 Wellcome Library, London. 228 Science Photo Library. 229 Corbis: Visuals Unlimited (ftr, tc, tl); Corbis: Dennis Kunkel Microscopy, Inc. / Visuals Unlimited (tr). 231 Getty Images: Hulton Archive. 232 Science & Society Picture Library: Science Museum. 233 Getty Images: Buyenlarge. 234 Scala, Florence: White Images. 237 Corbis. 238–239 Corbis: Burstein Collection. 240 Science Photo Library: Dept. of Microbiology, Biozentrum. 242 Getty Images: Universal History Archive. 245 U.S. National Library of Medicine, History of Medicine Division. 247 Science & Society Picture Library: Science Museum. 249 Corbis: Bettmann. 250–251 Science & Society Picture Library: Science Museum (c). 250 U.S. National Library of Medicine, History of Medicine Division (bl). 253 Getty Images: Davies. 254 Science & Society Picture Library: Science Museum. 257 Library of Congress. 258 Corbis: Bettmann. 261 Alamy: BSIP SA. 262 Getty Images: Esther Bubley / Time & Life Pictures. 265 U.S. National Library of Medicine, History of Medicine Division. 267 Alamy: ZUMA Press, Inc. 268 Wellcome Images: Yorgos Nikas, (bl); Wellcome Images: K. Hodivala-Dilke & M. Stone (br); Wellcome Images: Annie Cavanagh (cl); Wellcome Images: Steven Pollard (cr). 269 Science Photo Library: Steve Gschmeissner (br); Wellcome Images: Anne Weston, LRI, CRUK, (bl, tl); Wellcome Images: Dr. Yi Feng, University of Bristol (tr). 270 Science & Society Picture Library: Science Museum. 273 Getty Images: Steve Allen. 274 Science & Society Picture Library: Science Museum. 276 Science & Society Picture Library: Science Museum (bl, cr); Wellcome Library, London: (cl). 277 Science Photo Library: James King-Holmes (br); Science & Society Picture Library: Science Museum (bl, t); Wellcome Images: (cl); 279 Getty Images: Universal History Archive. 282 Courtesy of St Christopher's Hospice, London. 284–285 The Bridgeman Art Library: Musée de l'Assistance Publique, Hopitaux de Paris, France / Archives Charmet. 286 Corbis. 288 U.S. National Library of Medicine, History of Medicine Division. 289 Science Photo Library: AMI Images. 290 Getty Images: Archive Photos (br). 292 Getty Images: Evans / Three Lions. 293 Science & Society Picture Library: Science Museum. 294 Getty Images: Charles H. Phillips / Time Life Pictures. 297 Corbis: Bettmann. 298 Corbis: Mediscan. 300–301 Science & Society Picture Library: Science Museum (c). 300 Corbis: Bettmann (bl). 302 Science & Society Picture Library: Science Museum. 303 Getty Images: Universal History

Archive. **304 Wellcome Library, London:** (tr). **308 Science Photo Library:** Arno Massee. **310 Corbis:** Zephyr / Science Photo Library (cr); **Getty Images:** Dirk Freder (cl); **Science Photo Library:** Zephyr (br); **Science Photo Library:** CNRI (bl). **311 Alamy:** Chad Ehlers (br); **Science Photo Library:** GJLP (bl); **Science Photo Library:** Wellcome Dept. of Cognitive Neurology (tr); **Wellcome Images:** Mark Lythgoe & Chloe Hutton (tl). **313 Getty Images:** Gamma-Keystone. **314 Rex Features:** Sipa Press. **317 Science Photo Library:** Colin Cuthbert. **318–319 Rex Features:** Image Broker. **321 Corbis:** Hero Images. **322 The Bridgeman Art Library:** Société d'Histoire de la Pharmacie, Paris, France / Archives Charmet. **325 Science Photo Library:** Thierry Berrod / Mona Lisa Production. **326–327 Scala, Florence:** White Images. **328 Getty Images:** Michel Clement / AFP. **330 Getty Images:** BSIP / UIG. **333 Getty Images:** Patrick Lin / AFP. **334–335 (background) Science & Society Picture Library:** Science Museum. **334 akg-images:** Paul Almasy (cr); **Corbis:** Wavebreak Media Ltd. (cla); **Science & Society Picture Library:** Science Museum (cl). **335 Wellcome Library, London:** (cl, cr). **336 Science Photo Library:** Riccardo Cassiani-Ingoni. **339 Corbis:** Thomas Deerinck / Visuals Unlimited. **340 Science Photo Library:** A. Barrington Brown. **343 Corbis:** Karen Kasmauski.

344 Corbis: Tek Image / Science Photo Library. **346 Science Photo Library:** David McCarthy. **348 Alamy:** INTERFOTO. **351 Corbis:** epa. **352 Rex Features:** Intuitive Surgical. **354–355 Science Photo Library:** Peter Menzel. **356 The Bridgeman Art Library:** Musée du Val-de-Grace, Paris, France / Archives Charmet. **358 Science & Society Picture Library:** Science Museum. **361 Getty Images:** DreamPictures. **362–363 Science & Society Picture Library:** Science Museum (c). **362 Wellcome Library, London:** (c). **365 Corbis:** David Scharf / Science Faction. **369 Corbis:** epa. **370–371 Science Photo Library:** Riccardo Cassiani-Ingoni. **372 Corbis:** Dan McCoy, Rainbow / Science Faction. **374–375 The Art Archive: British Museum / Jacqueline Hyde. 377 Corbis:** SuperStock. **380–381 Corbis:** Hulton-Deutsch Collection. **382 Getty Images:** Adam Pretty. **384 Corbis:** Yang Liu. **387 Getty Images:** Jeff J. Mitchell. **388–389 (background) Getty Images:** BSIP / UIG. **388 Science Photo Library:** (cr); Wellcome Images: Hugh Sturrock (cla); Wellcome Library, London: (cr). **389 Corbis:** Studio Patellani (cl); Wellcome Library, London: (cr).

All other images © Dorling Kindersley
For further information see: www.dkimages.com